HOLE IN THE HEART

GRAPHIC
MEDICINE

Susan Merrill Squier and Ian Williams,
General Editors

Editorial Collective
MK Czerwiec (Northwestern University)
Michael J. Green (Penn State University
  College of Medicine)
Kimberly R. Myers (Penn State University
  College of Medicine)
Scott T. Smith (Penn State University)

Books in the Graphic Medicine series are
inspired by a growing awareness of the
value of comics as an important resource
for communicating about a range of issues
broadly termed "medical." For healthcare
practitioners, patients, families, and
caregivers dealing with illness and disability,
graphic narrative enlightens complicated or
difficult experience. For scholars in literary,
cultural, and comics studies, the genre
articulates a complex and powerful analysis
of illness, medicine, and disability and a
rethinking of the boundaries of "health." The
series includes original comics from artists
and non-artists alike, such as self-reflective
"graphic pathographies" or comics used in
medical training and education, as well as
monographic studies and edited collections
from scholars, practitioners, and medical
educators.

Other titles in the series:

MK Czerwiec, Ian Williams, Susan Merrill
Squier, Michael J. Green, Kimberly R.
Myers, and Scott T. Smith, *Graphic
Medicine Manifesto*

Ian Williams, *The Bad Doctor: The Troubled
Life and Times of Dr. Iwan James*

Peter Dunlap-Shohl, *My Degeneration:
A Journey Through Parkinson's*

Aneurin Wright, *Things to Do in a
Retirement Home Trailer Park: . . . When
You're 29 and Unemployed*

Dana Walrath, *Aliceheimers: Alzheimer's
Through the Looking Glass*

Lorenzo Servitje and Sherryl Vint, eds.,
*The Walking Med: Zombies and the Medical
Image*

Hole in the Heart

Bringing Up Beth

HENNY BEAUMONT

The Pennsylvania State University Press
University Park, Pennsylvania

Note to the North American edition:

This book was originally published in the United Kingdom and contains a number of Britishisms that might require clarification for North American readers. For example, the DSA is the British Down's Syndrome Association, equivalent to the National Down Syndrome Society (NDSS) in the United States and the CDSS in Canada. OFSTED is the Office for Standards in Education, Children's Services and Skills. Finally, in the United Kingdom, the preferred spelling is Down's syndrome, with an apostrophe, while North American preferred usage is Down syndrome, without an apostrophe. As for people with Down's, they should always be referred to as people first.

Library of Congress Cataloging-in-Publication Data

Names: Beaumont, Henny, author, artist.
Title: Hole in the heart : bringing up Beth / Henny Beaumont.
Other titles: Graphic medicine.
Description: University Park, Pennsylvania : The Pennsylvania State University Press, [2016] |
Series: Graphic medicine | Reprint of: Hole in the heart / Henny Beaumont. Brighton : Myriad, 2016.
Identifiers: LCCN 2016027143 | ISBN 9780271077406 (pbk. : alk. paper)
Summary: "A memoir, in graphic novel format, of the author's emotions and the challenges and decisions she faces in raising a child with Down syndrome"—Provided by publisher.
Subjects: | MESH: Beaumont Epstein, Beth. | Down Syndrome | Child | Family Relations--psychology | Infant | Adolescent | Great Britain | Graphic Novels | Popular Works | Personal Narratives
Classification: LCC RC571 | NLM WS 17 | DDC 616.85/88420092 [B]—dc23
LC record available at https://lccn.loc.gov/2016027143

Published by
The Pennsylvania State University Press,
University Park, PA 16802-1003

First published by Myriad Editions,
www.myriadeditions.com

The Pennsylvania State University Press is a member of the Association of American University Presses.

It is the policy of The Pennsylvania State University Press to use acid-free paper. Publications on uncoated stock satisfy the minimum requirements of American National Standard for Information Sciences— Permanence of Paper for Printed Library Material, ANSI Z39.48–1992.

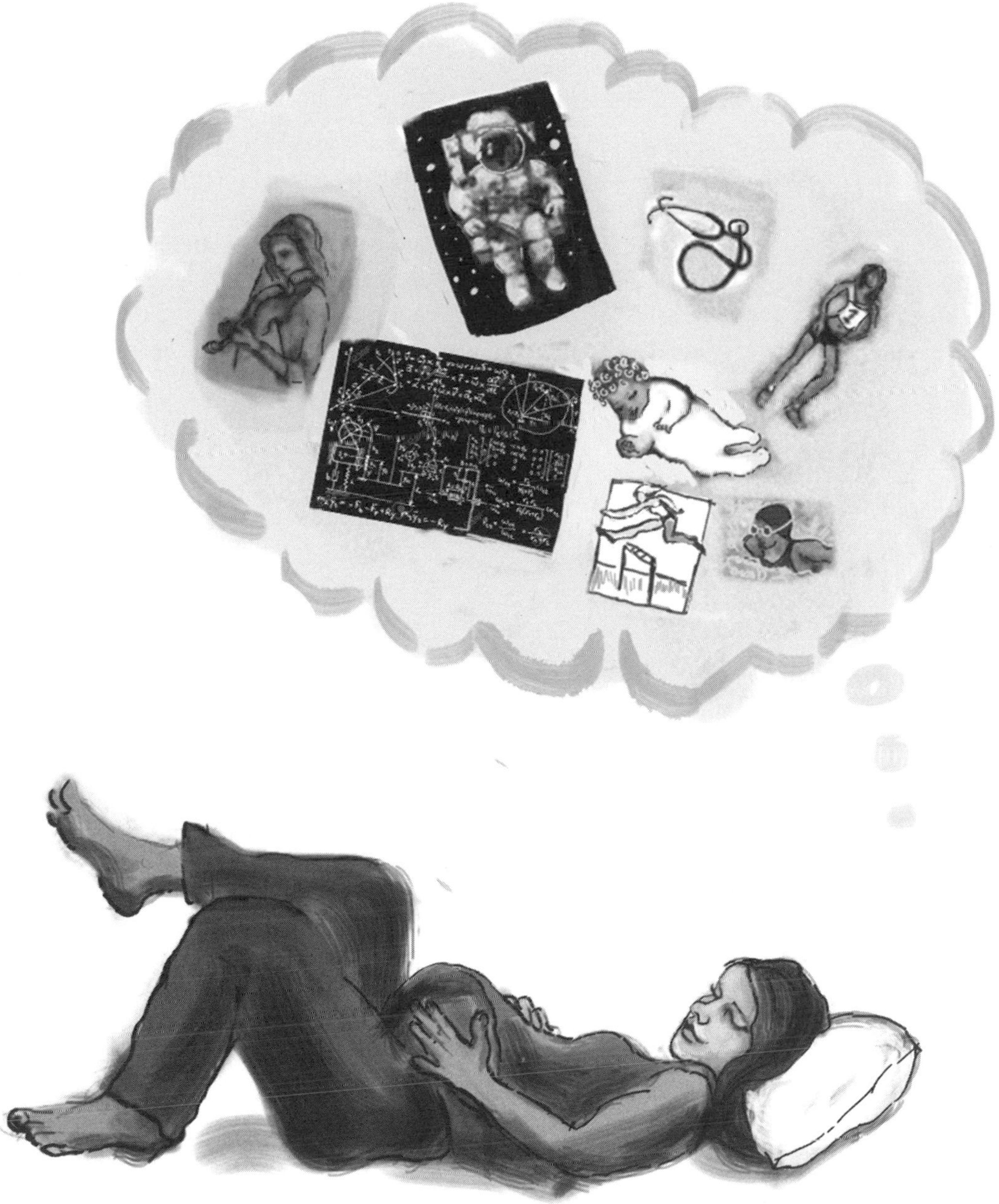

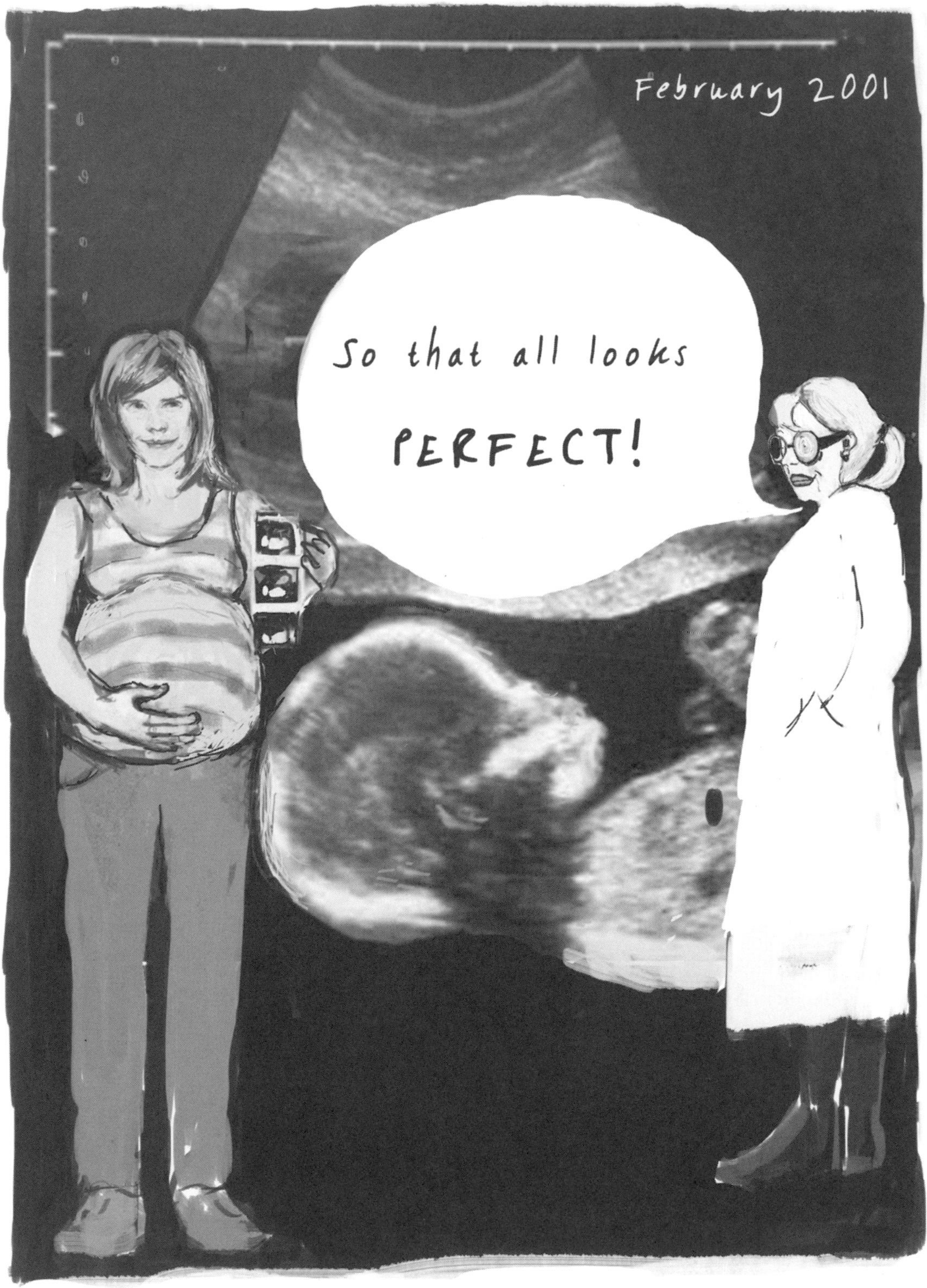
February 2001
So that all looks PERFECT!

For Steve, Matty, Bridie, Beth and Karl

Part One

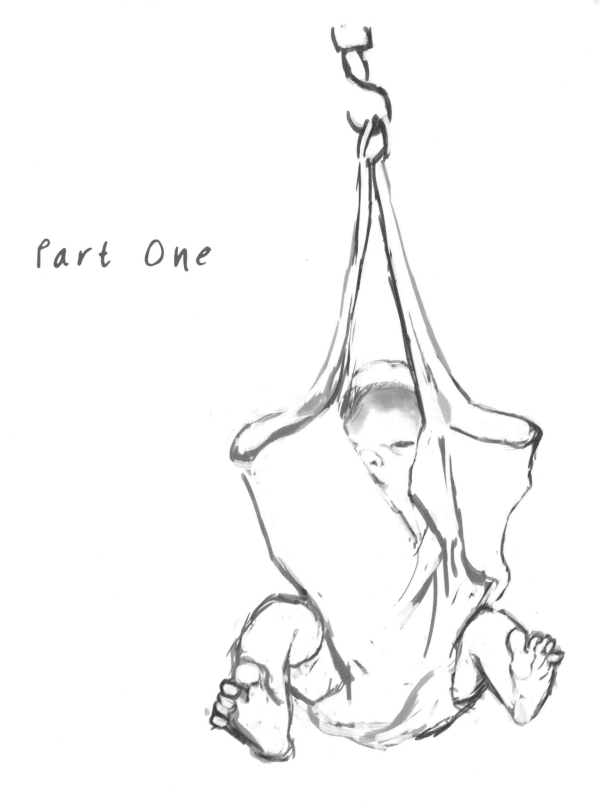

25 March 2001

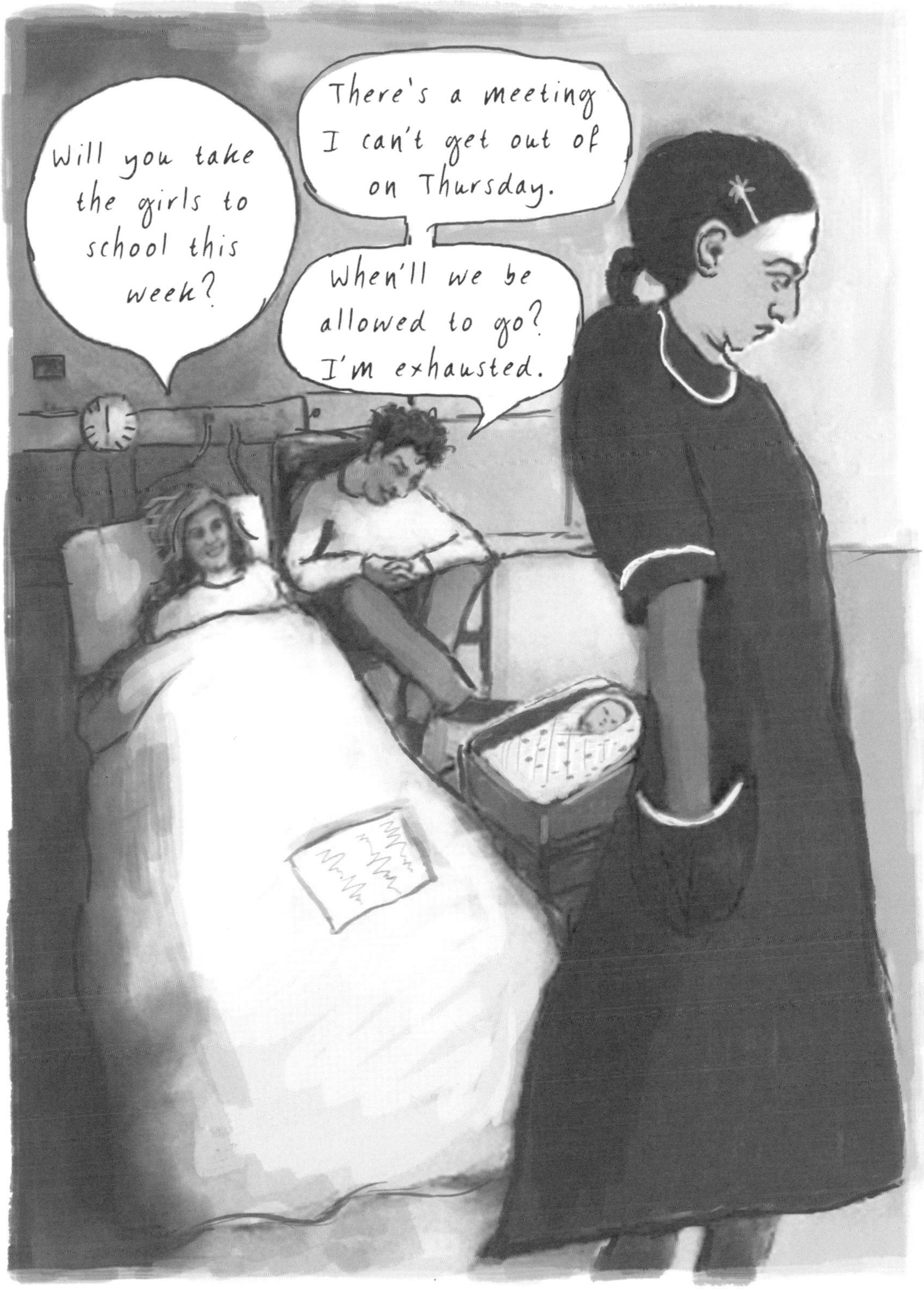
Will you take the girls to school this week?
There's a meeting I can't get out of on Thursday.
When'll we be allowed to go? I'm exhausted.

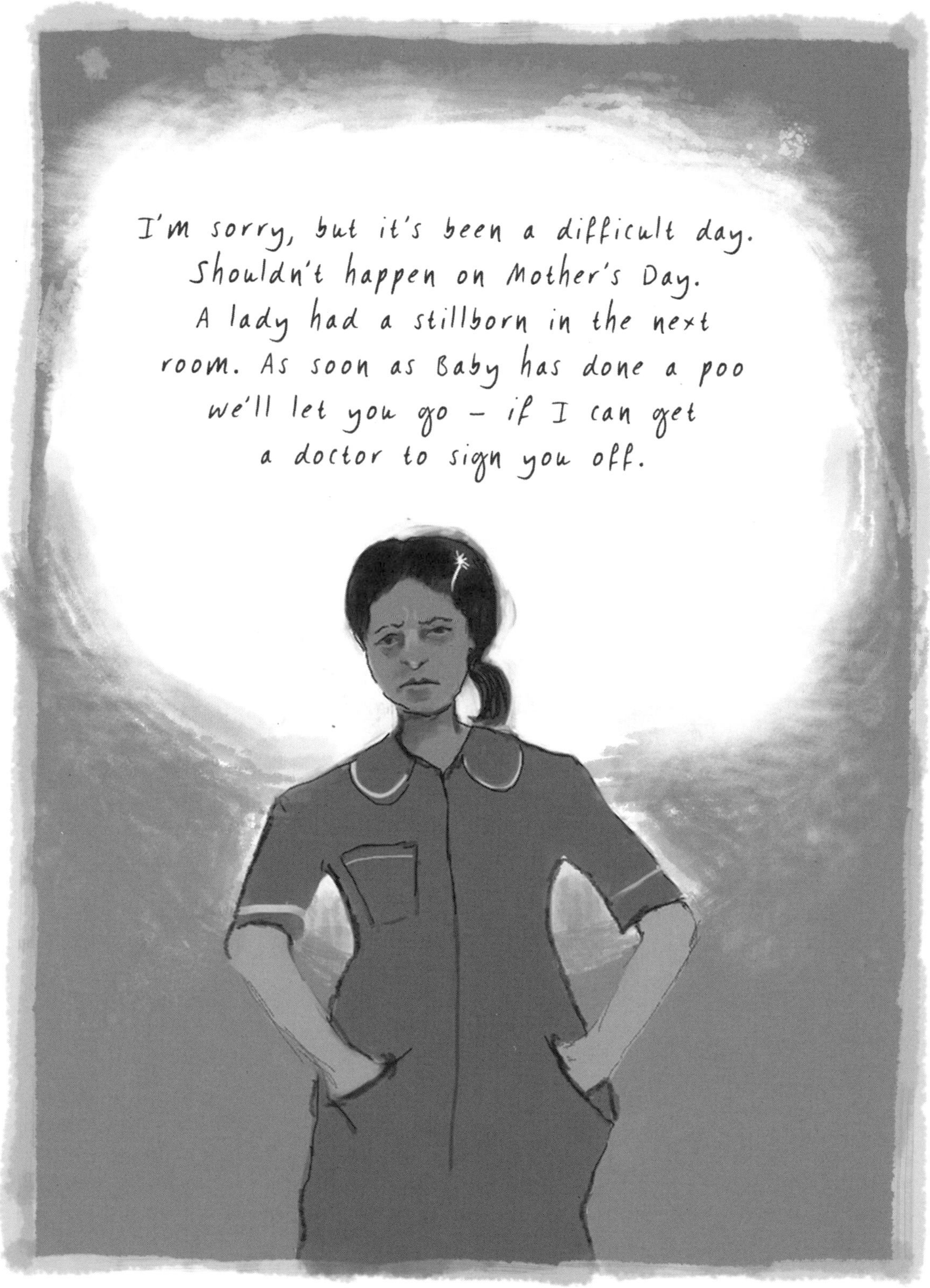
I'm sorry, but it's been a difficult day. Shouldn't happen on Mother's Day. A lady had a stillborn in the next room. As soon as Baby has done a poo we'll let you go – if I can get a doctor to sign you off.

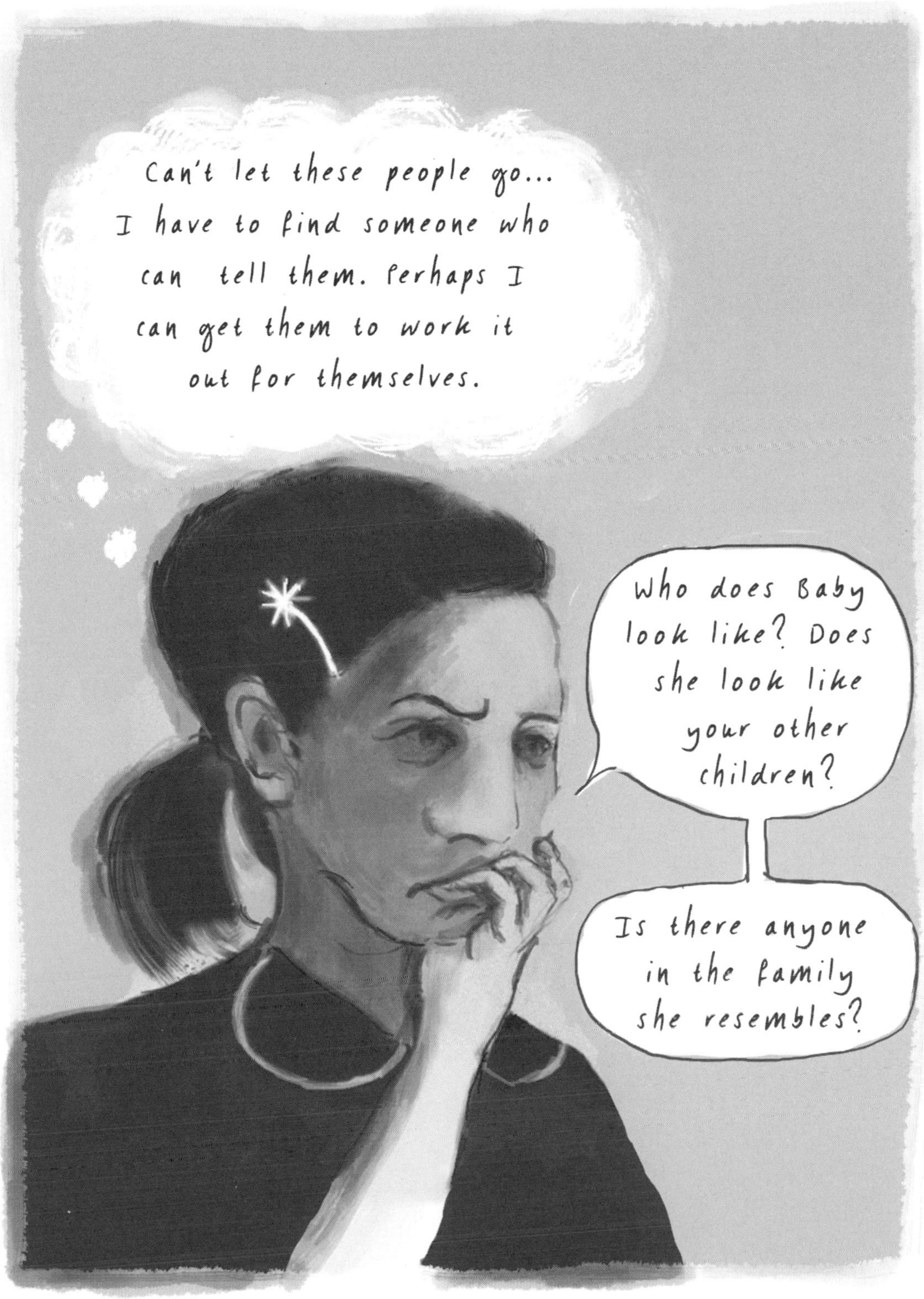
Can't let these people go... I have to find someone who can tell them. Perhaps I can get them to work it out for themselves.
Who does Baby look like? Does she look like your other children?
Is there anyone in the family she resembles?

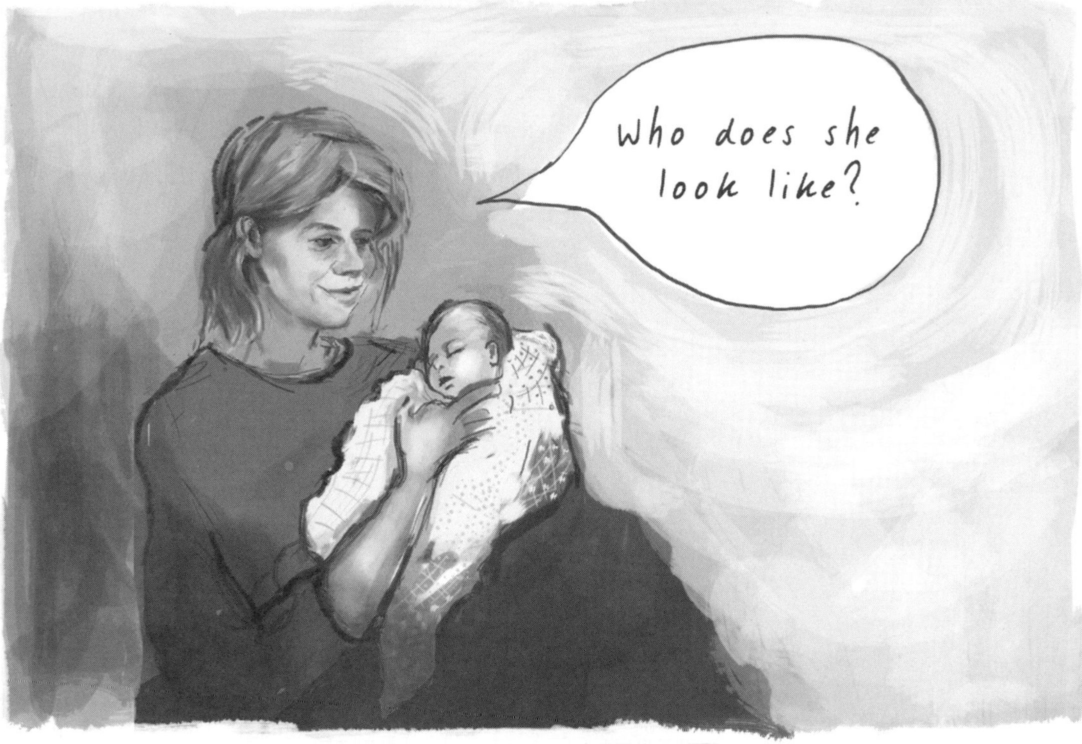
Who does she look like?

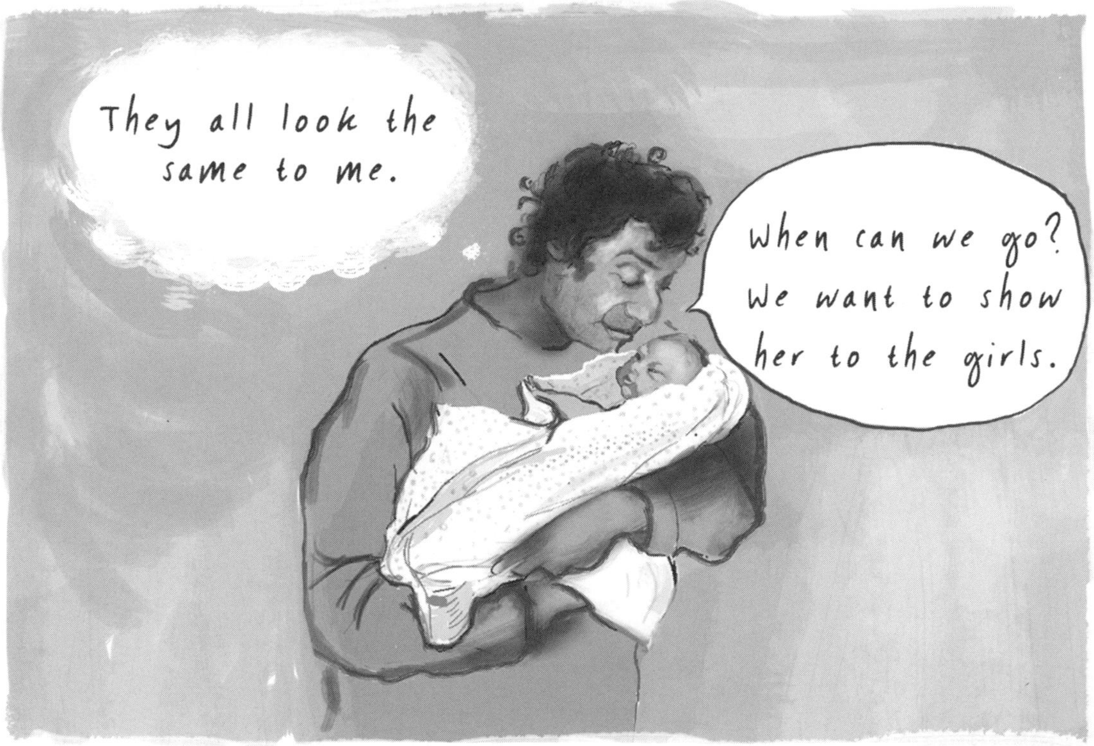
They all look the same to me.
When can we go? We want to show her to the girls.

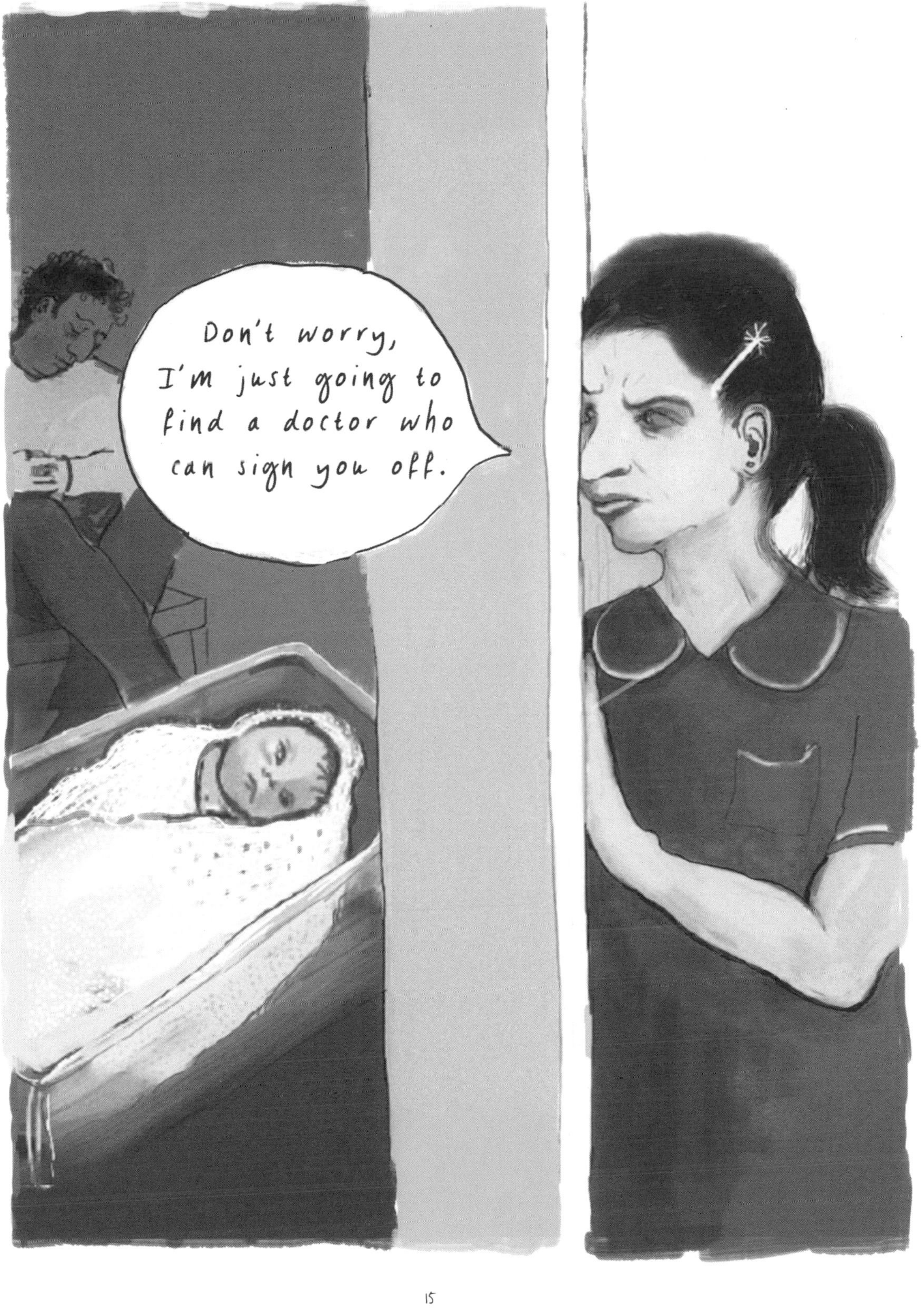
Don't worry, I'm just going to find a doctor who can sign you off.

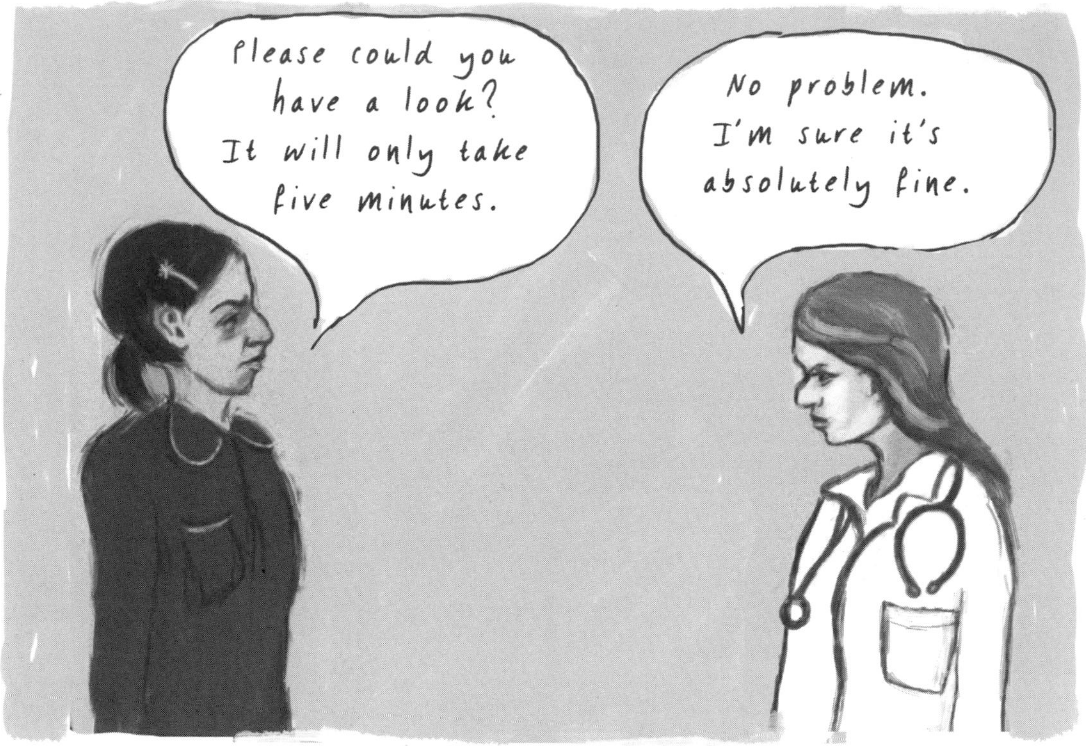
Please could you have a look? It will only take five minutes.
No problem. I'm sure it's absolutely fine.

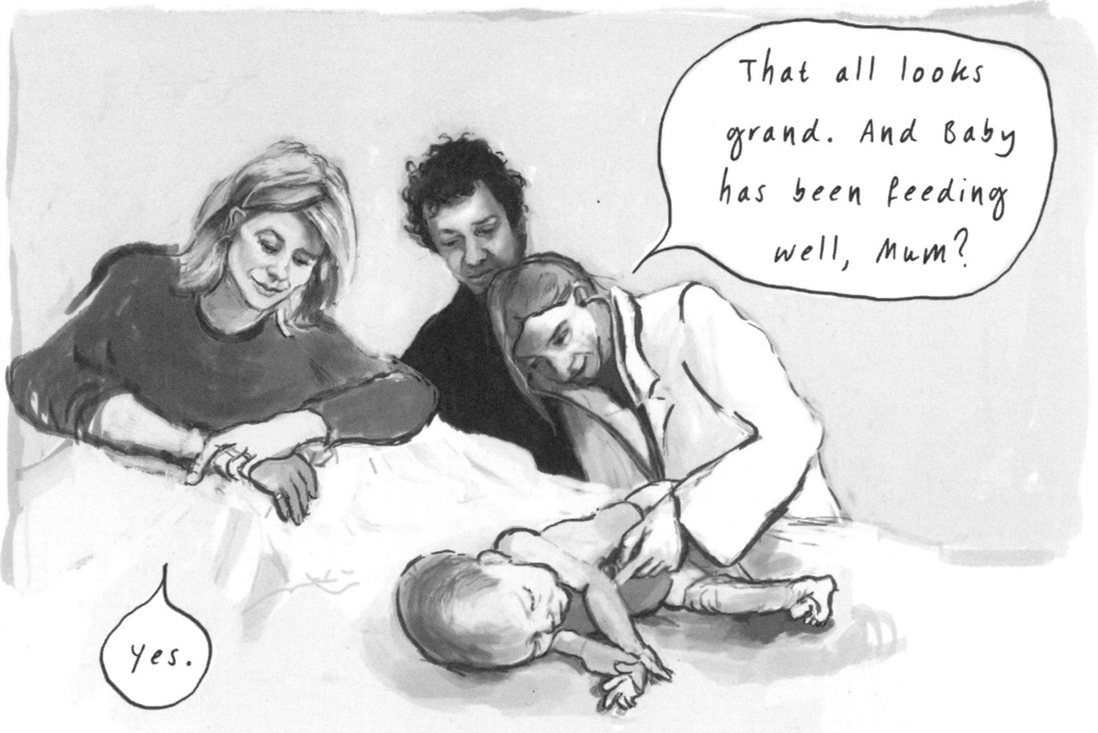
That all looks grand. And Baby has been feeding well, Mum?
Yes.

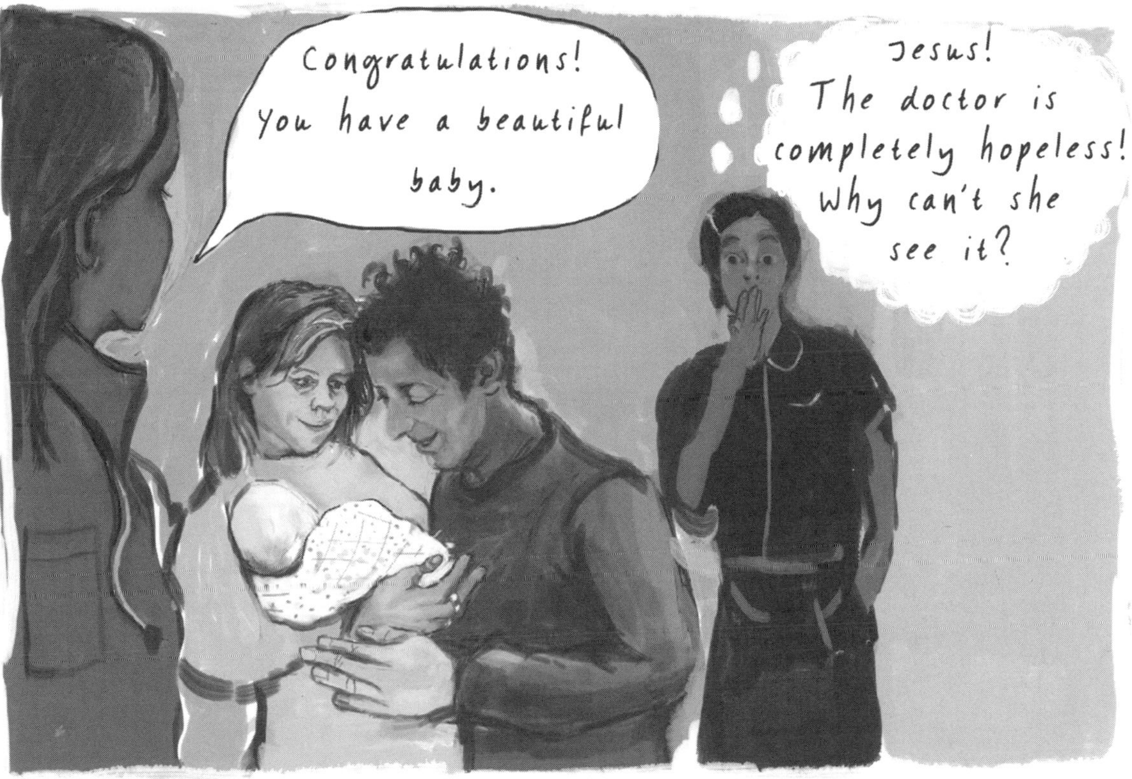
Congratulations! You have a beautiful baby.
Jesus! The doctor is completely hopeless! Why can't she see it?

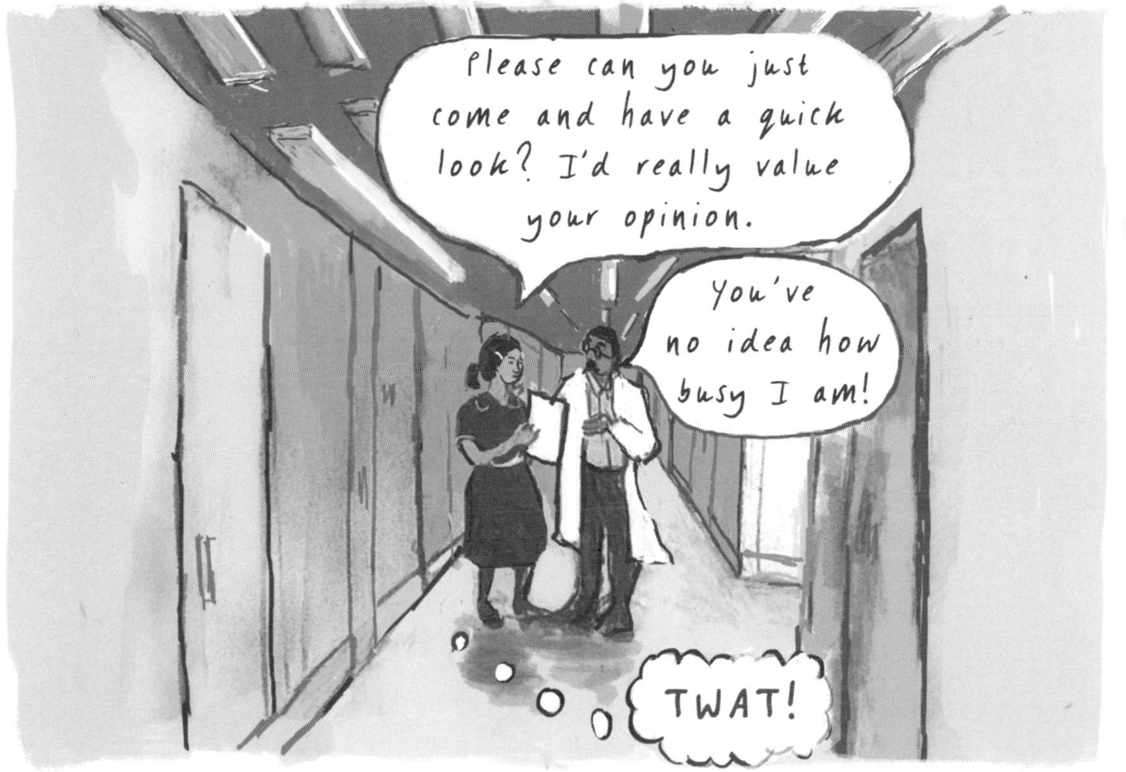
Please can you just come and have a quick look? I'd really value your opinion.
You've no idea how busy I am!
TWAT!

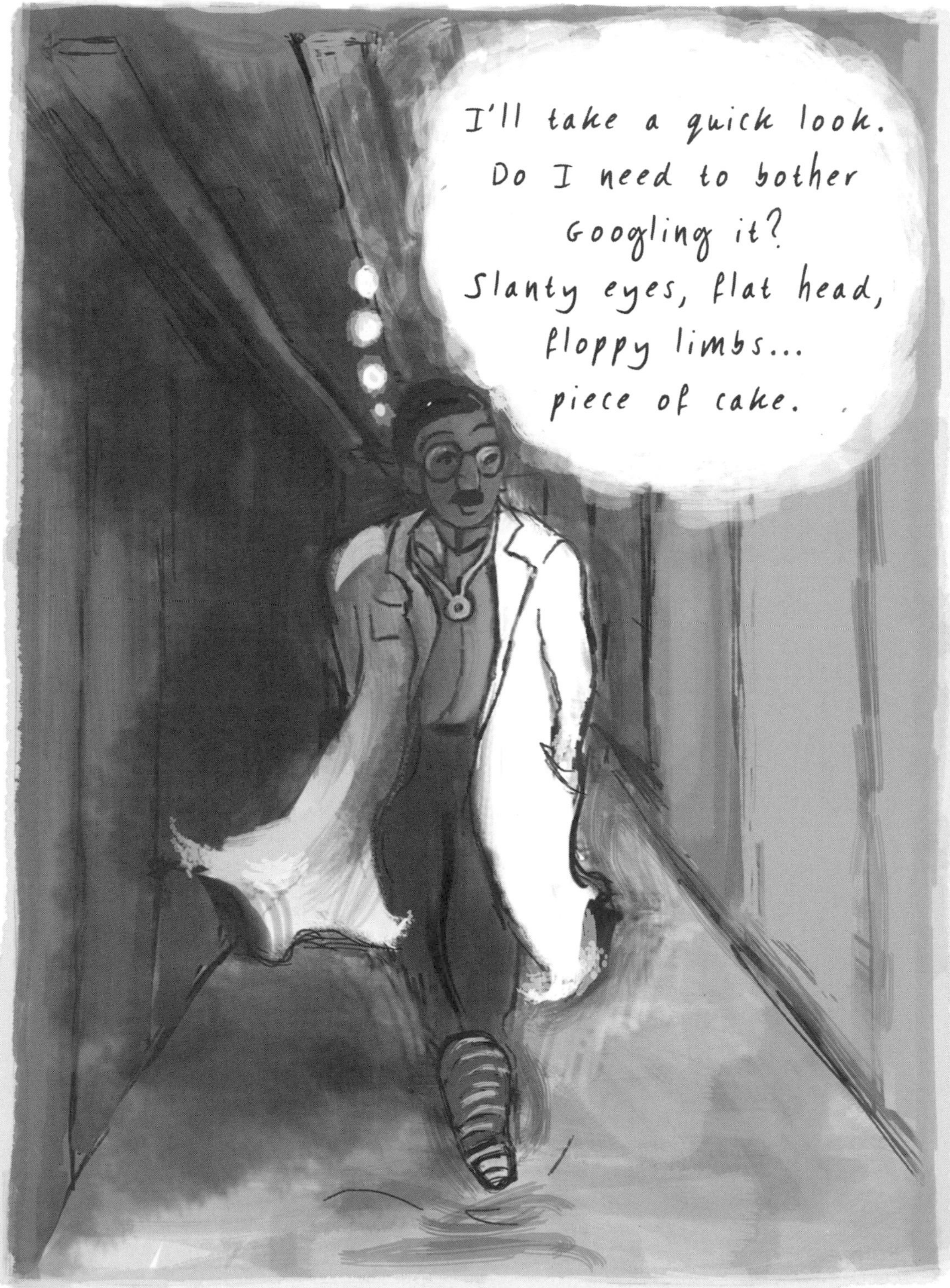
I'll take a quick look. Do I need to bother Googling it? Slanty eyes, flat head, floppy limbs... piece of cake.

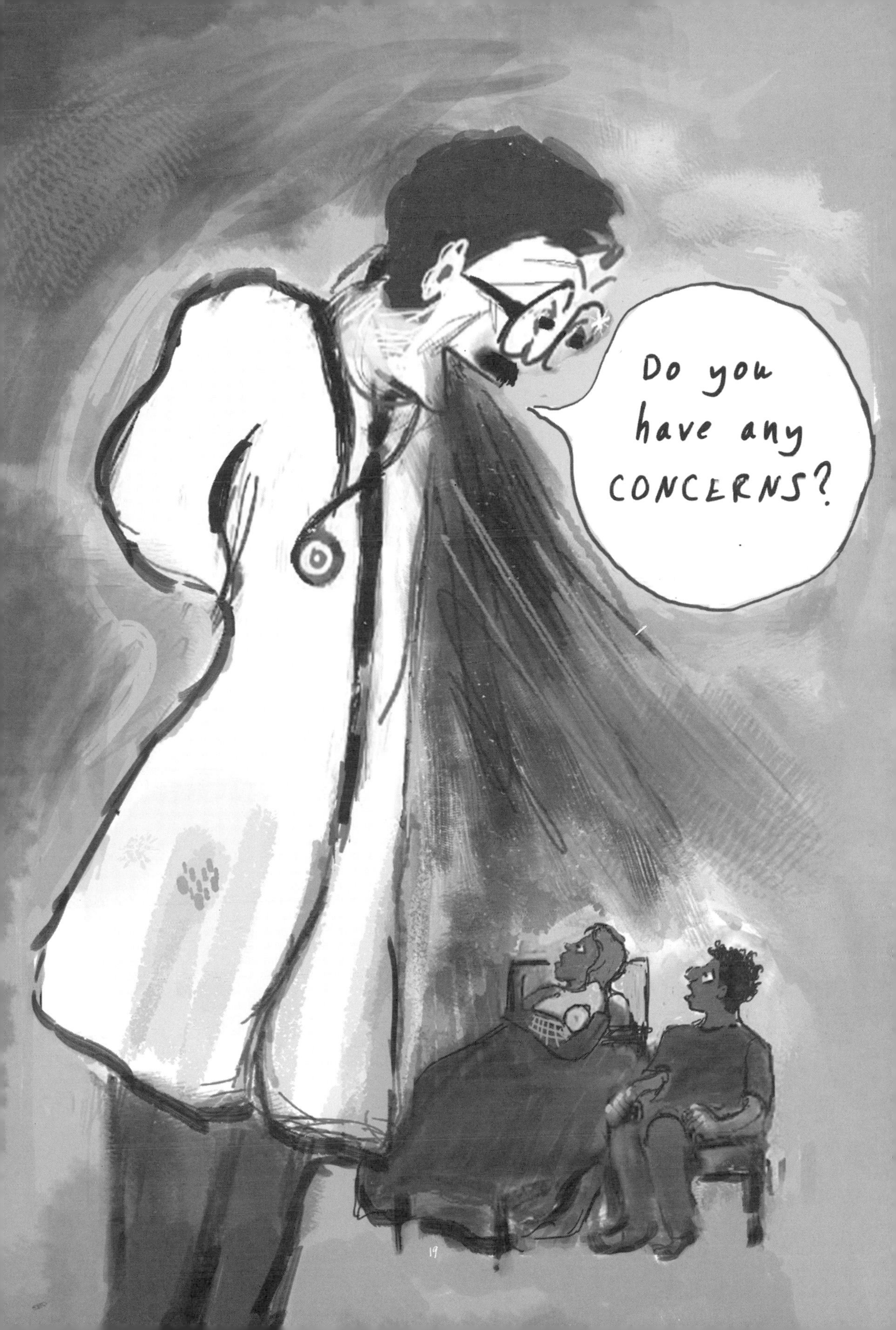
Do you have any CONCERNS?

Do you have any concerns?

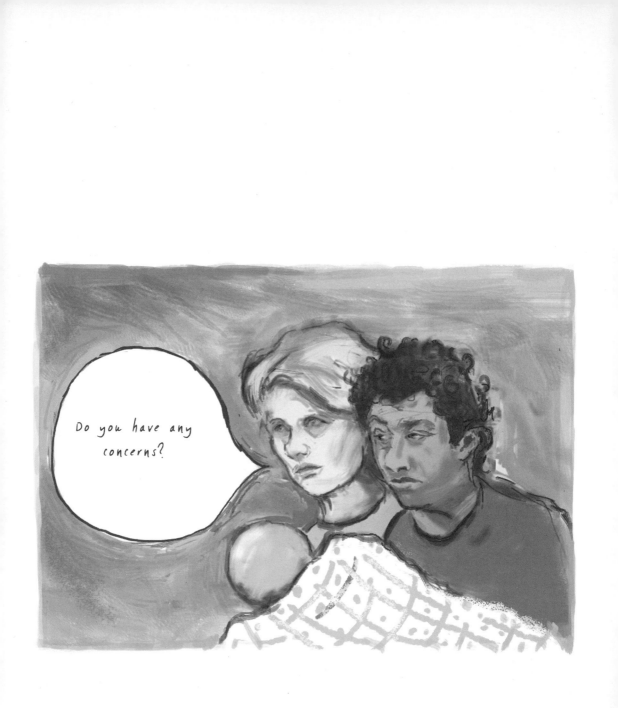

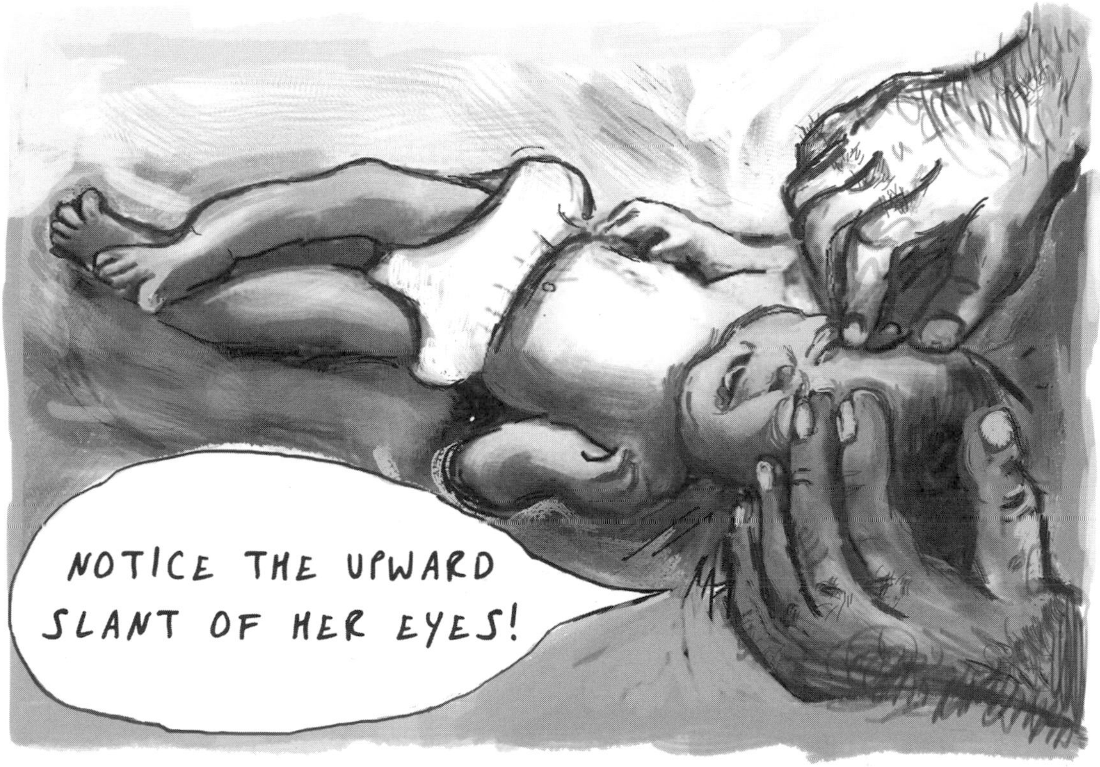
NOTICE THE UPWARD SLANT OF HER EYES!

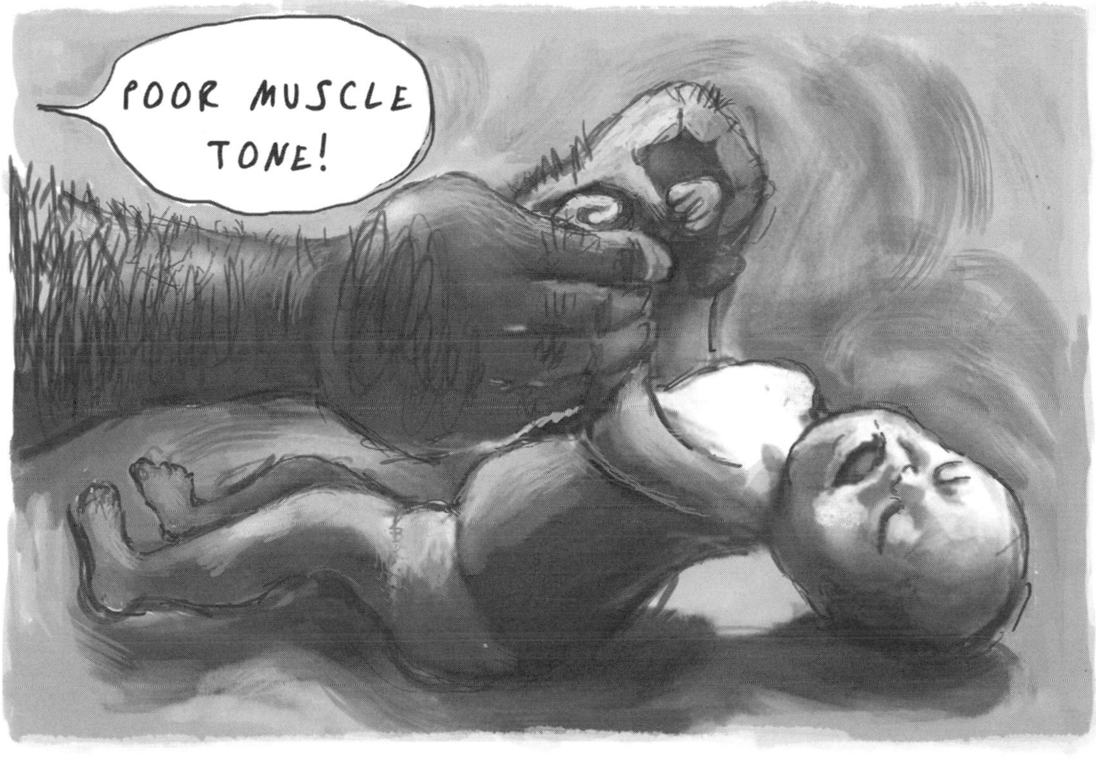
POOR MUSCLE TONE!

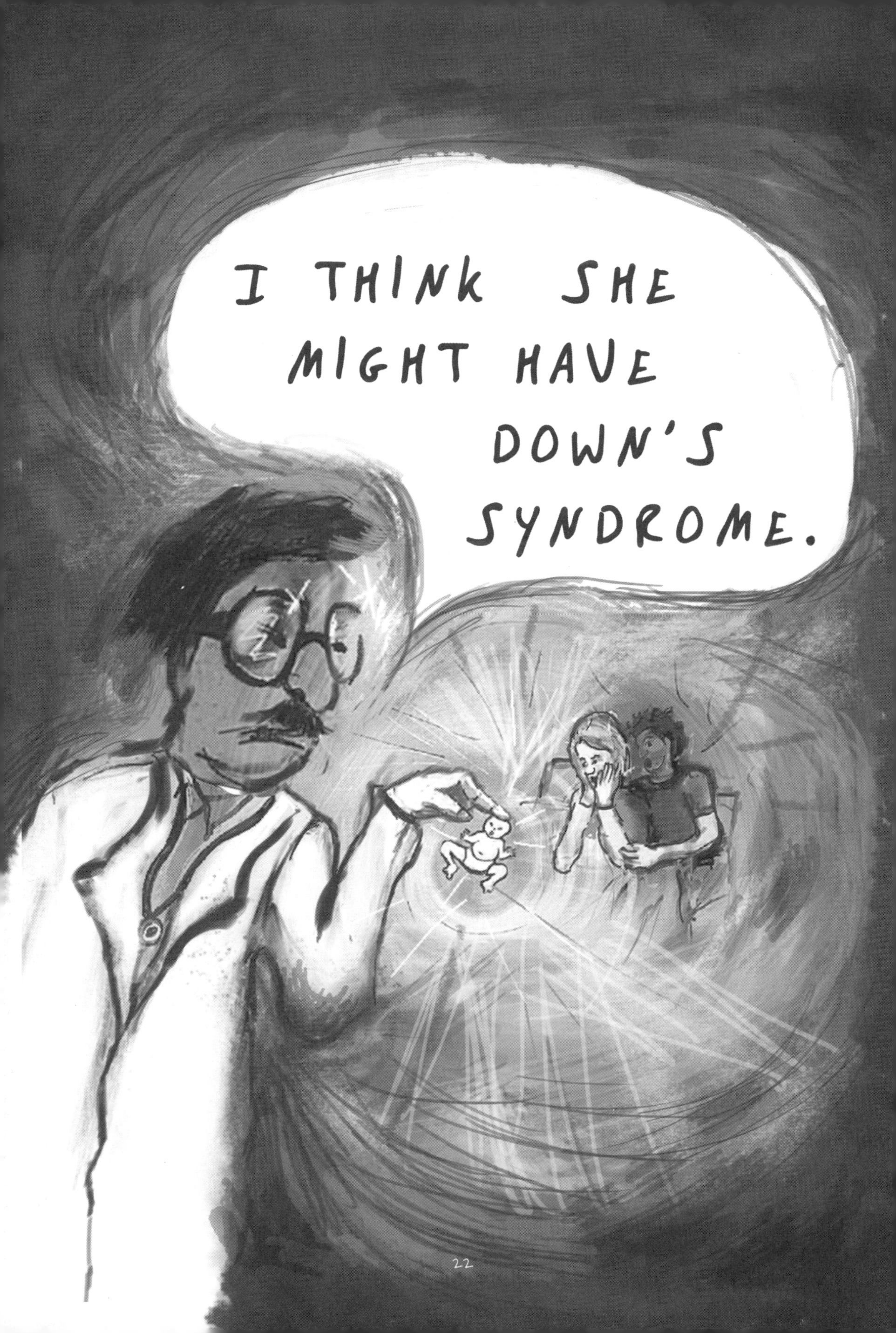
I THINK SHE MIGHT HAVE DOWN'S SYNDROME.

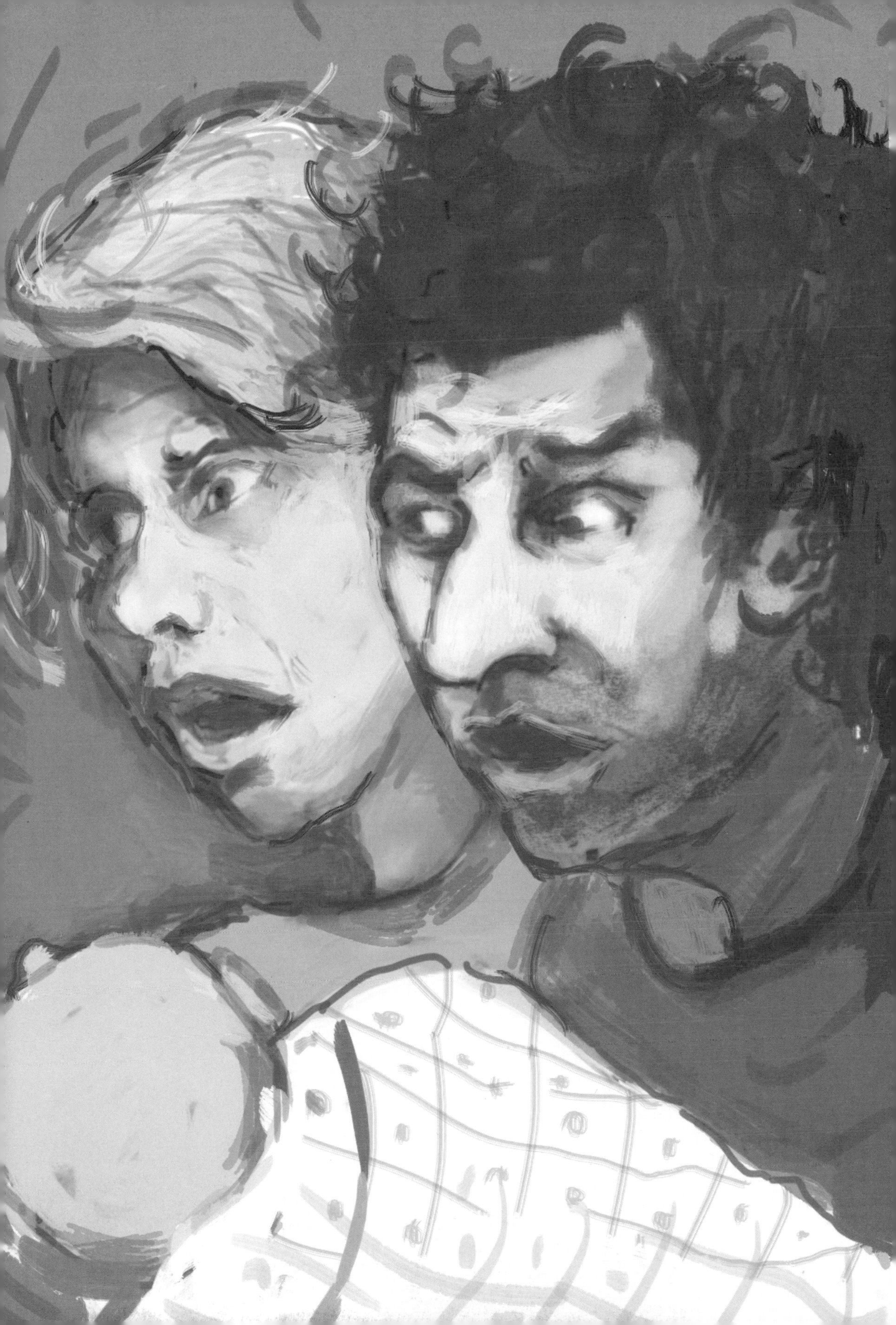

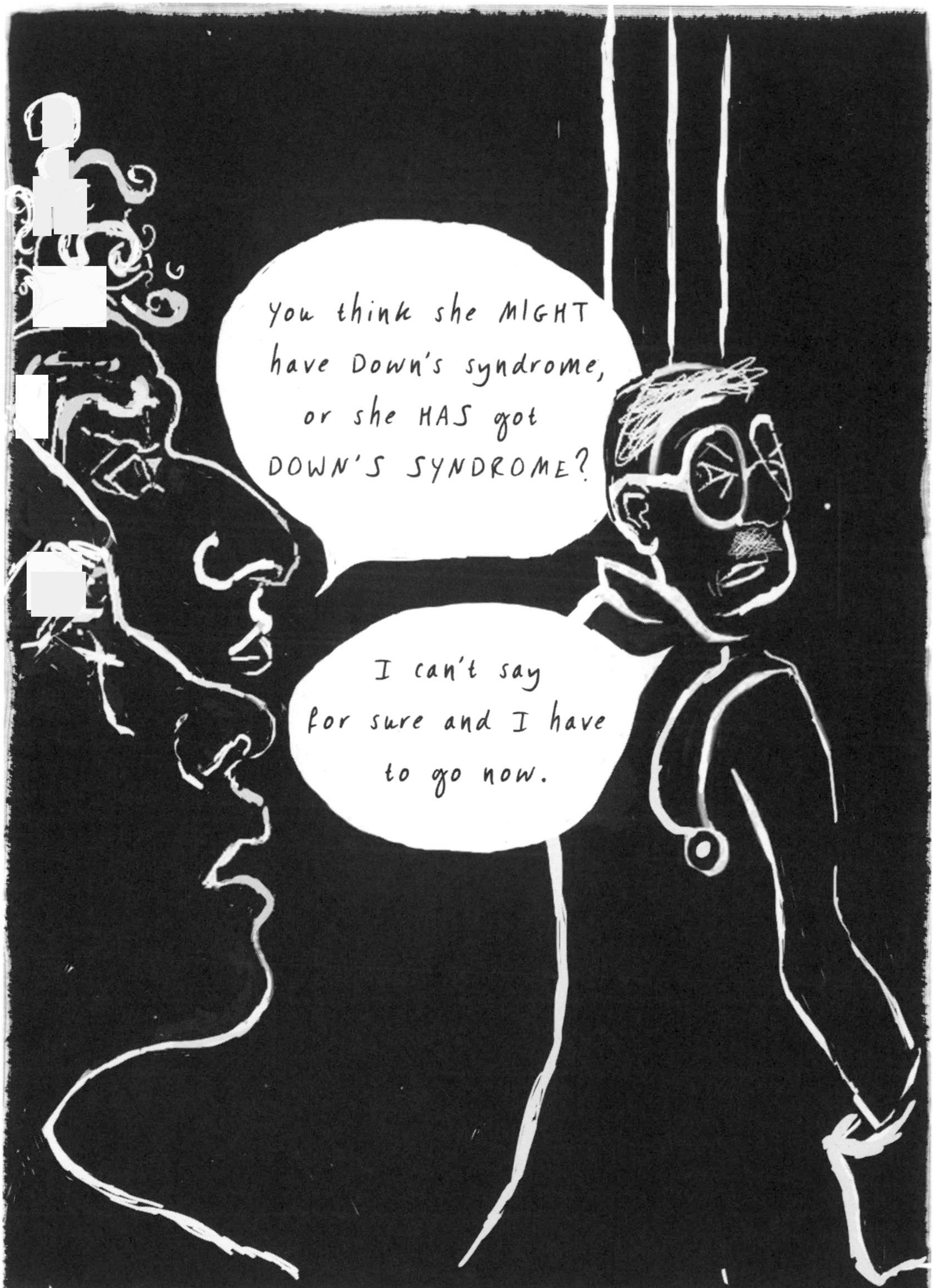
You think she MIGHT have Down's syndrome, or she HAS got DOWN'S SYNDROME?
I can't say for sure and I have to go now.

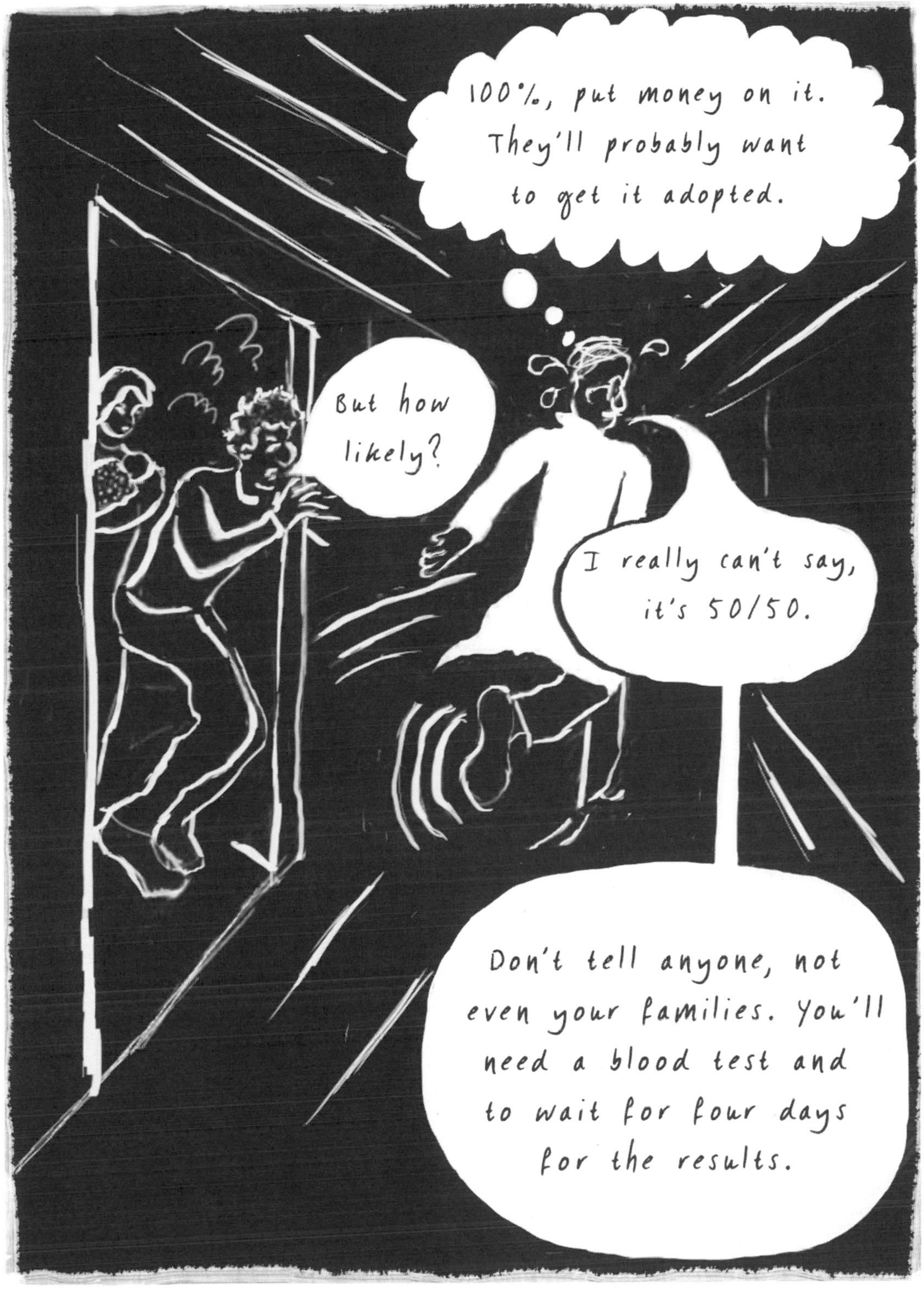
100%, put money on it. They'll probably want to get it adopted.
But how likely?
I really can't say, it's 50/50.
Don't tell anyone, not even your families. You'll need a blood test and to wait for four days for the results.

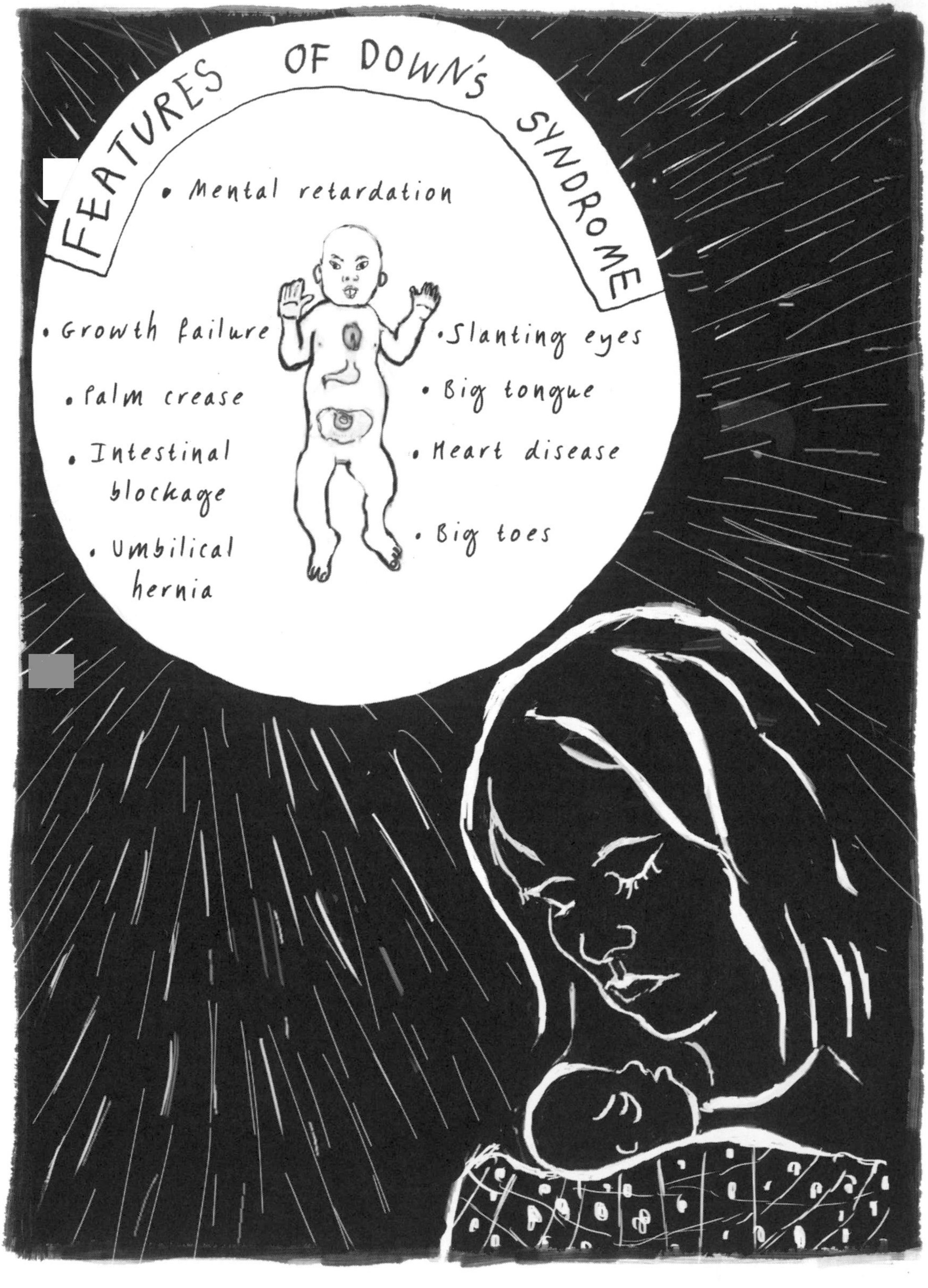
FEATURES OF DOWN'S SYNDROME
• Mental retardation
• Growth failure
• Palm crease
• Intestinal blockage
• Umbilical hernia
• Slanting eyes
• Big tongue
• Heart disease
• Big toes

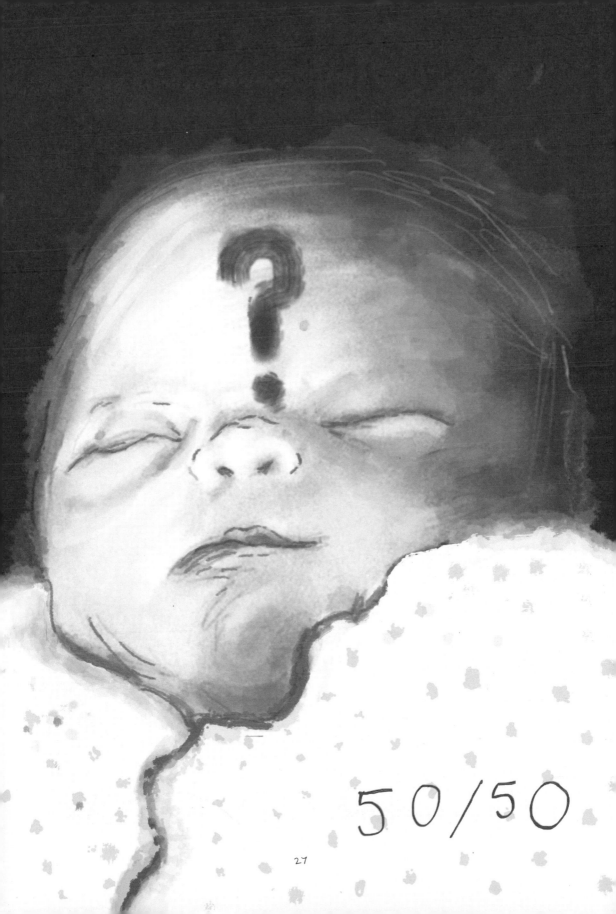

50/50

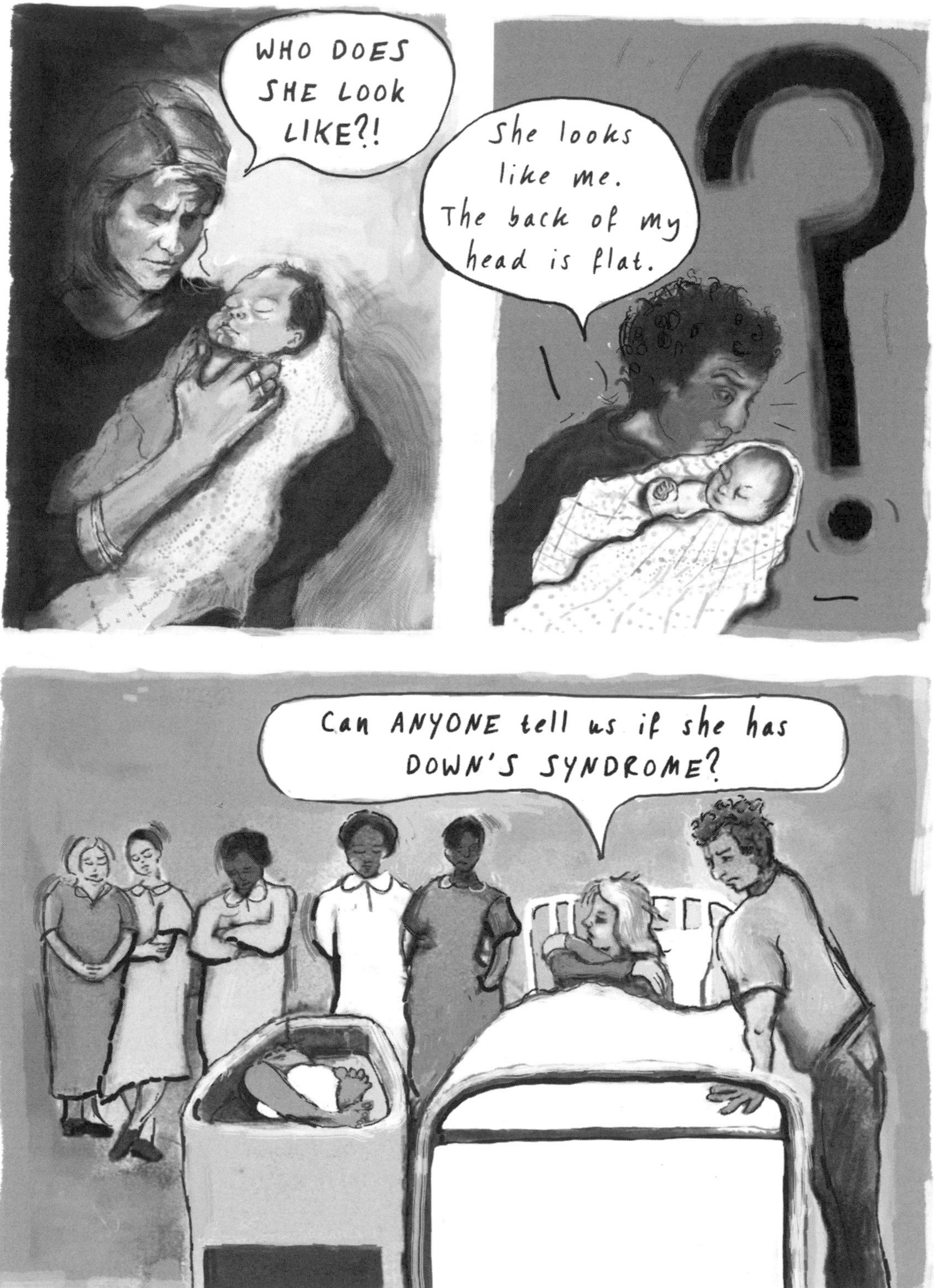
WHO DOES SHE LOOK LIKE?!
She looks like me. The back of my head is flat.
Can ANYONE tell us if she has DOWN'S SYNDROME?

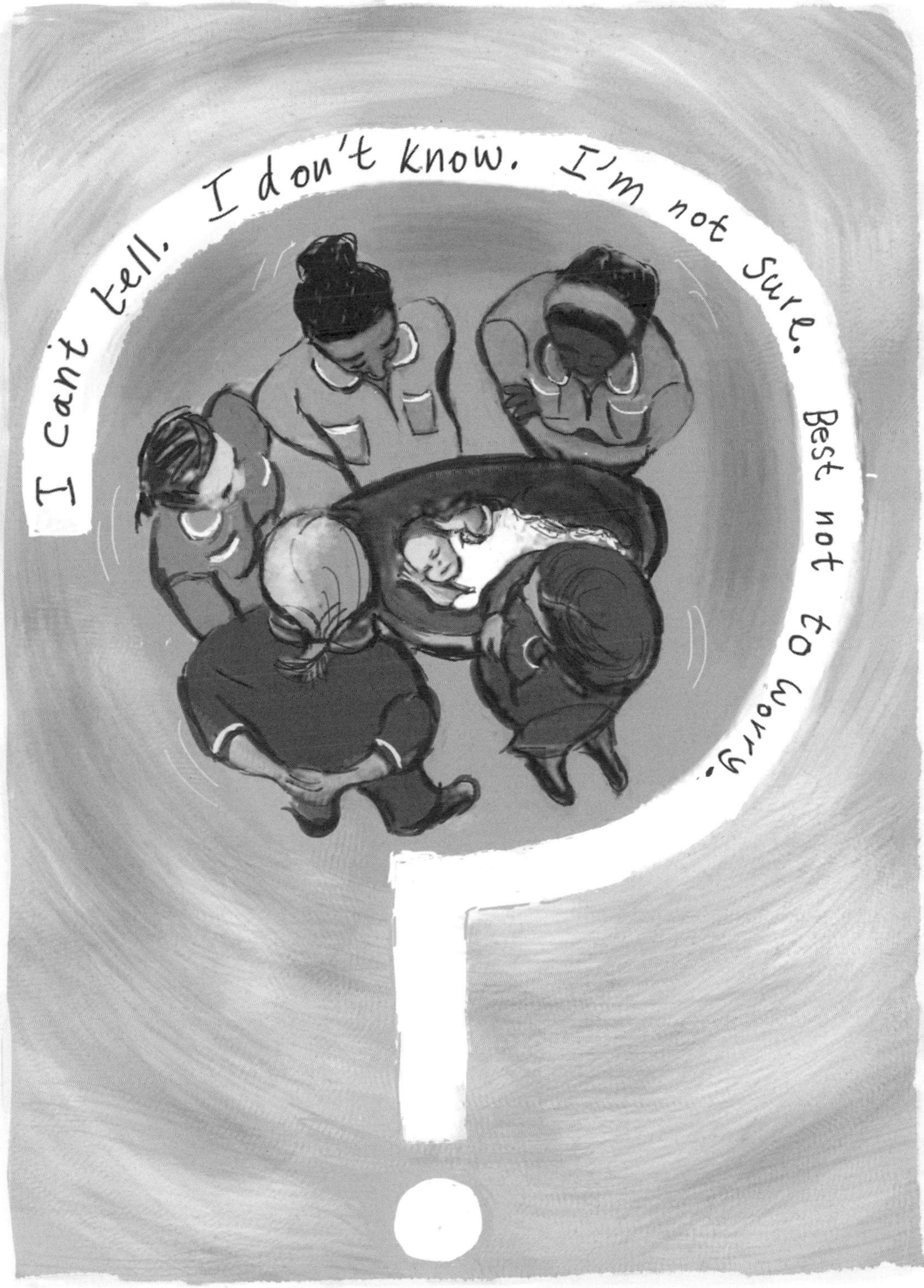
I can't tell. I don't know. I'm not sure. Best not to worry.

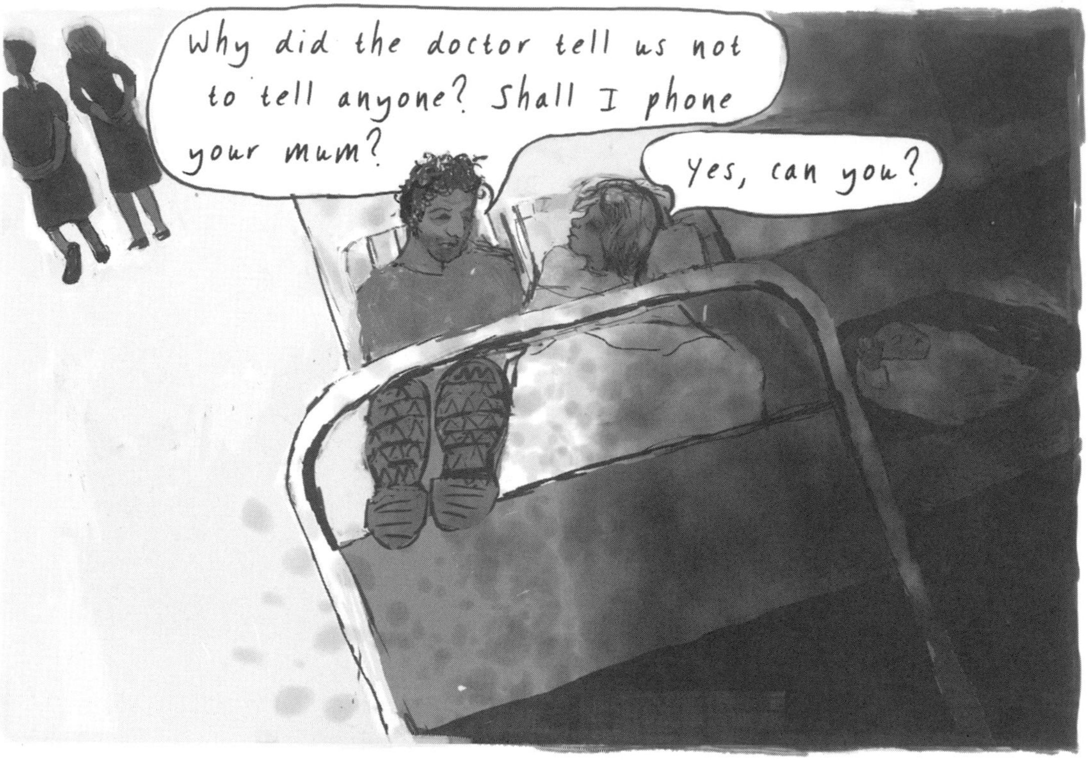
Why did the doctor tell us not to tell anyone? Shall I phone your mum?
Yes, can you?

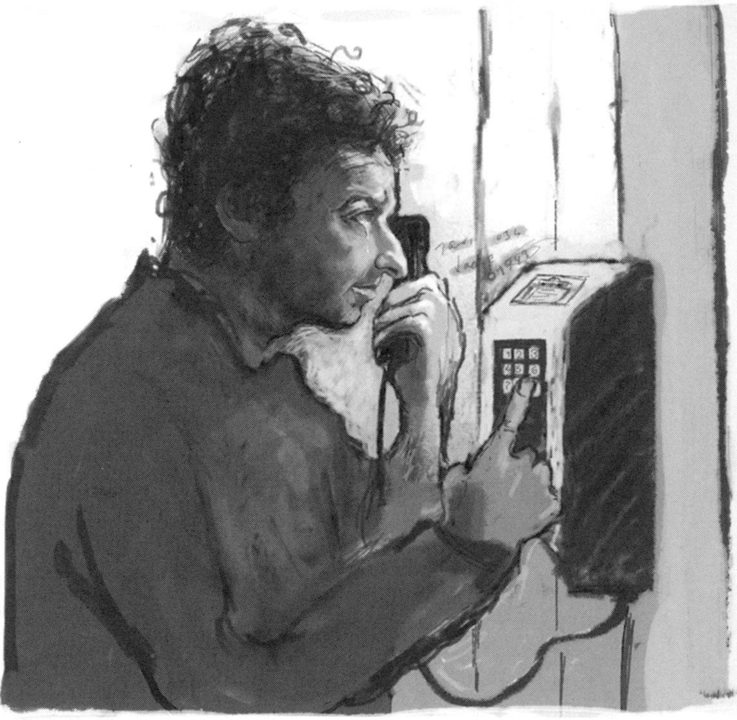

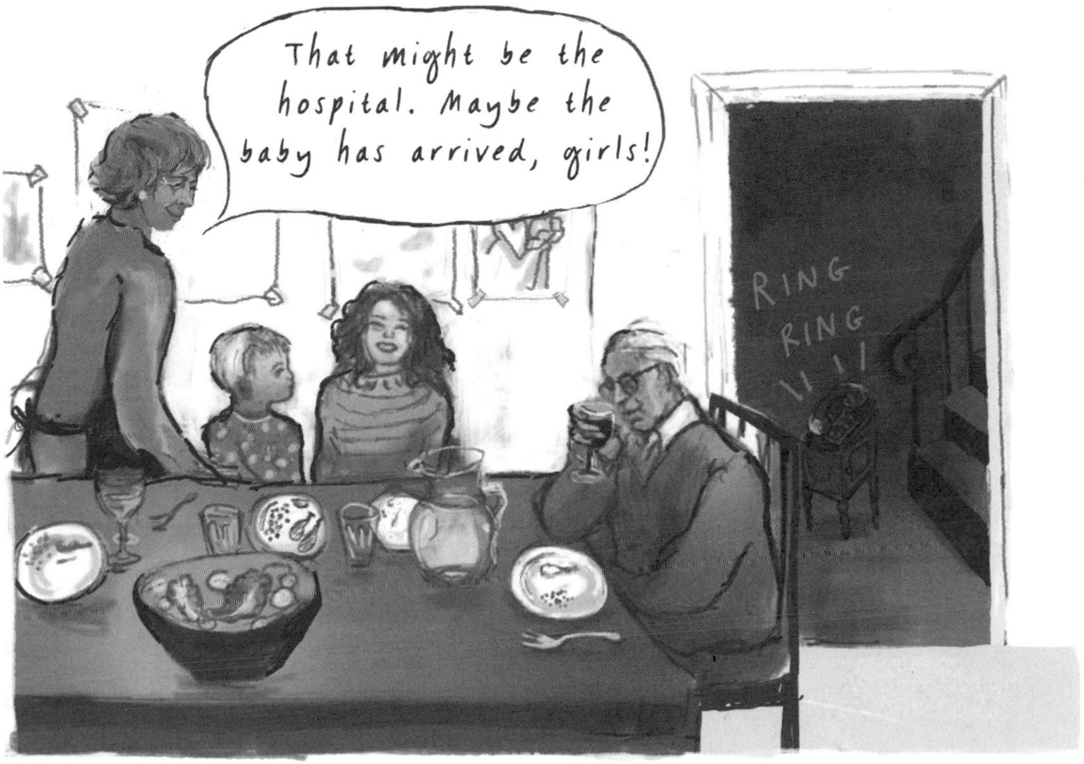
That might be the hospital. Maybe the baby has arrived, girls!
RING RING !!!

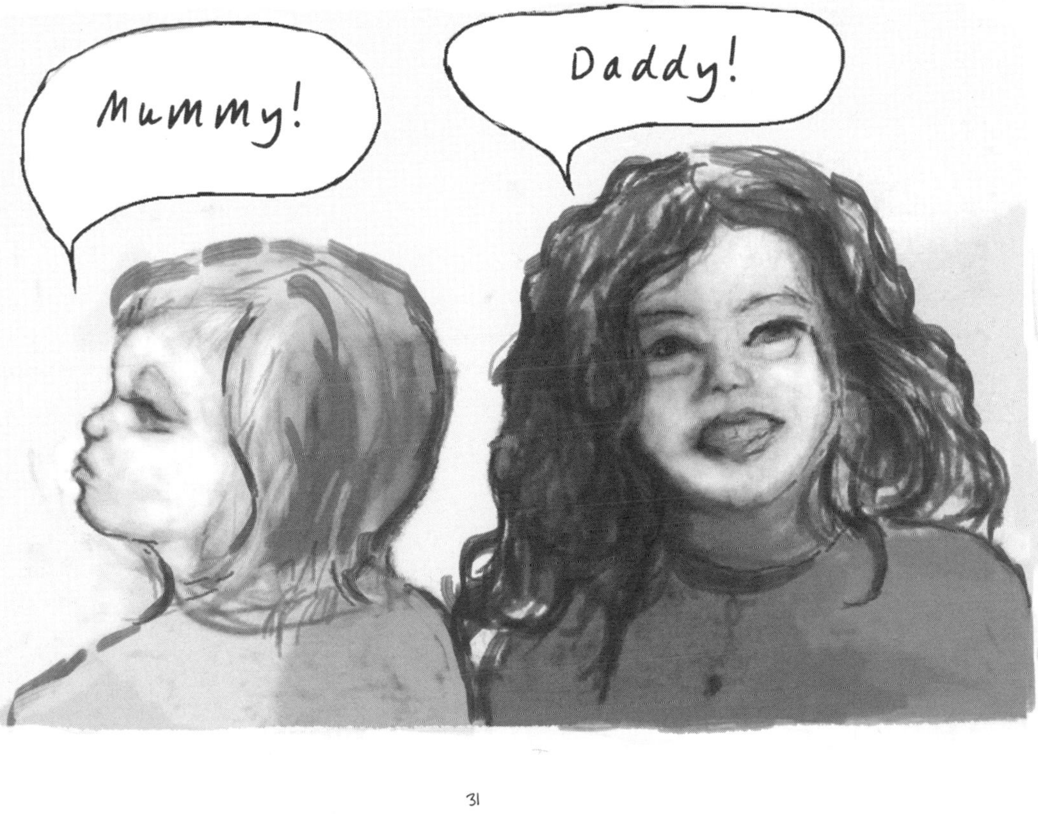
Mummy!
Daddy!

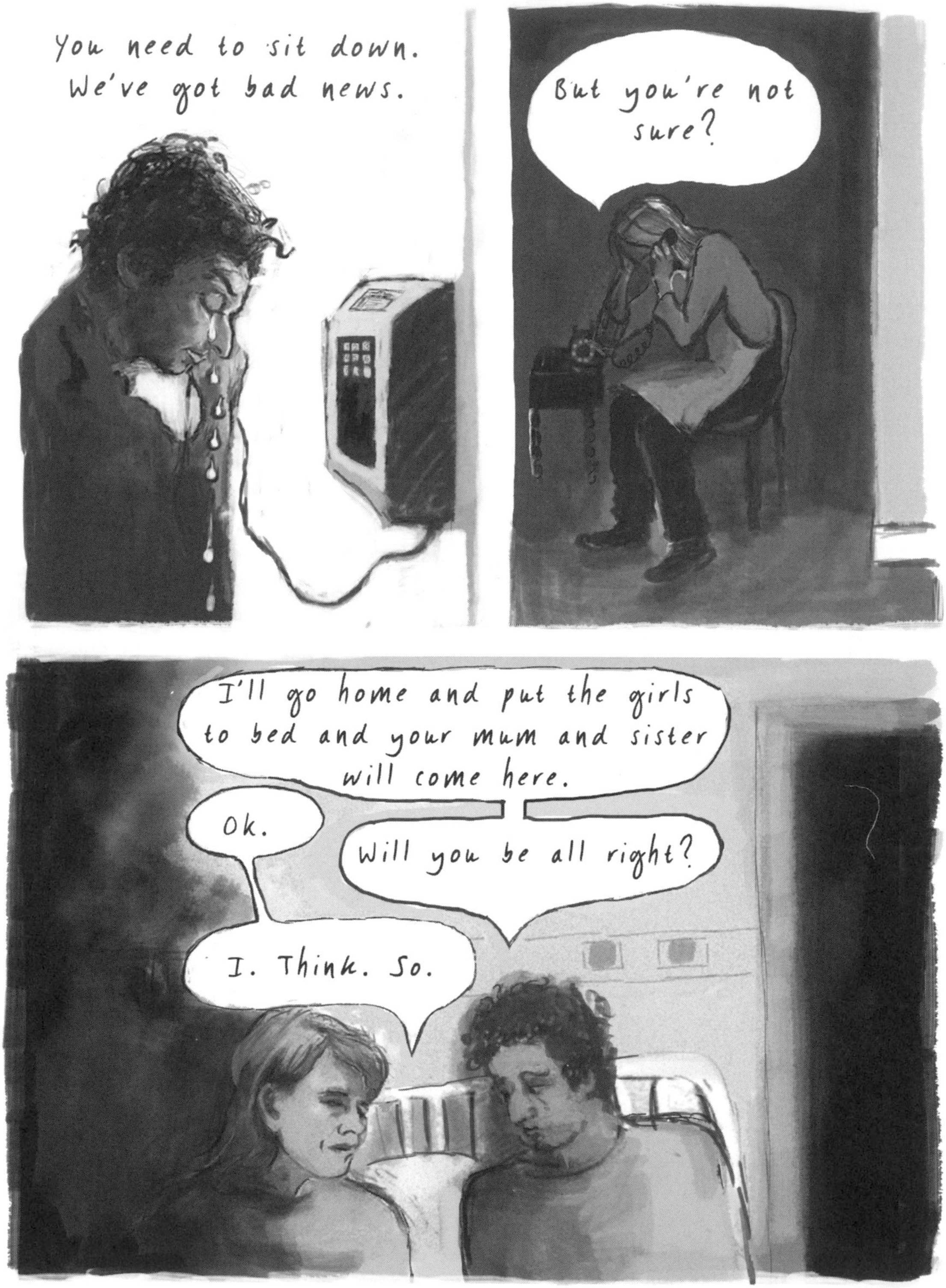
You need to sit down. We've got bad news.
But you're not sure?
I'll go home and put the girls to bed and your mum and sister will come here.
Ok.
Will you be all right?
I. Think. So.

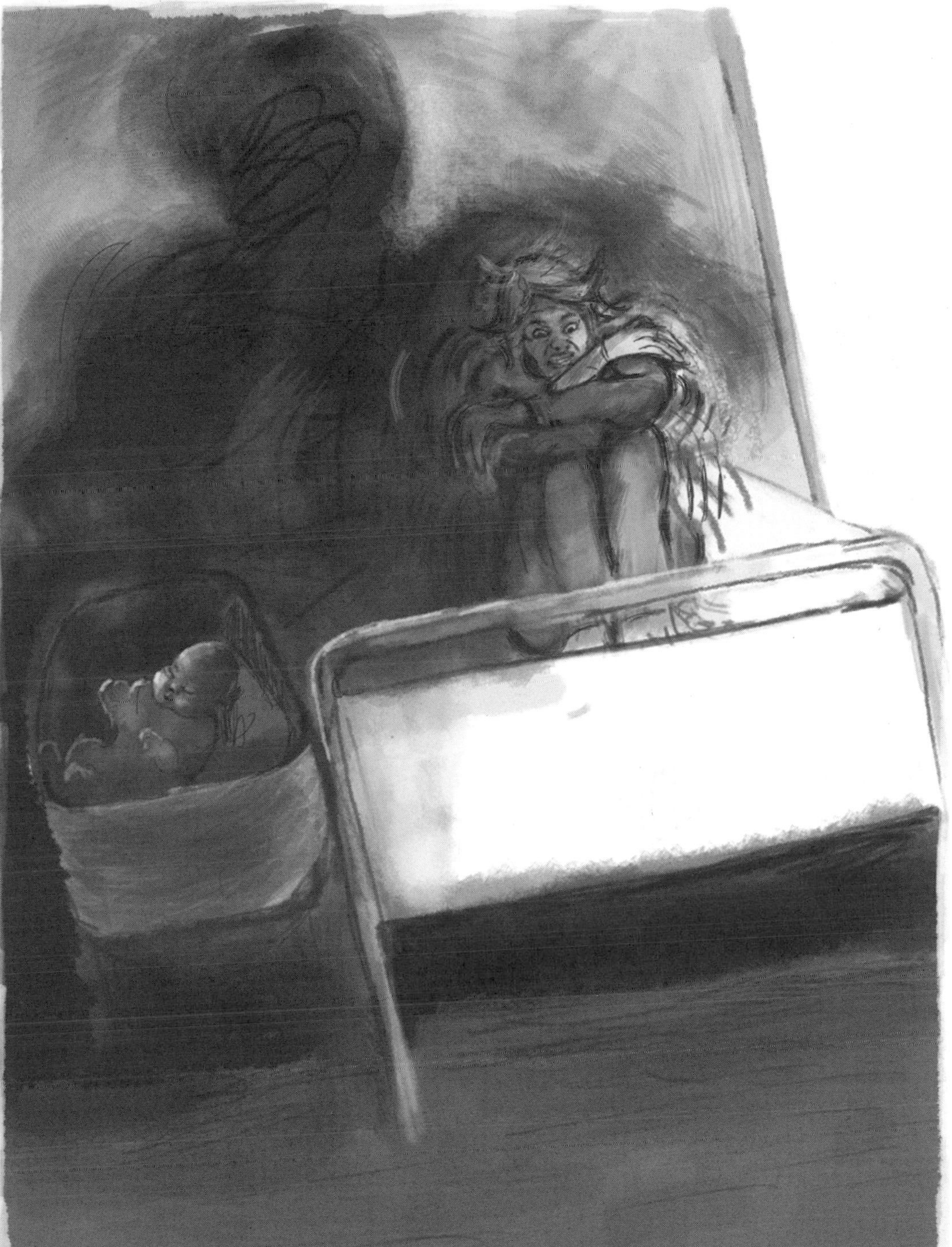

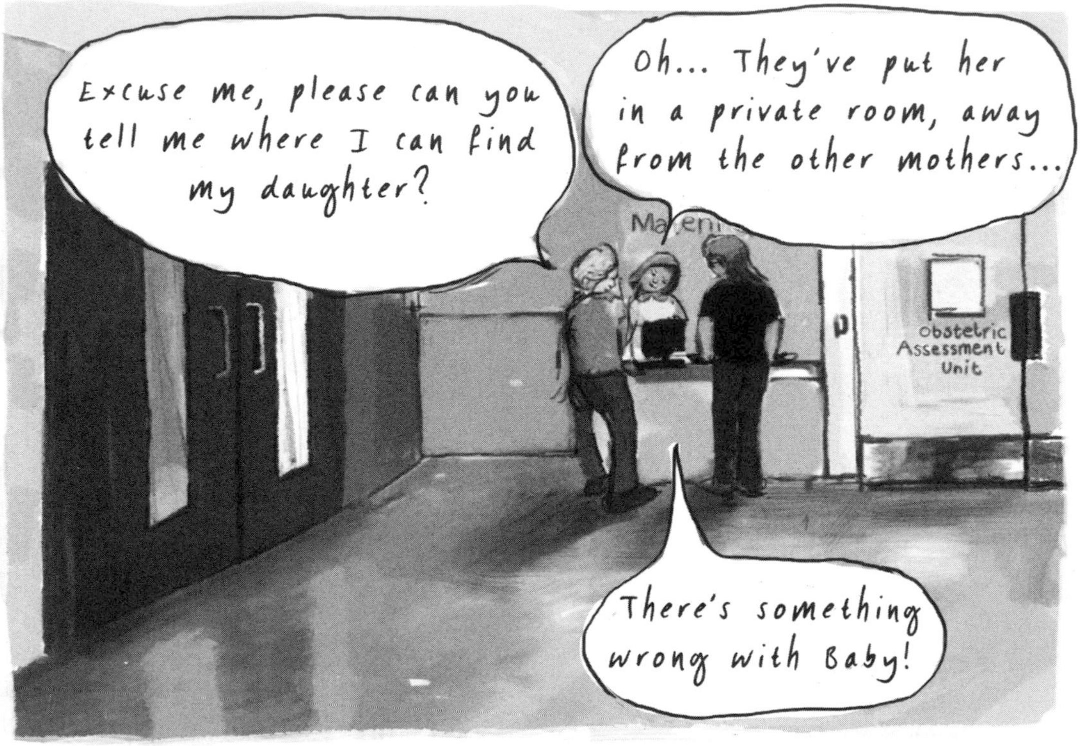
Excuse me, please can you tell me where I can find my daughter?
Oh... They've put her in a private room, away from the other mothers...
Obstetric Assessment Unit
There's something wrong with Baby!

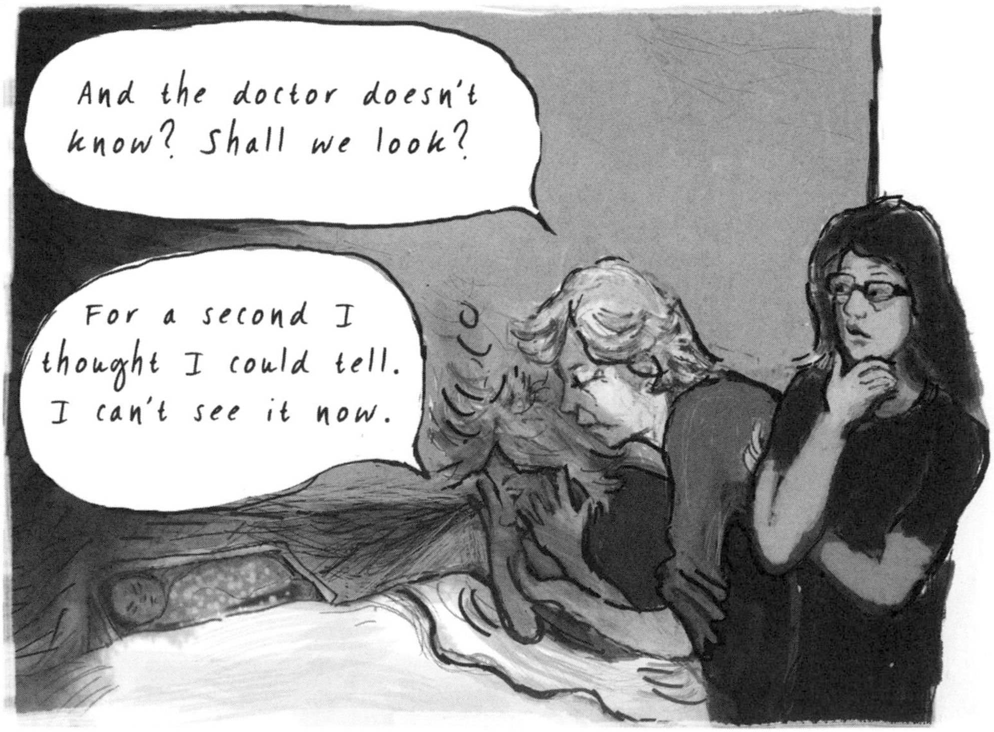
And the doctor doesn't know? Shall we look?
For a second I thought I could tell. I can't see it now.

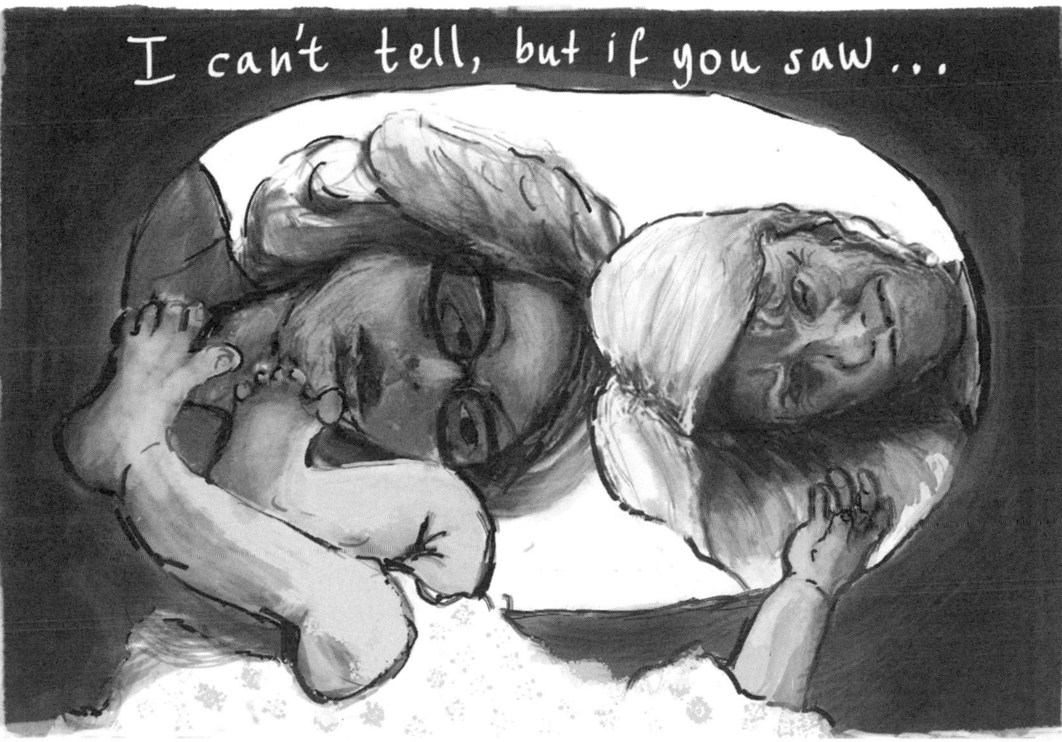
I can't tell, but if you saw...

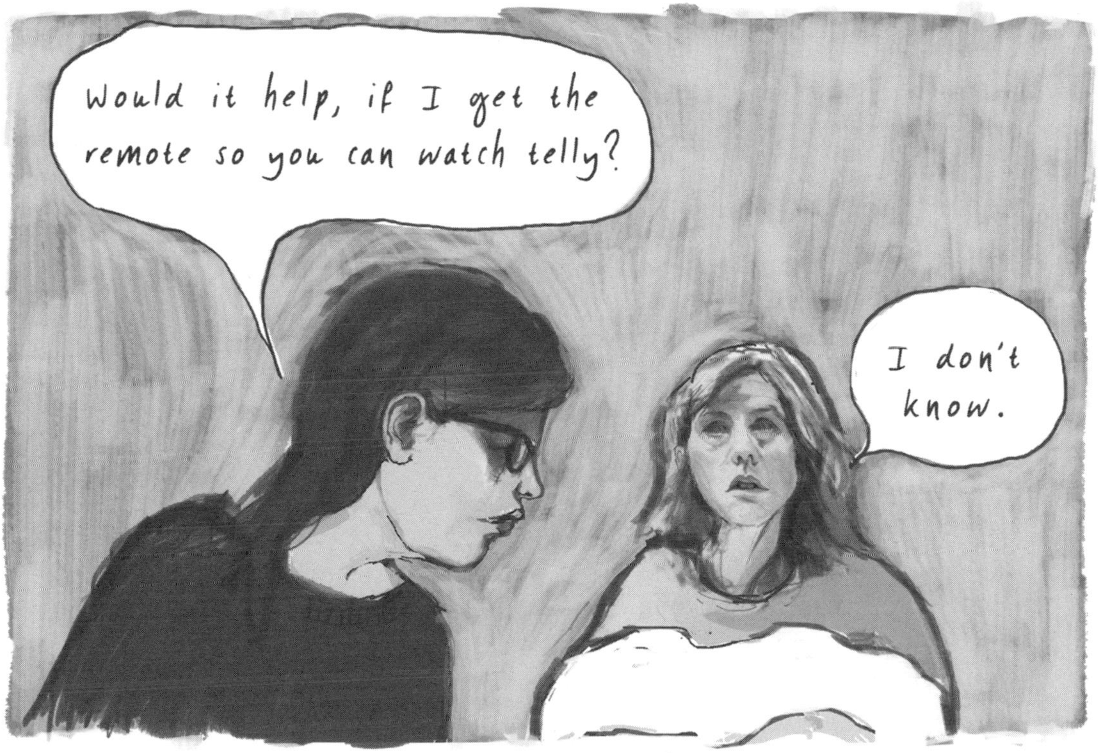
Would it help, if I get the remote so you can watch telly?
I don't know.

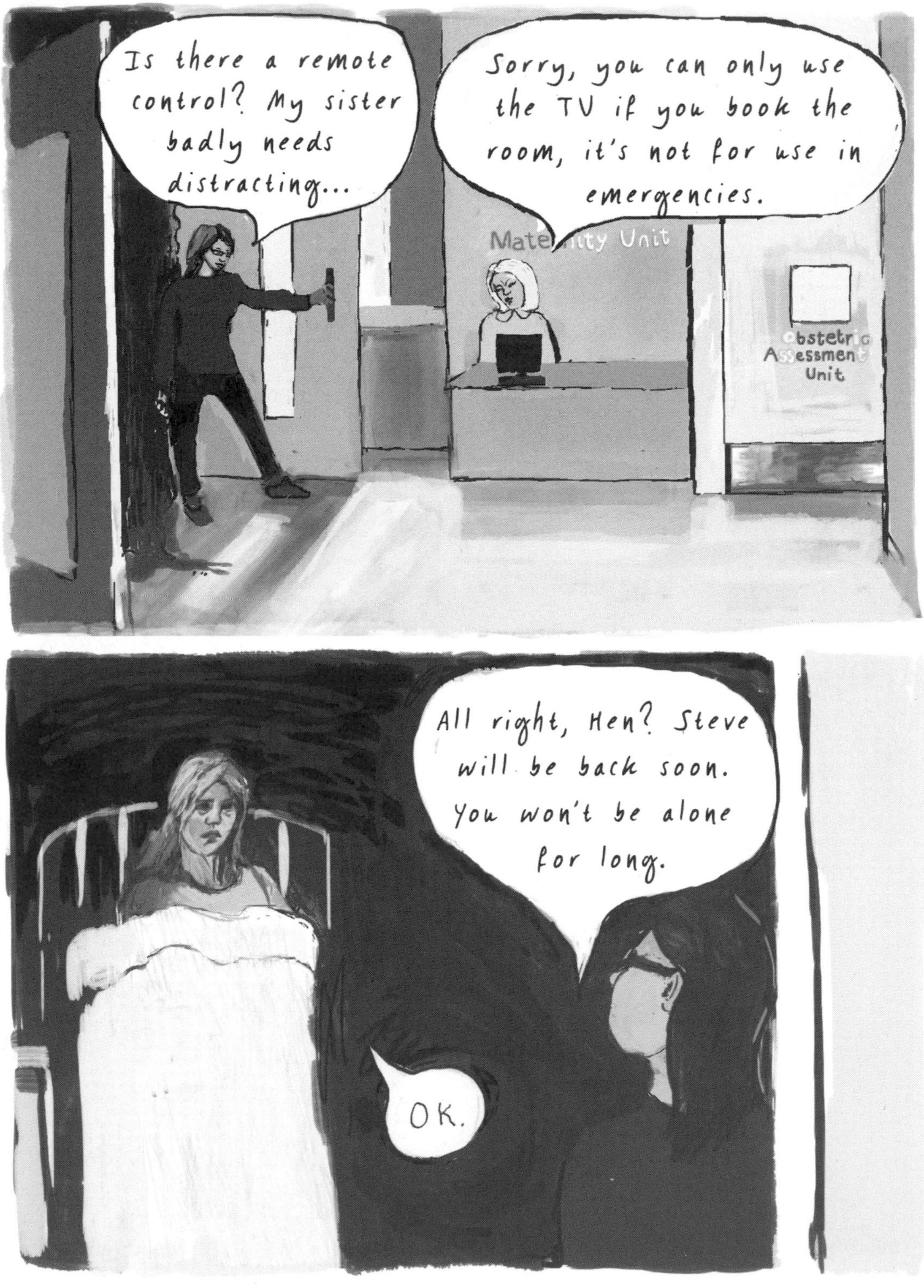
Is there a remote control? My sister badly needs distracting...
Sorry, you can only use the TV if you book the room, it's not for use in emergencies.
All right, Hen? Steve will be back soon. You won't be alone for long.
OK.

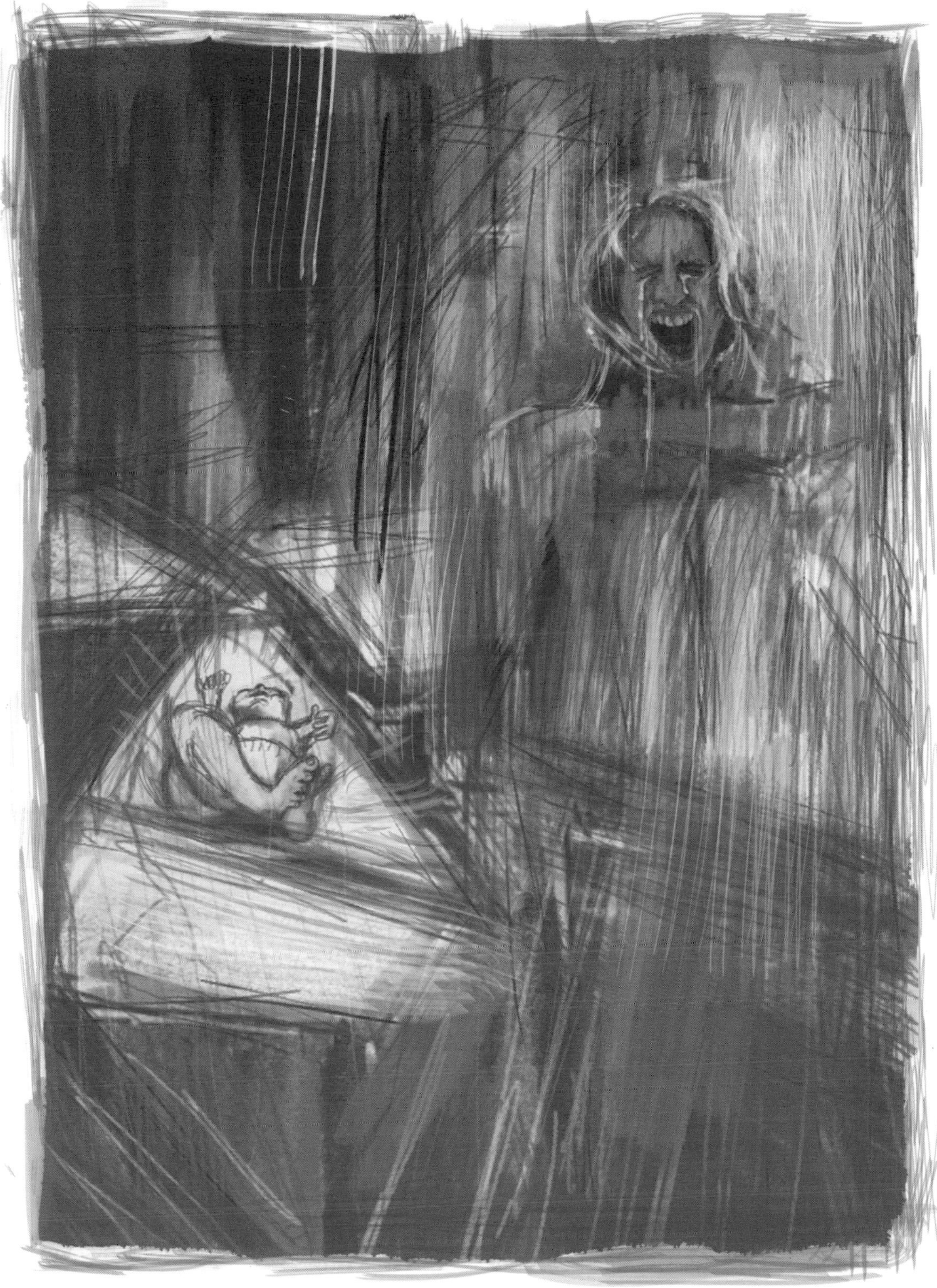

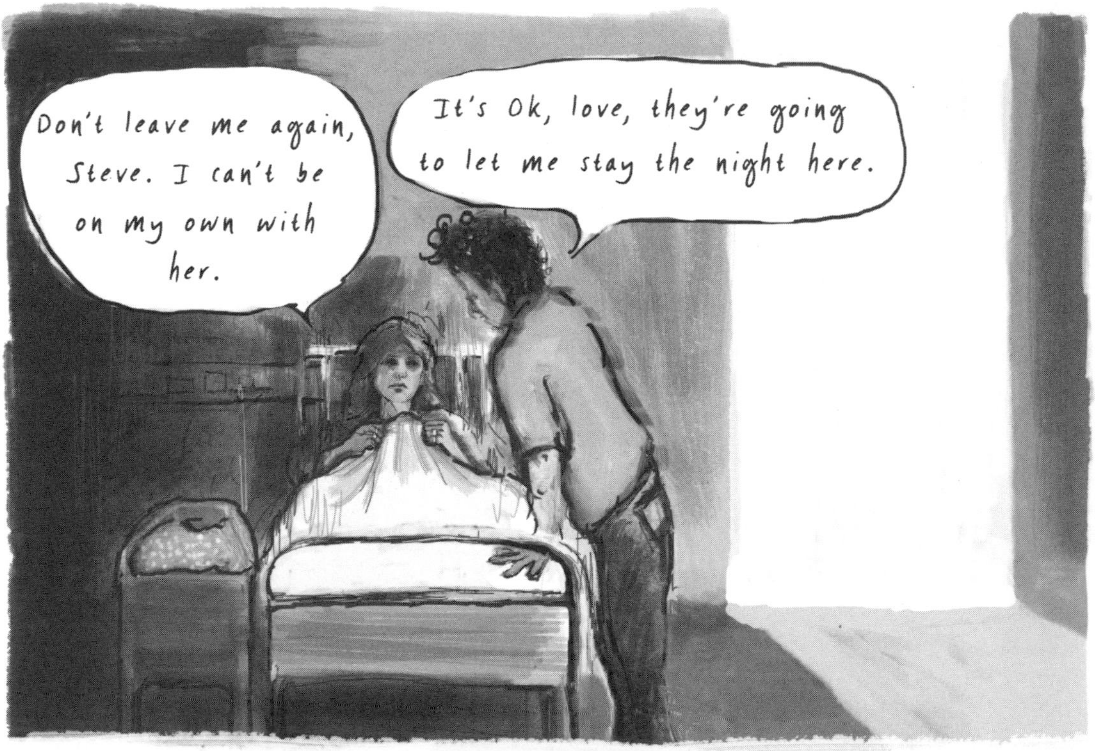
Don't leave me again, Steve. I can't be on my own with her.
It's Ok, love, they're going to let me stay the night here.

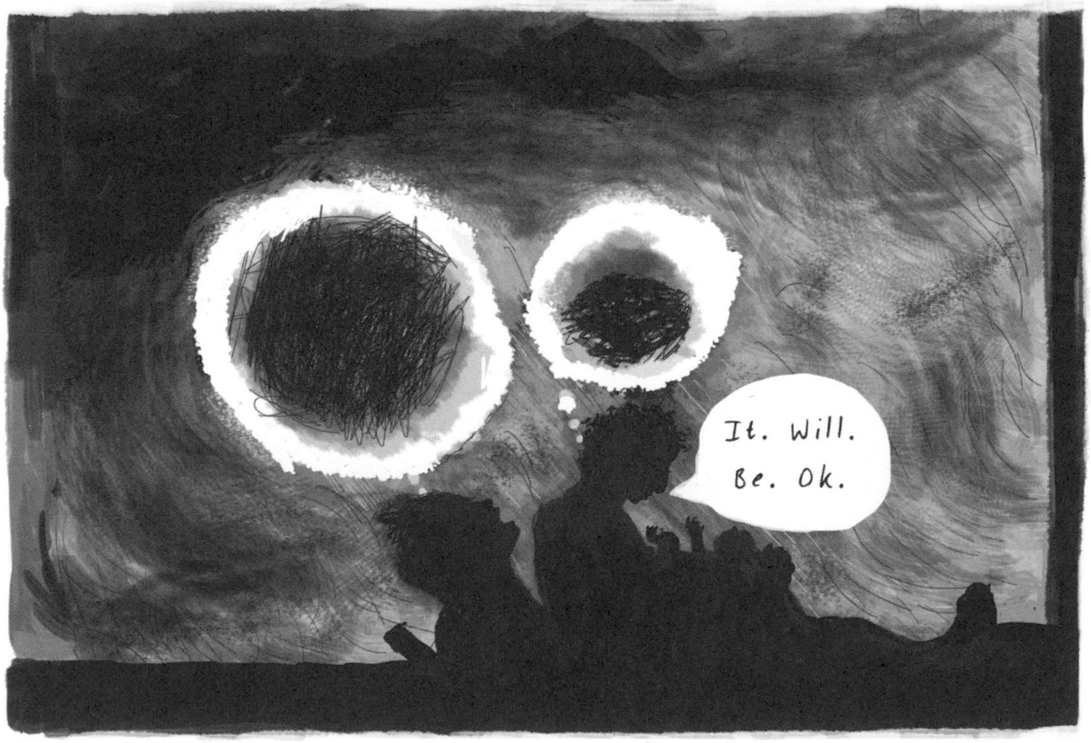
It. Will. Be. Ok.

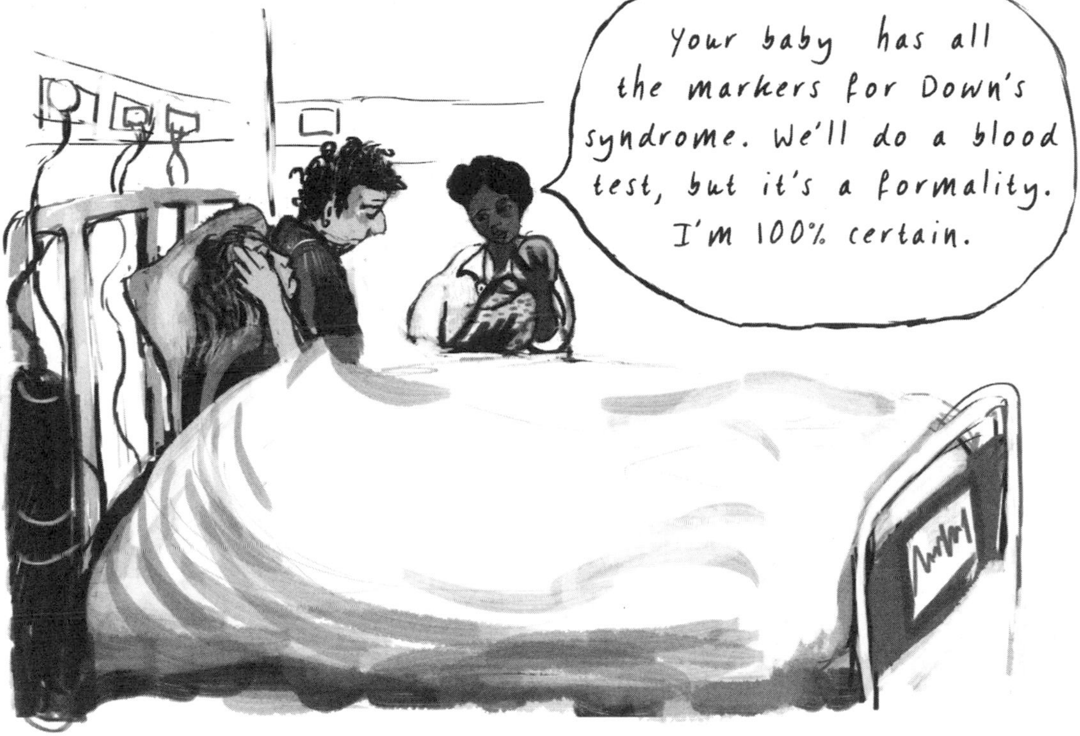
Your baby has all the markers for Down's syndrome. We'll do a blood test, but it's a formality. I'm 100% certain.

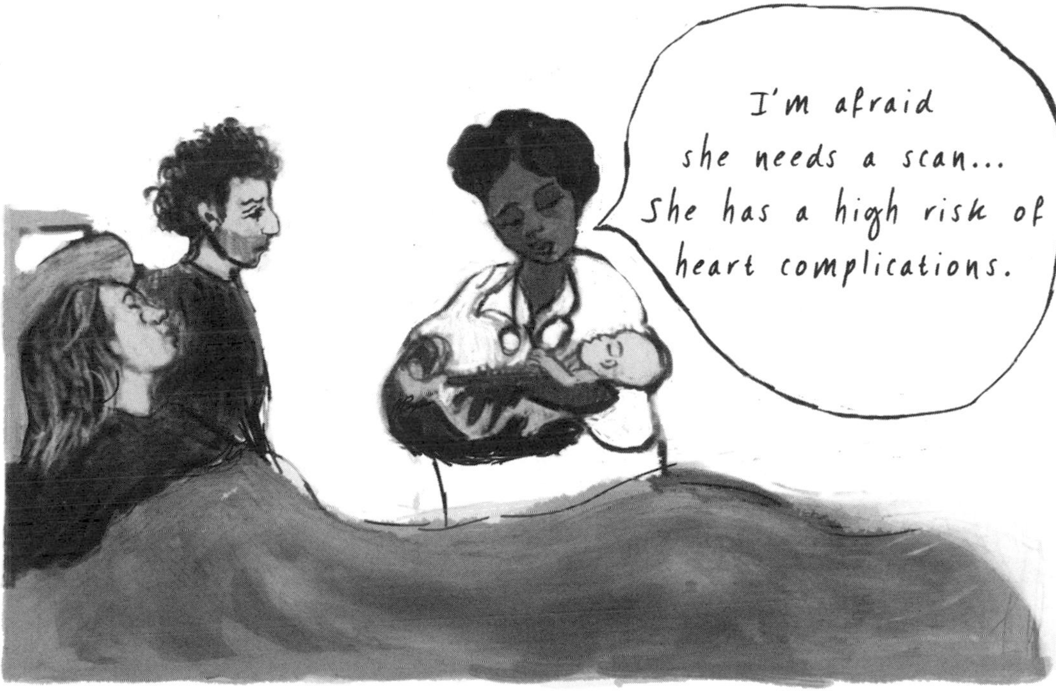
I'm afraid she needs a scan... She has a high risk of heart complications.

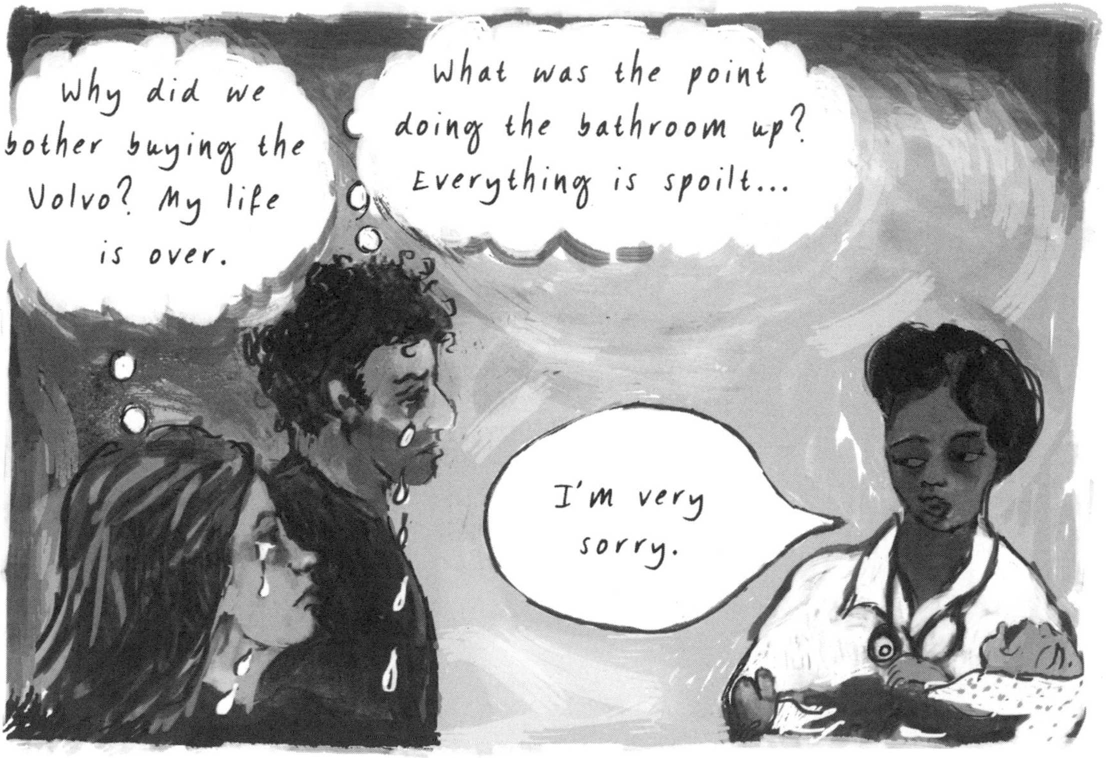
Why did we bother buying the Volvo? My life is over.
What was the point doing the bathroom up? Everything is spoilt...
I'm very sorry.

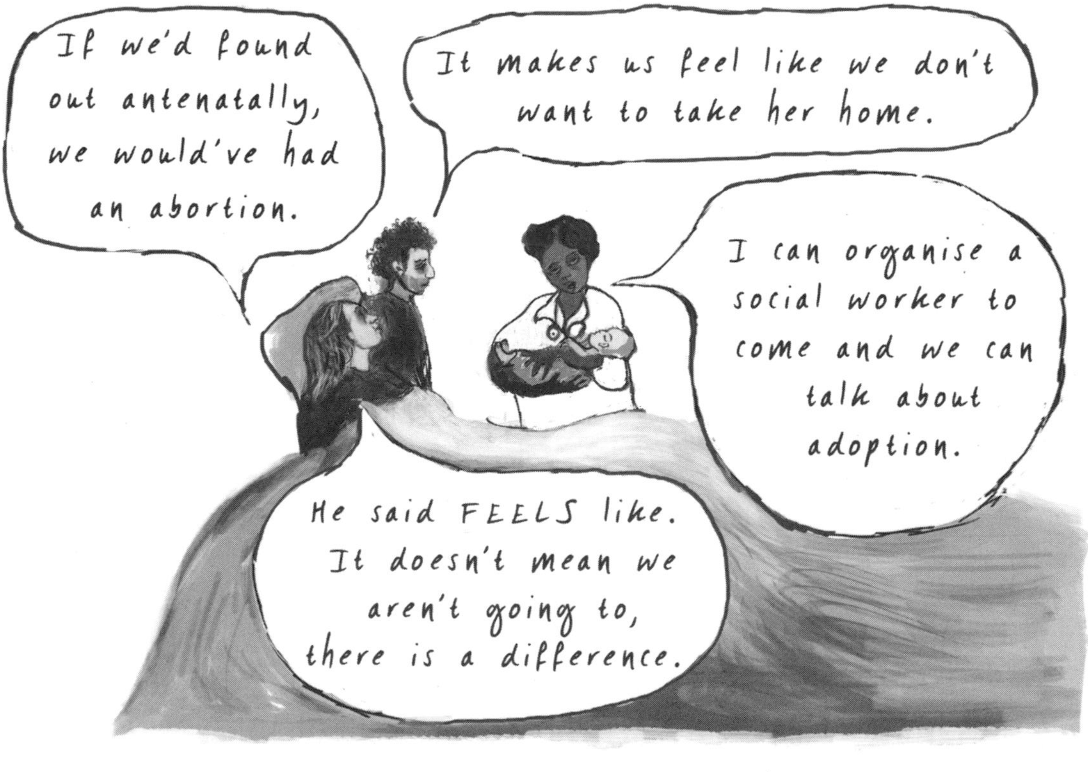
If we'd found out antenatally, we would've had an abortion.
It makes us feel like we don't want to take her home.
I can organise a social worker to come and we can talk about adoption.
He said FEELS like. It doesn't mean we aren't going to, there is a difference.

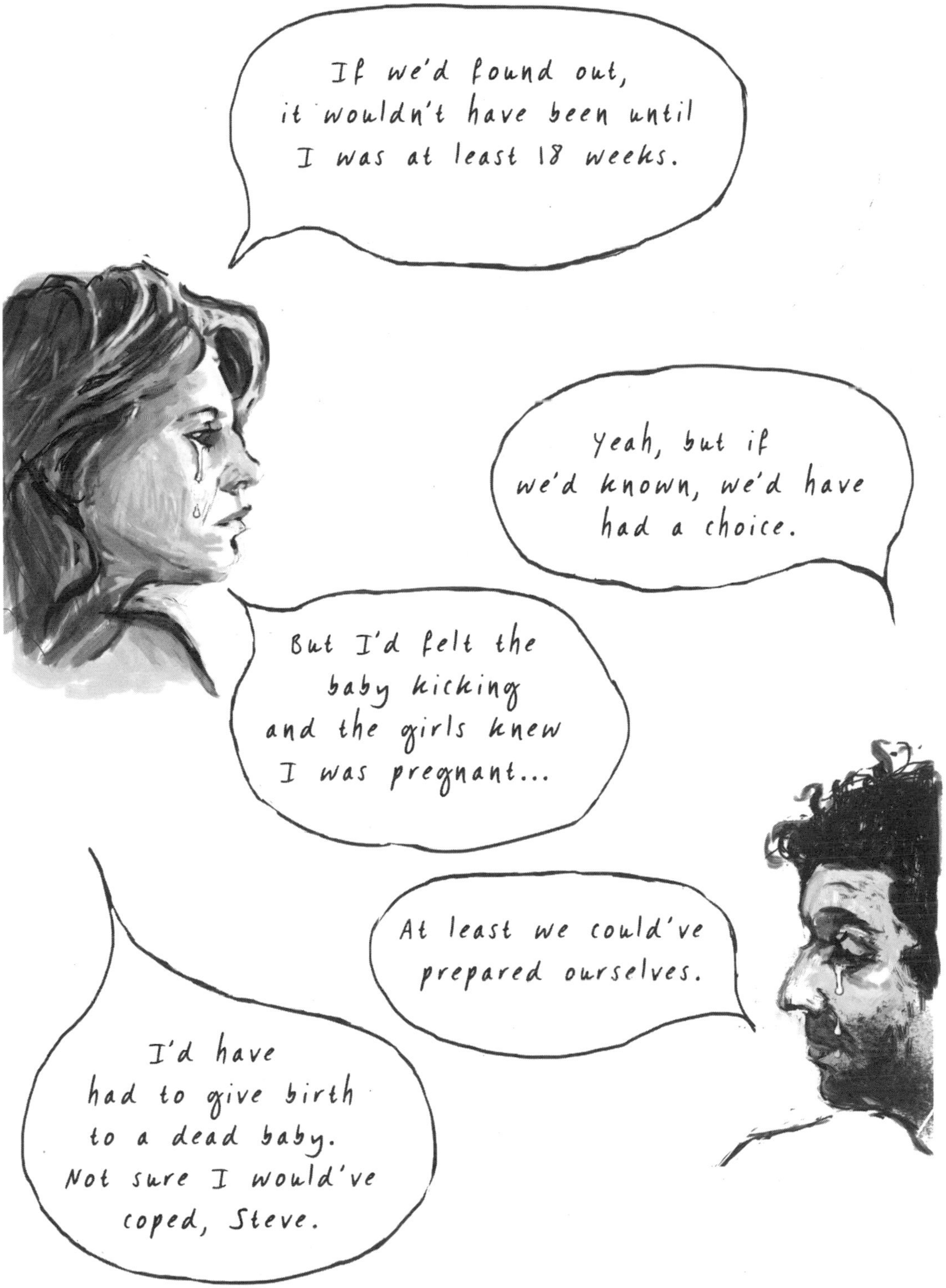
If we'd found out, it wouldn't have been until I was at least 18 weeks.
Yeah, but if we'd known, we'd have had a choice.
But I'd felt the baby kicking and the girls knew I was pregnant...
At least we could've prepared ourselves.
I'd have had to give birth to a dead baby. Not sure I would've coped, Steve.

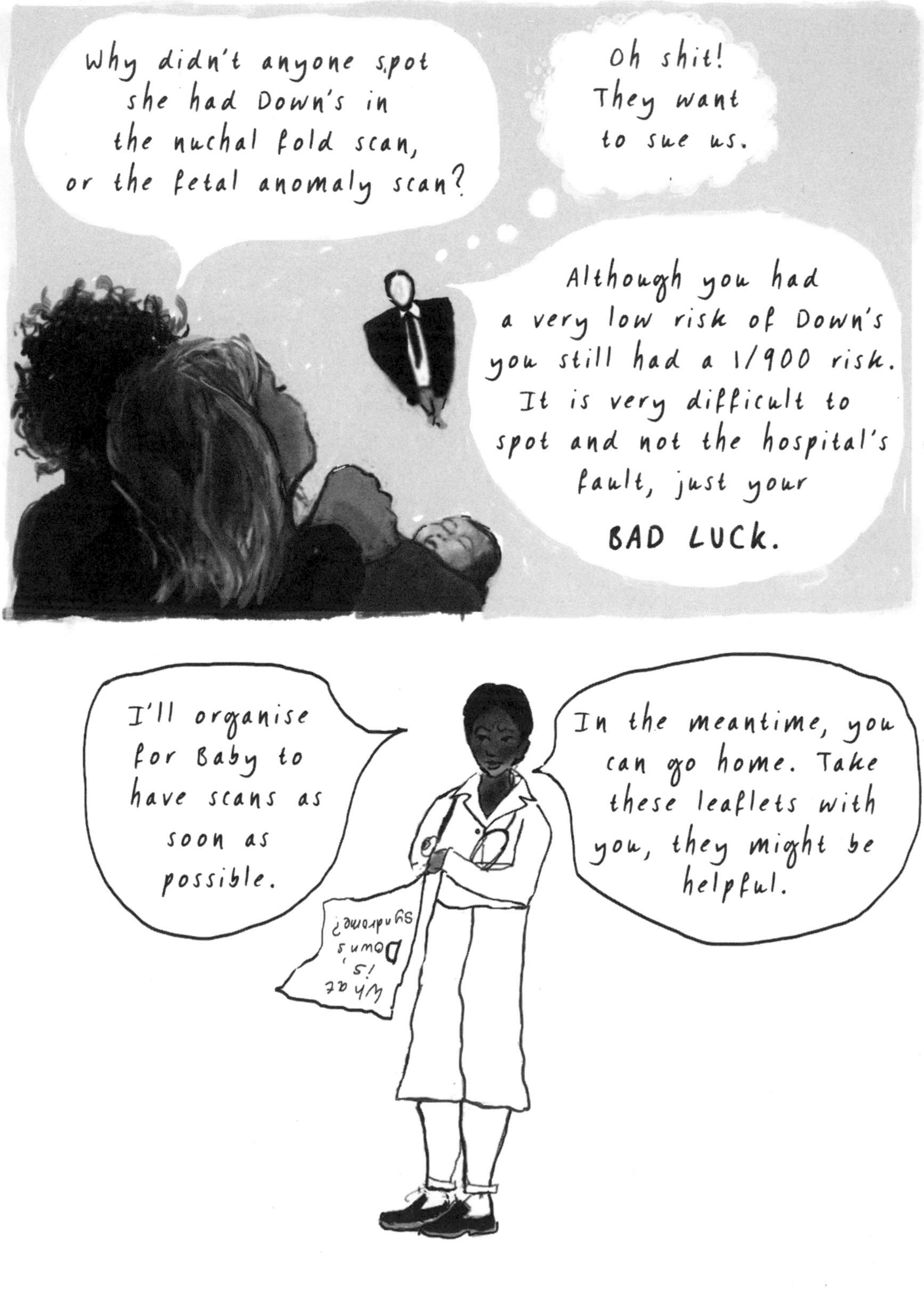
Why didn't anyone spot she had Down's in the nuchal fold scan, or the fetal anomaly scan?
Oh shit! They want to sue us.
Although you had a very low risk of Down's you still had a 1/900 risk. It is very difficult to spot and not the hospital's fault, just your BAD LUCK.
I'll organise for Baby to have scans as soon as possible.
In the meantime, you can go home. Take these leaflets with you, they might be helpful.
What is Down's Syndrome?

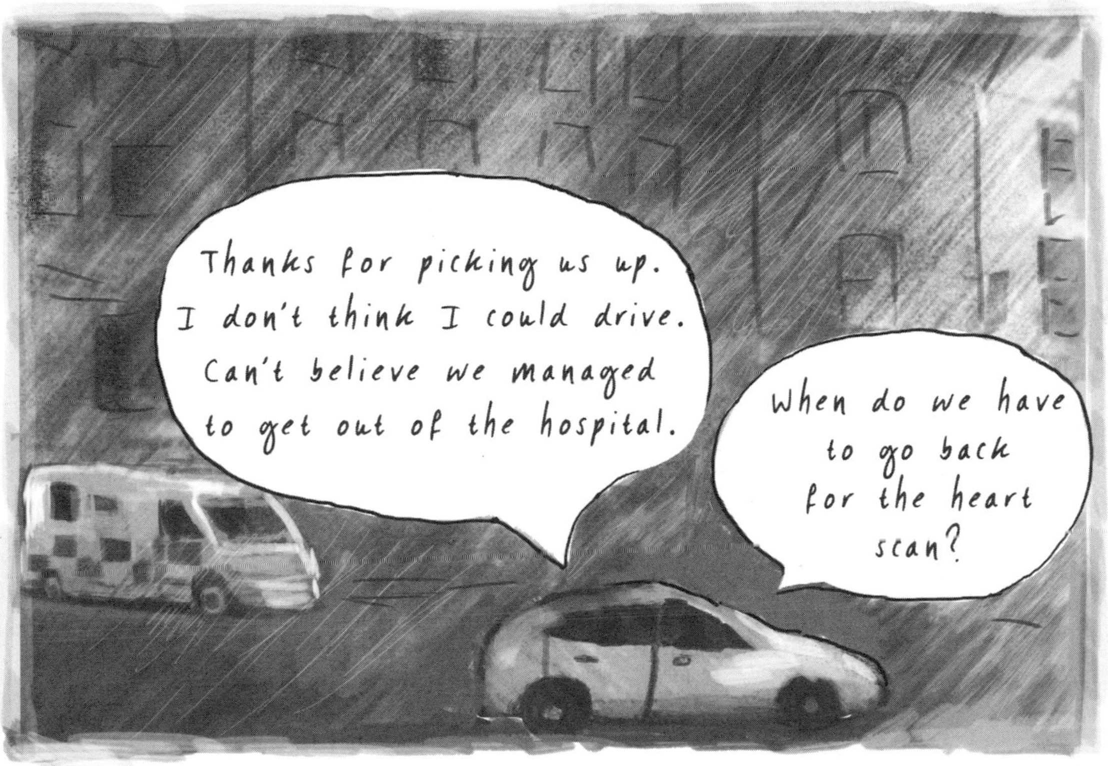
Thanks for picking us up. I don't think I could drive. Can't believe we managed to get out of the hospital.
When do we have to go back for the heart scan?

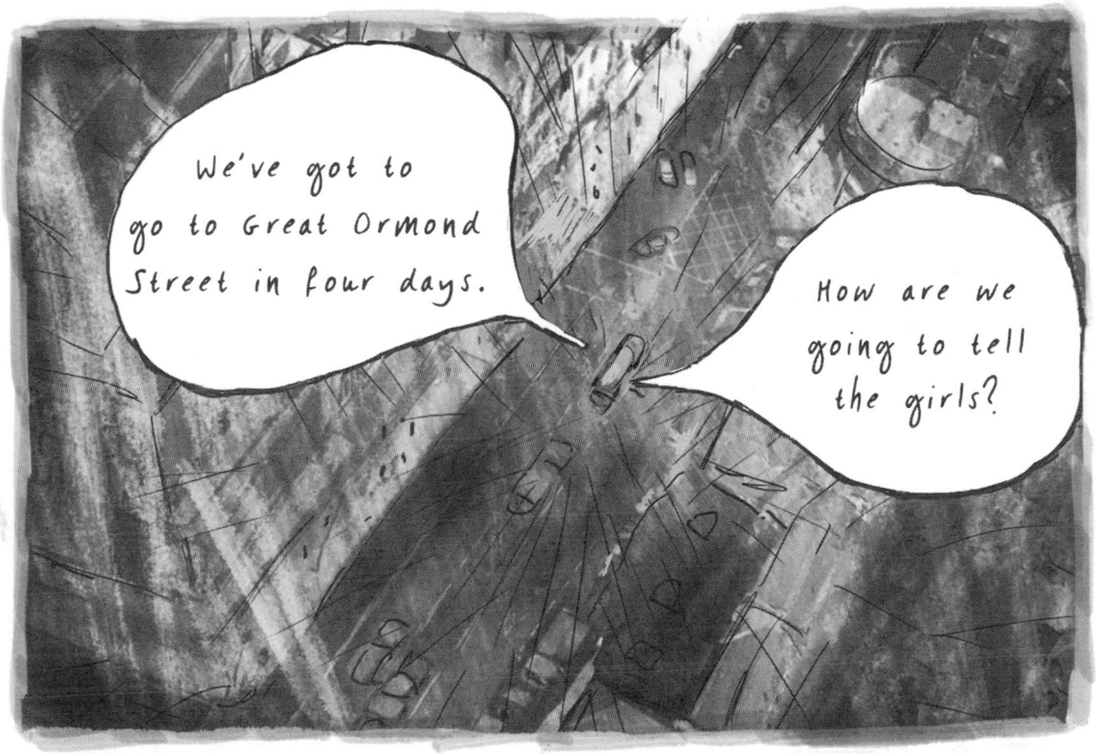
We've got to go to Great Ormond Street in four days.
How are we going to tell the girls?

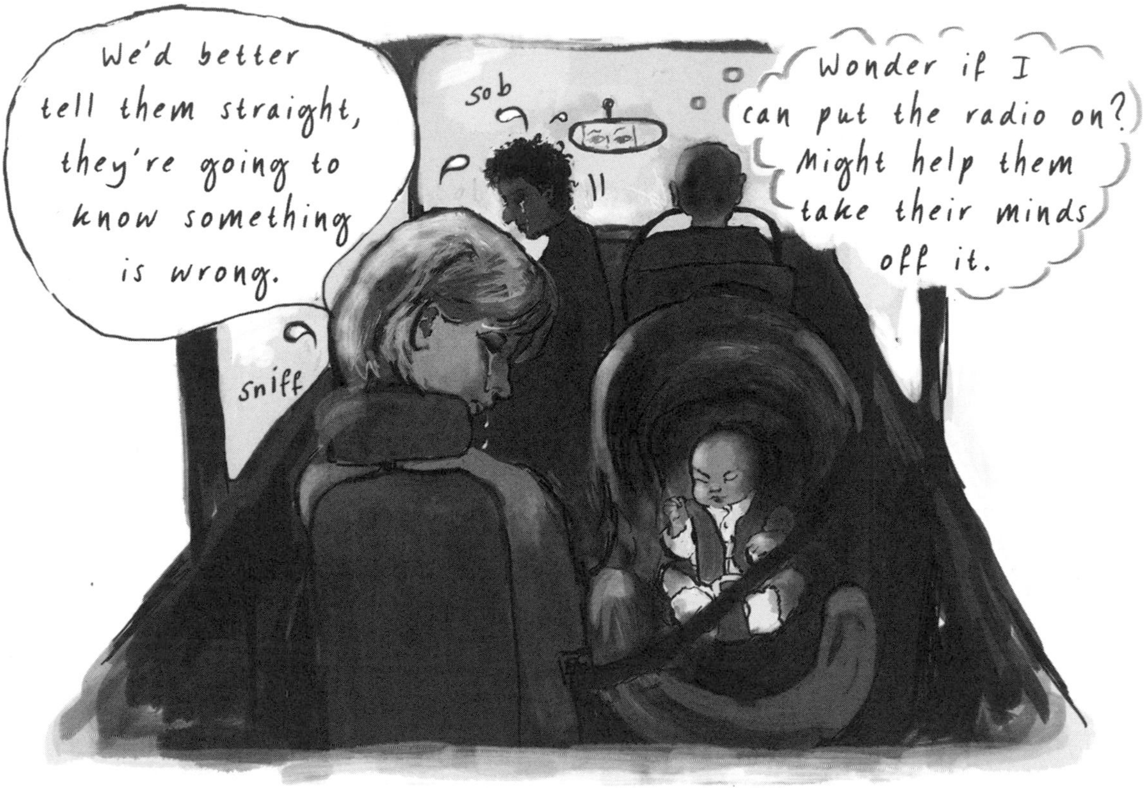
We'd better tell them straight, they're going to know something is wrong.
sob
sniff
Wonder if I can put the radio on? Might help them take their minds off it.

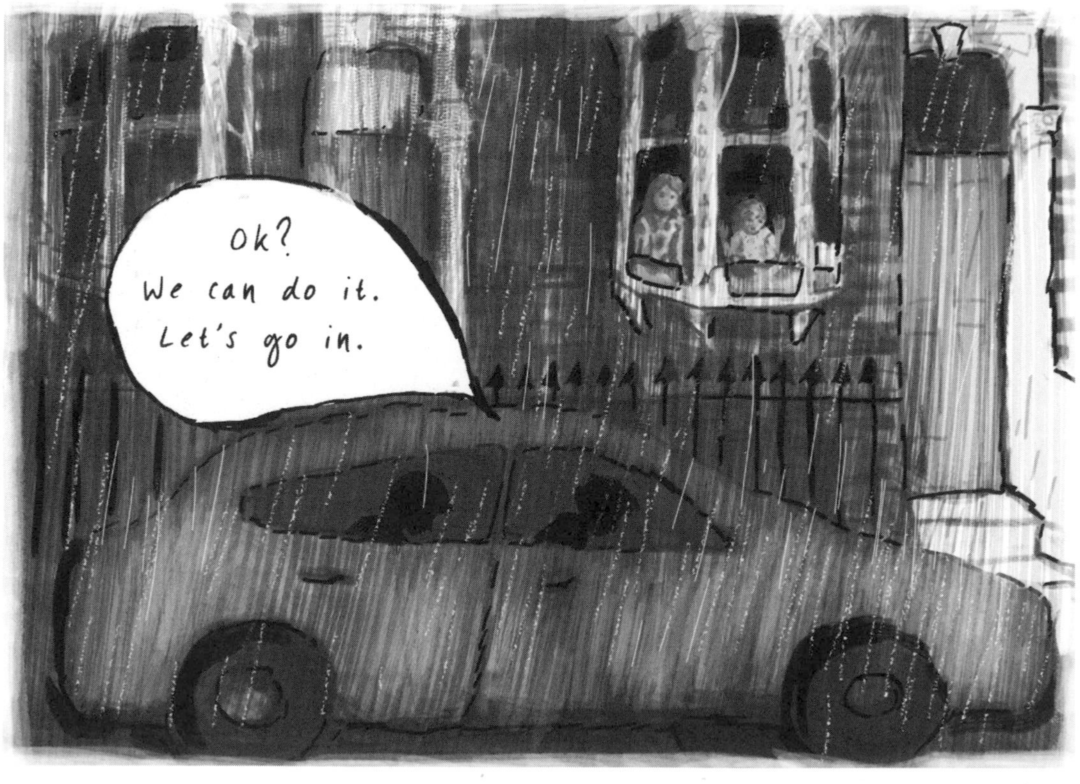
Ok? We can do it. Let's go in.

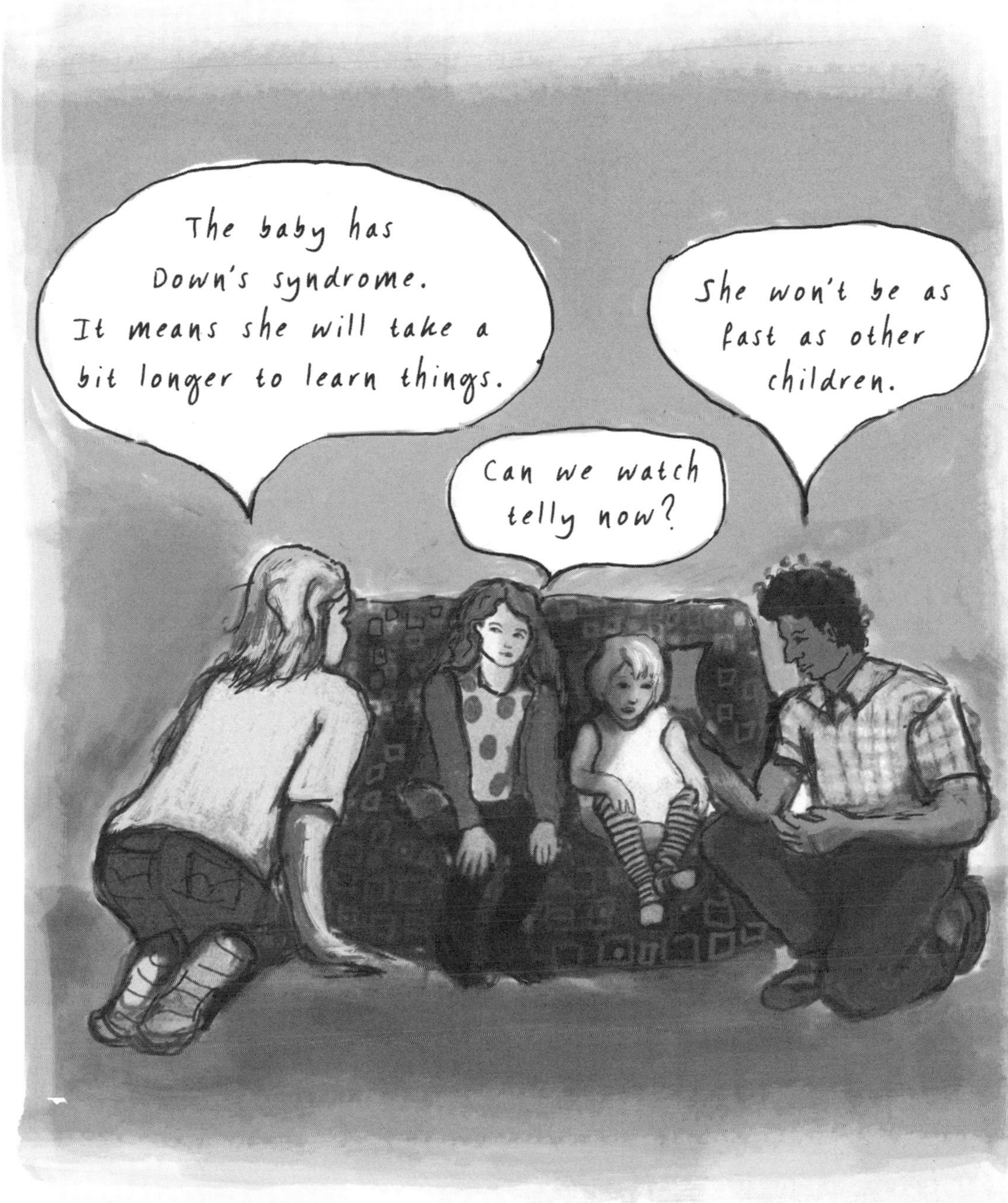
The baby has Down's syndrome. It means she will take a bit longer to learn things.
She won't be as fast as other children.
Can we watch telly now?

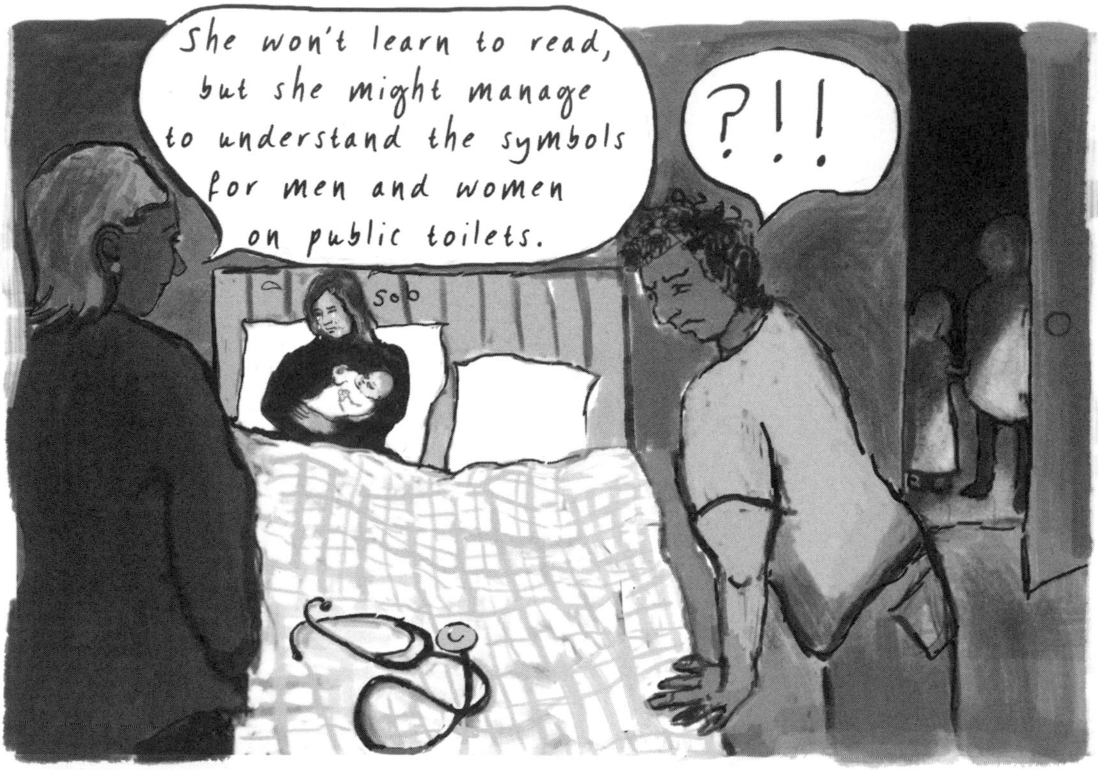
She won't learn to read, but she might manage to understand the symbols for men and women on public toilets.
?!!
SOB

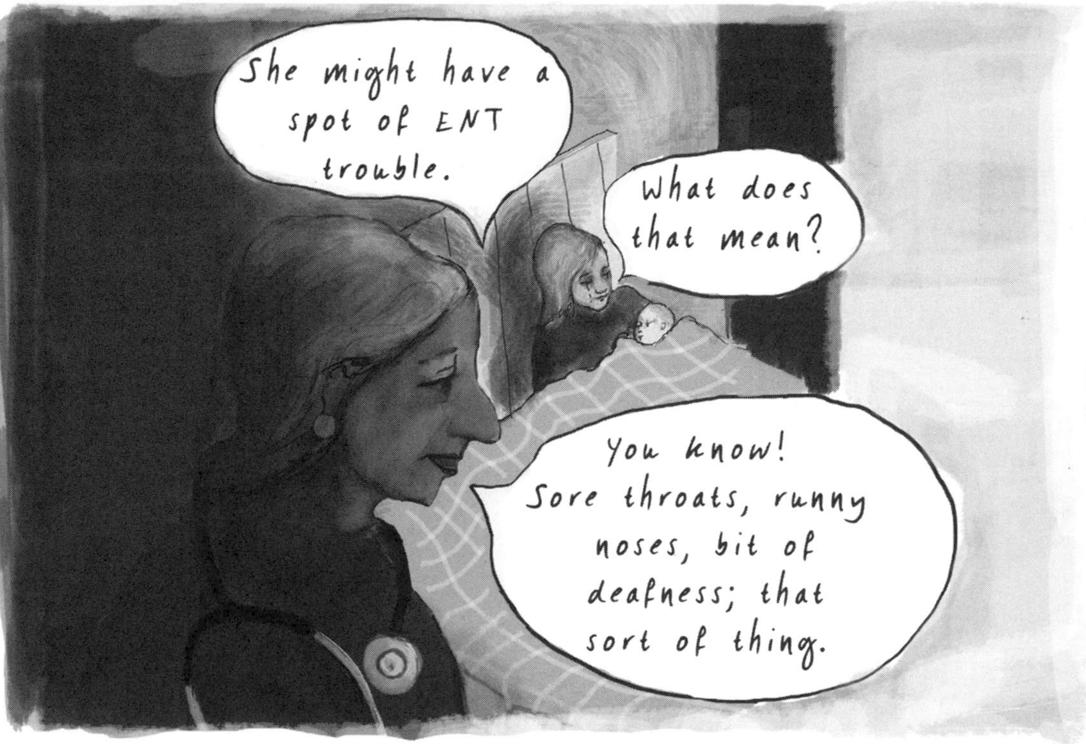
She might have a spot of ENT trouble.
What does that mean?
You know! Sore throats, runny noses, bit of deafness; that sort of thing.

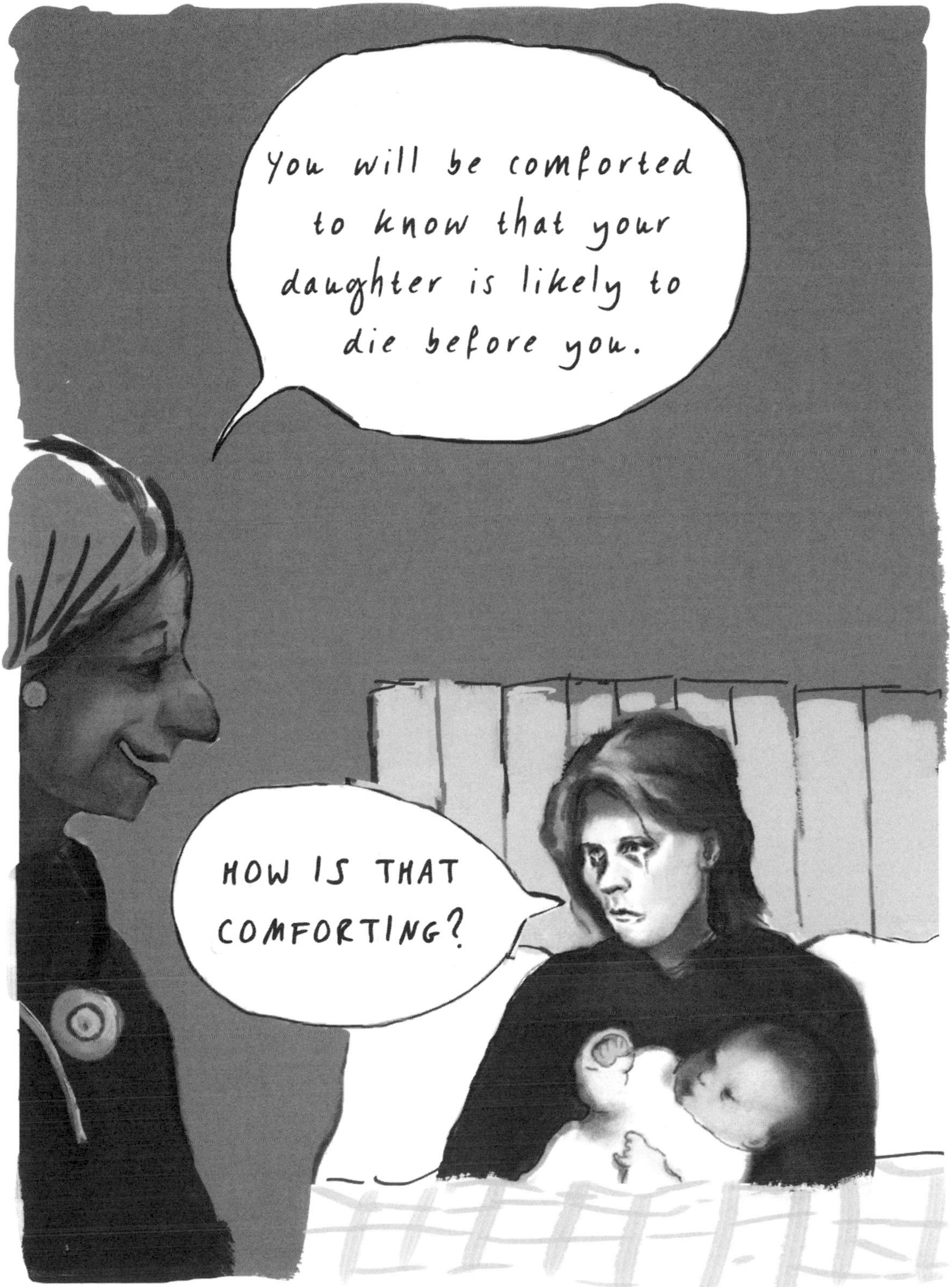
You will be comforted to know that your daughter is likely to die before you.
HOW IS THAT COMFORTING?

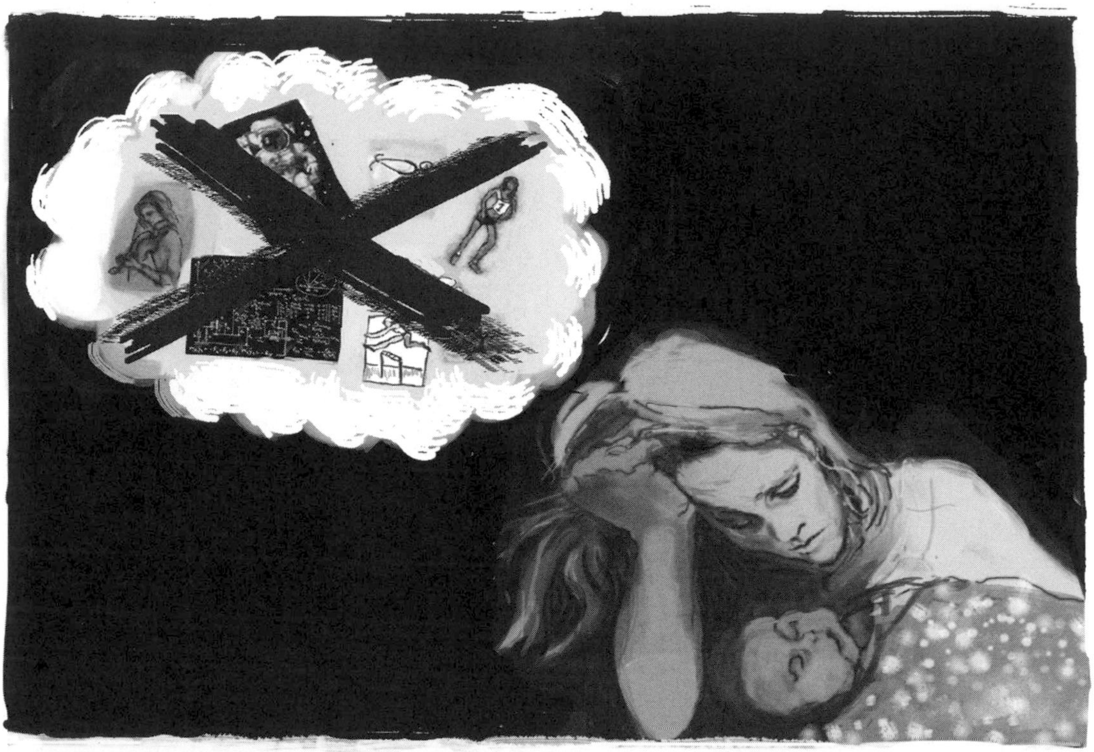

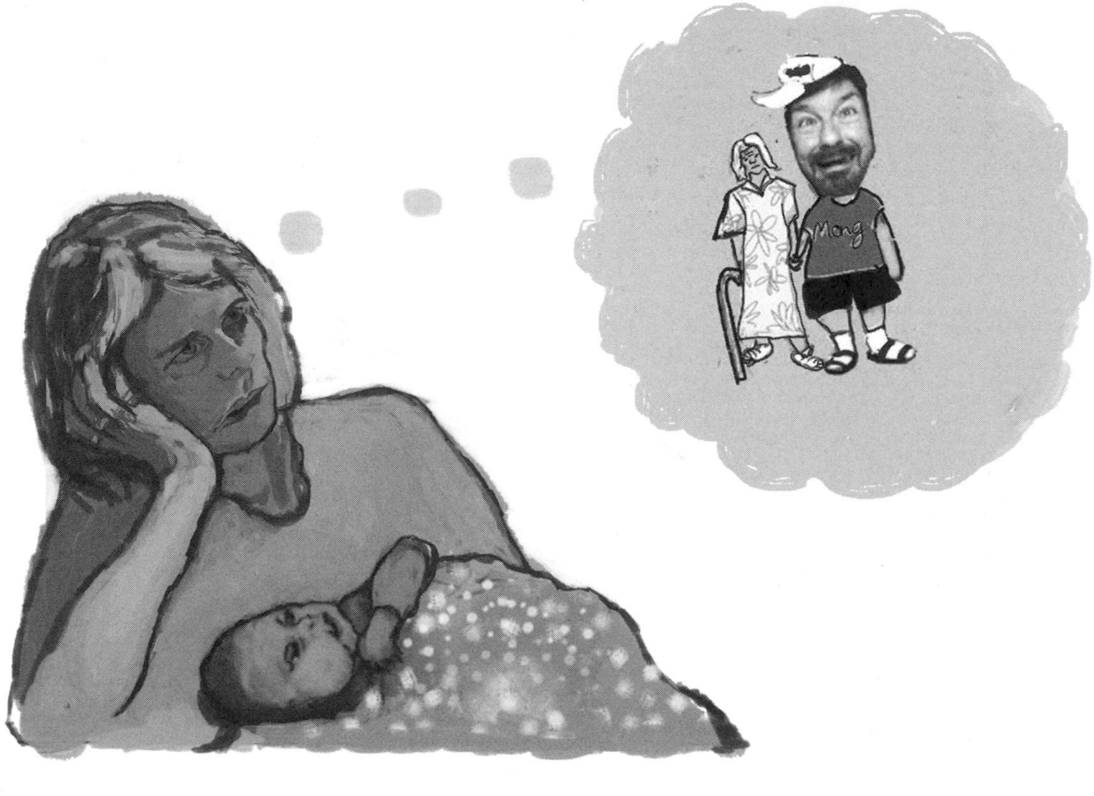
Mong

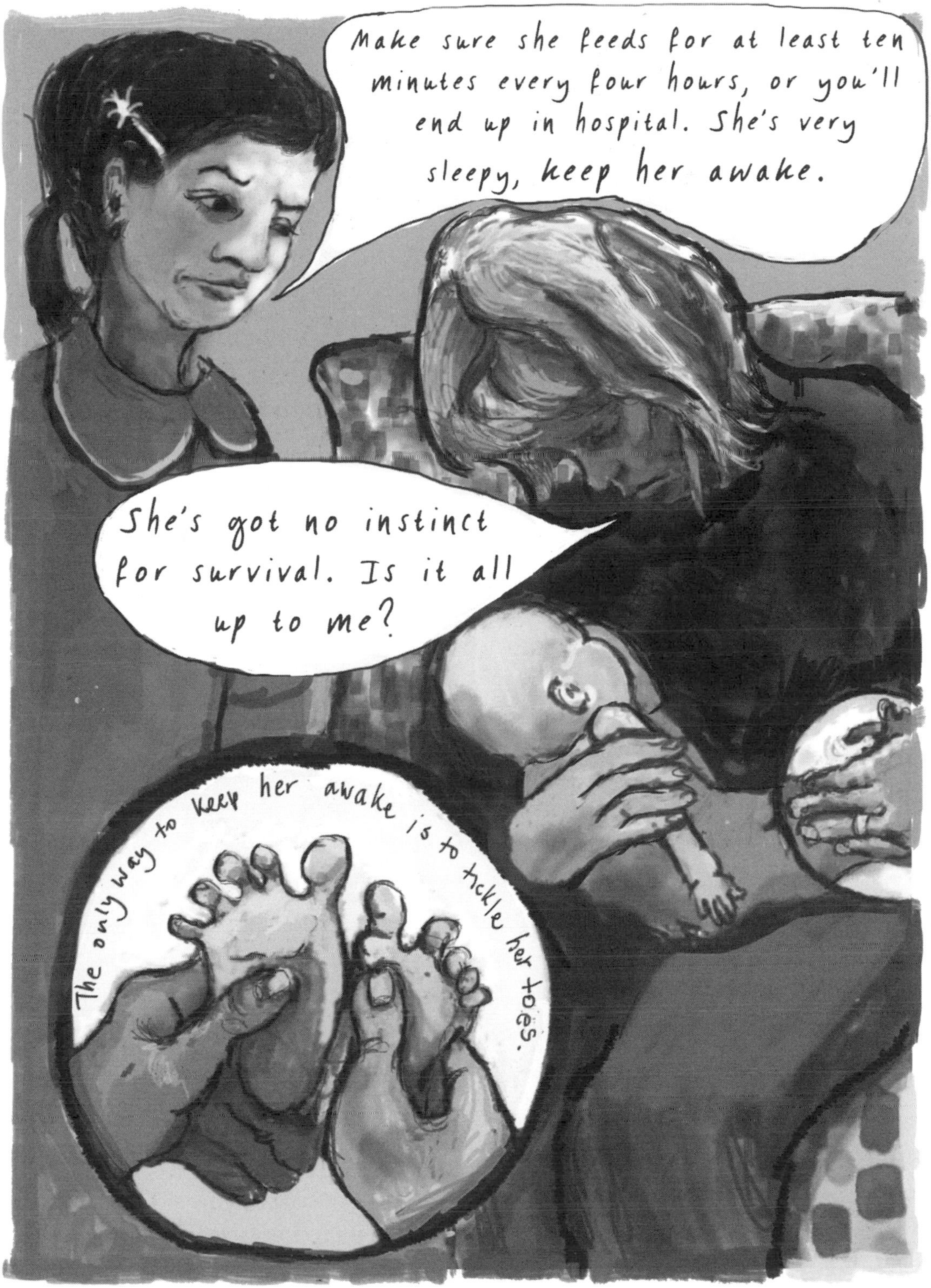

Make sure she feeds for at least ten minutes every four hours, or you'll end up in hospital. She's very sleepy, keep her awake.
She's got no instinct for survival. Is it all up to me?
The only way to keep her awake is to tickle her toes.

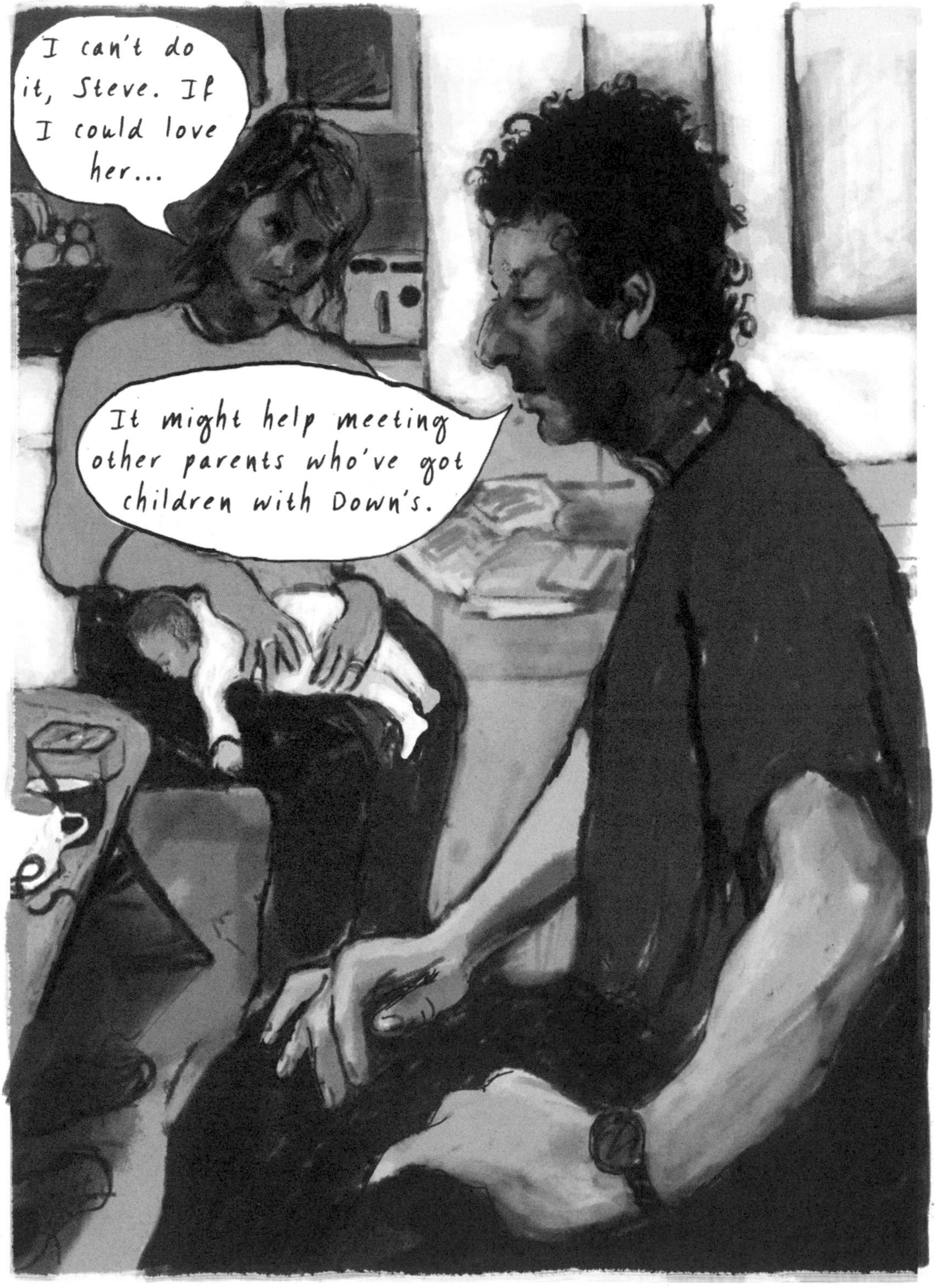
I can't do it, Steve. If I could love her...
It might help meeting other parents who've got children with Down's.

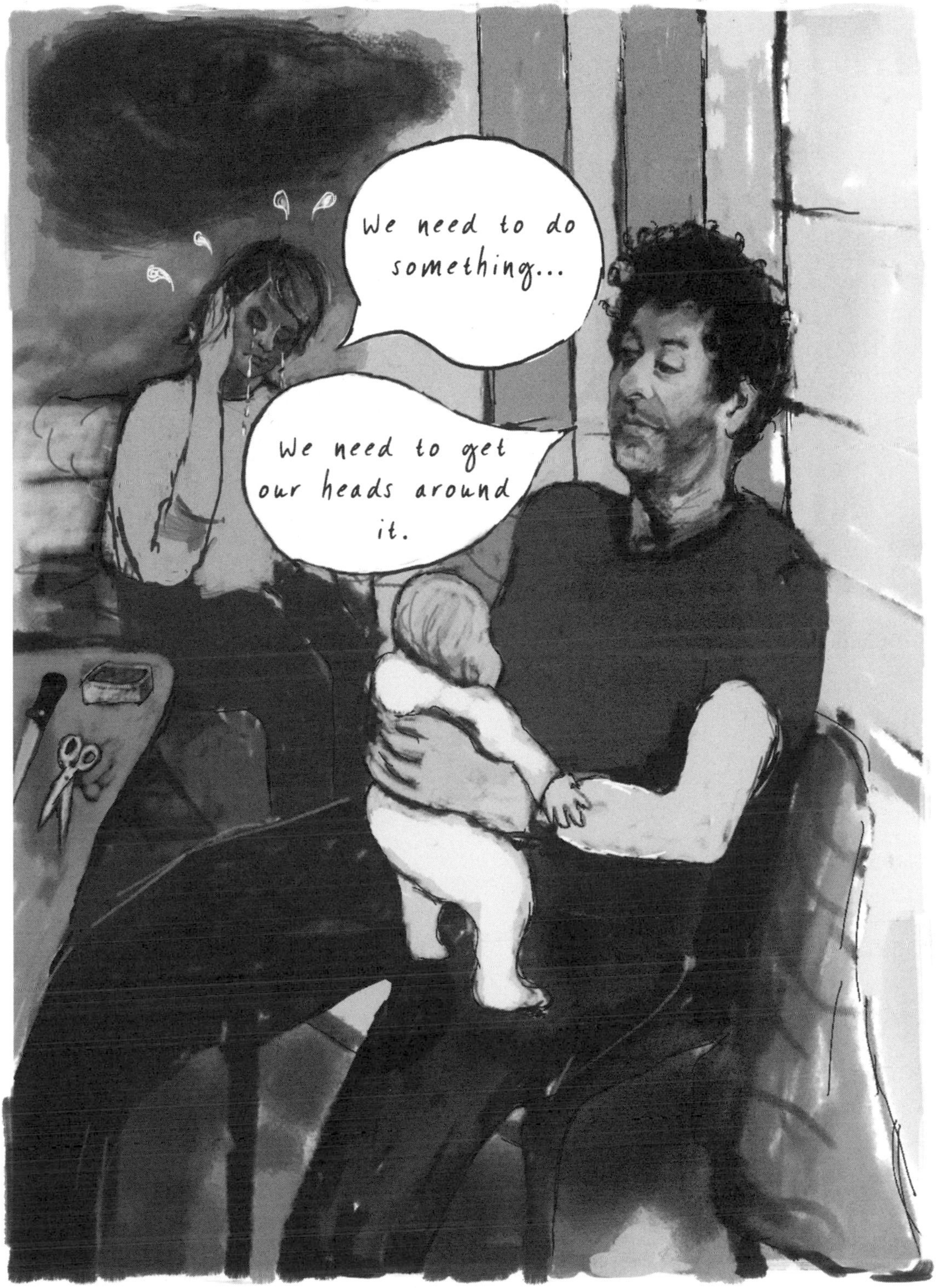
We need to do something...
We need to get our heads around it.

Nothing will help.

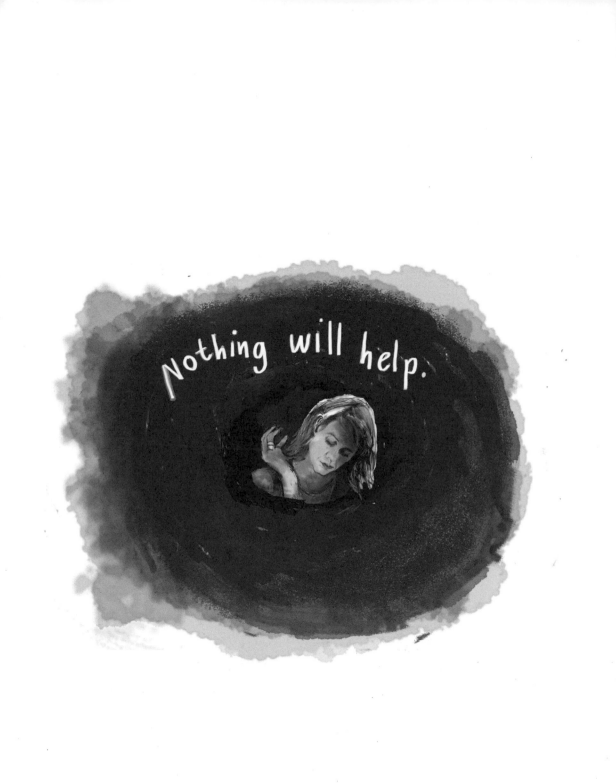

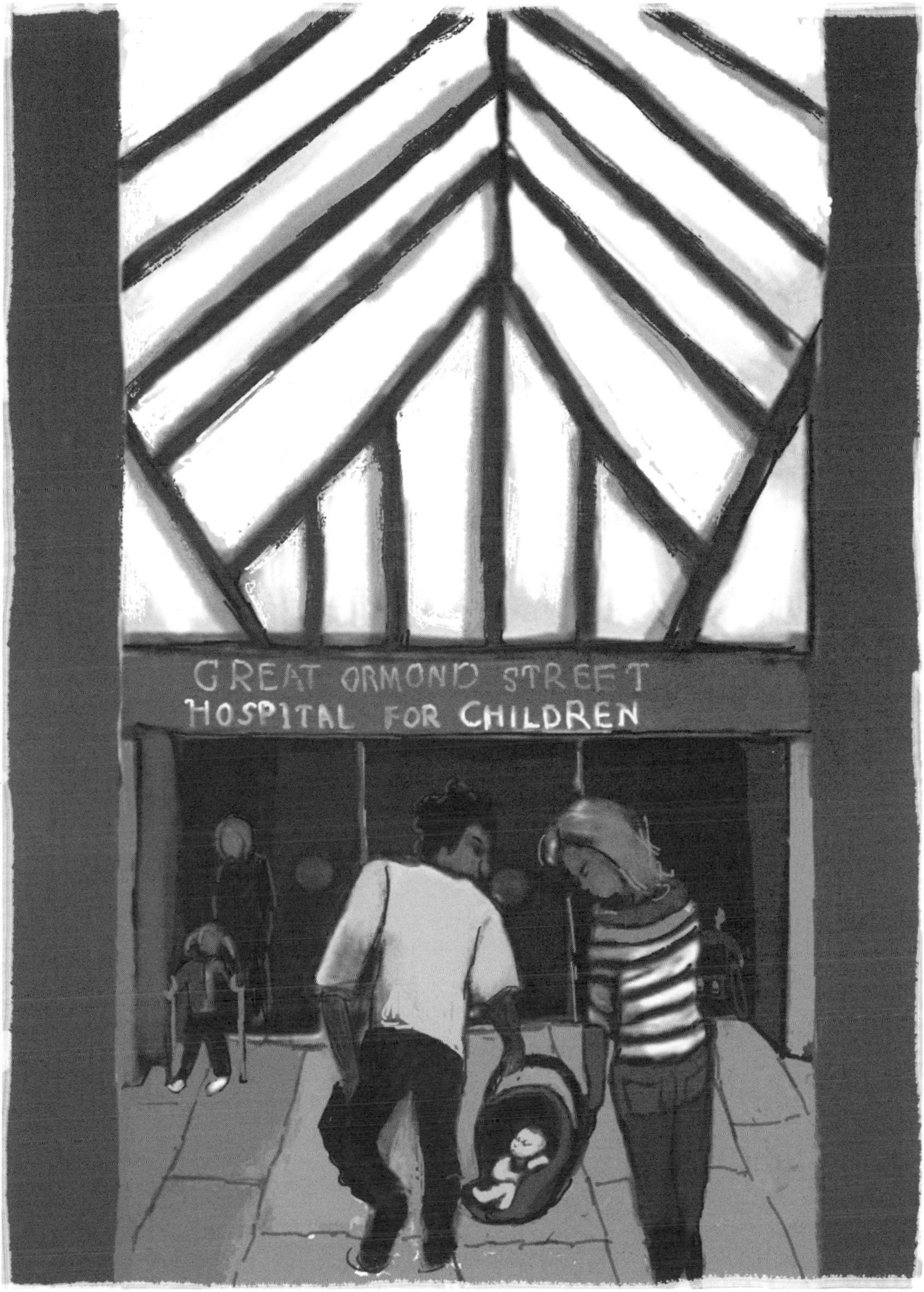
GREAT ORMOND STREET
HOSPITAL FOR CHILDREN

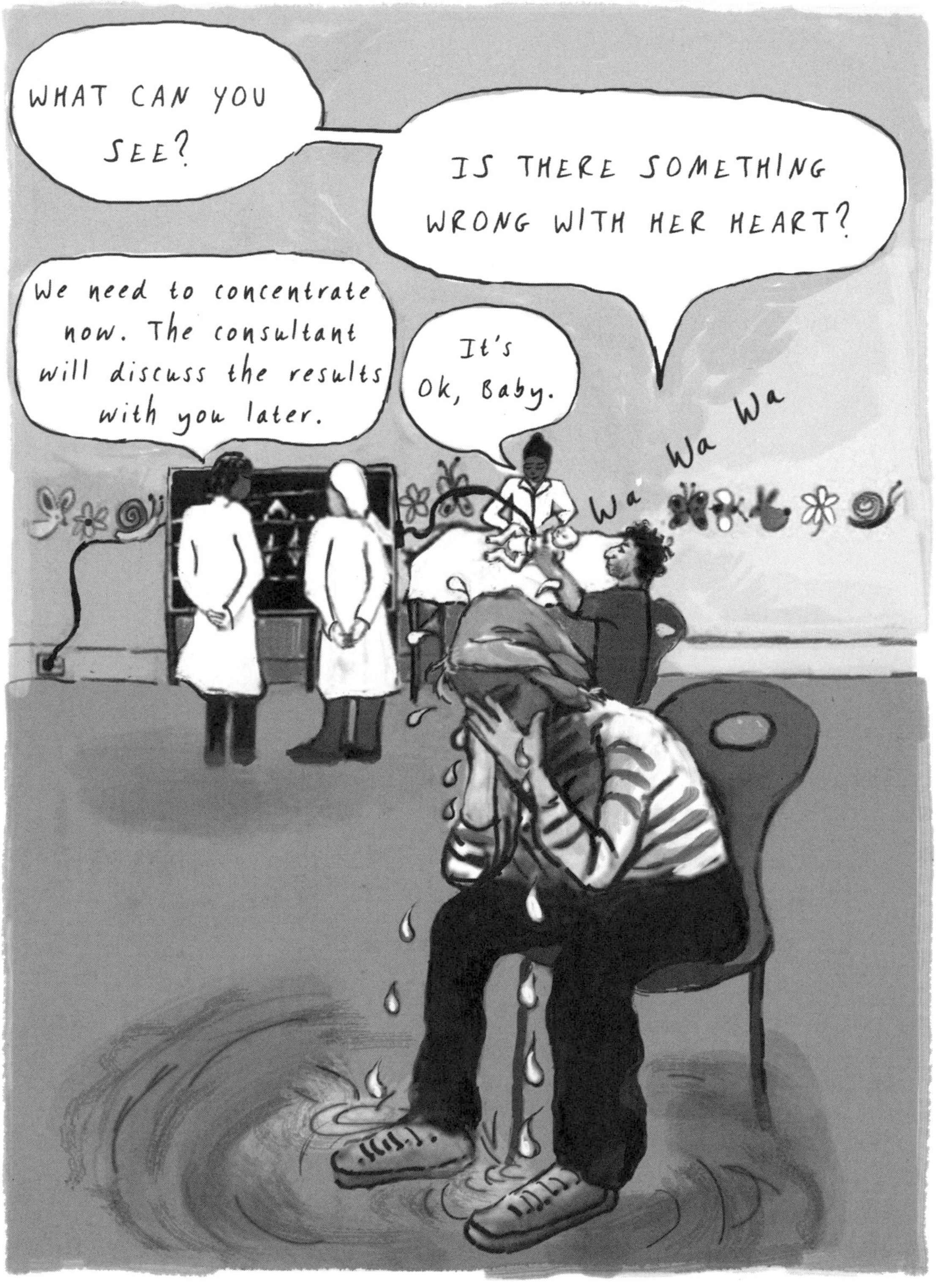
WHAT CAN YOU SEE?
IS THERE SOMETHING WRONG WITH HER HEART?
We need to concentrate now. The consultant will discuss the results with you later.
It's Ok, Baby.
Wa Wa Wa

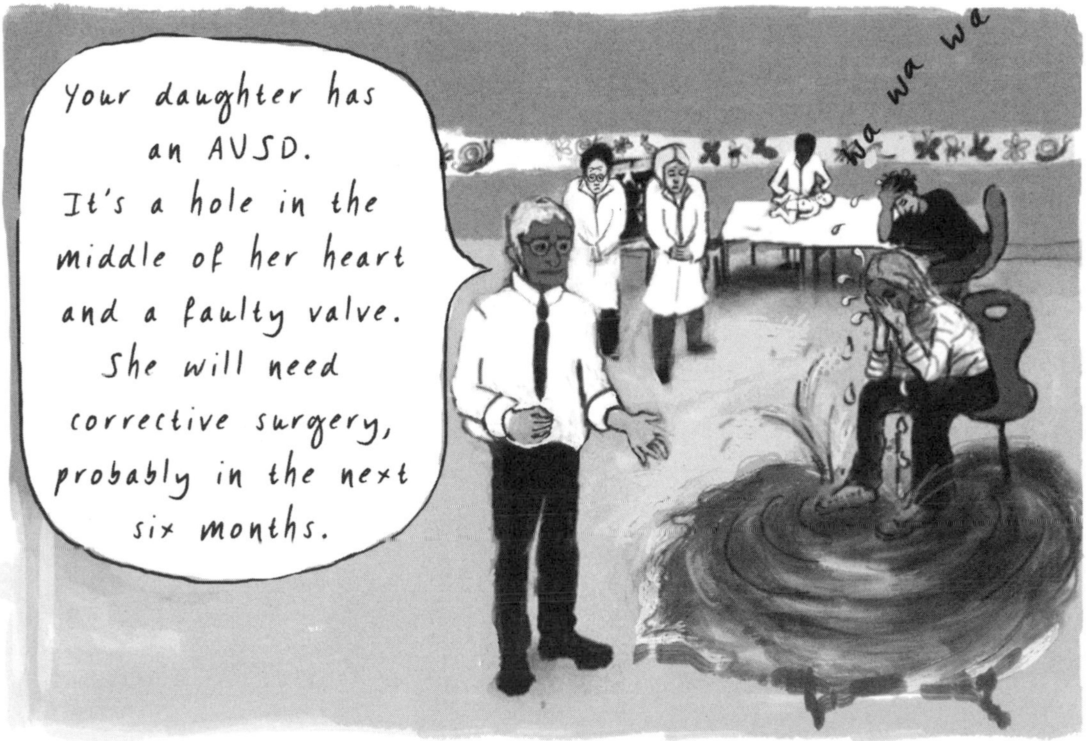
Your daughter has an AVSD. It's a hole in the middle of her heart and a faulty valve. She will need corrective surgery, probably in the next six months.
wa wa wa

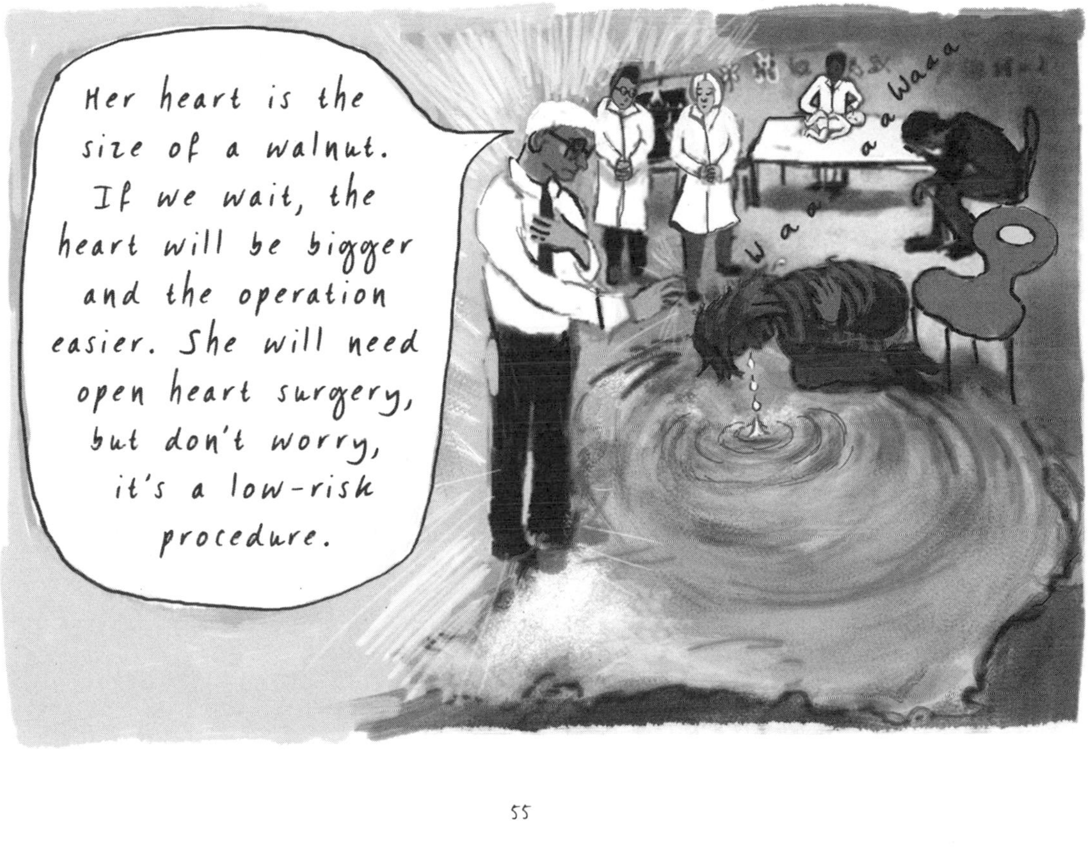
Her heart is the size of a walnut. If we wait, the heart will be bigger and the operation easier. She will need open heart surgery, but don't worry, it's a low-risk procedure.
Waa a a Waaa

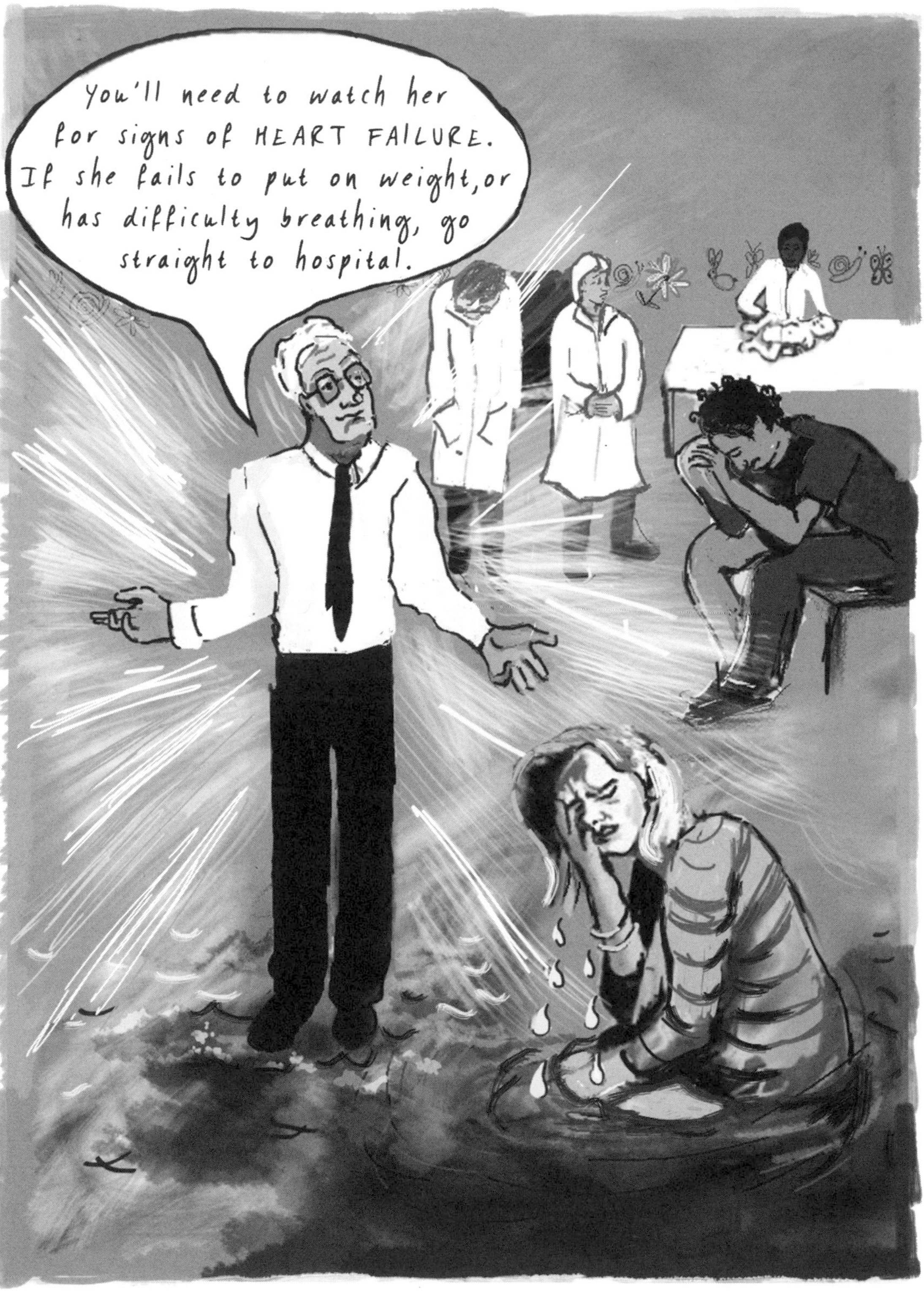
You'll need to watch her for signs of HEART FAILURE. If she fails to put on weight, or has difficulty breathing, go straight to hospital.

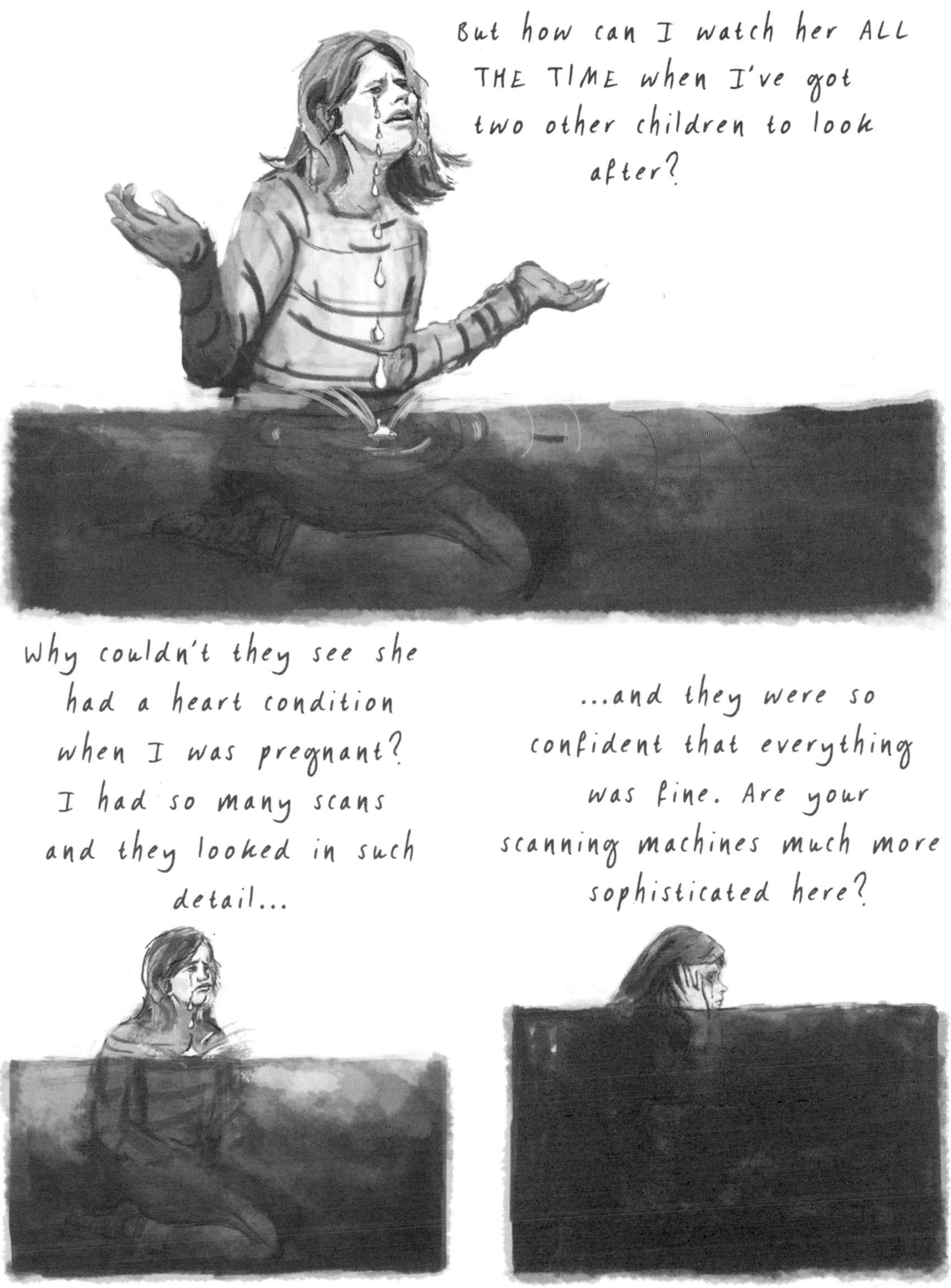
But how can I watch her ALL THE TIME when I've got two other children to look after?
Why couldn't they see she had a heart condition when I was pregnant? I had so many scans and they looked in such detail...
...and they were so confident that everything was fine. Are your scanning machines much more sophisticated here?

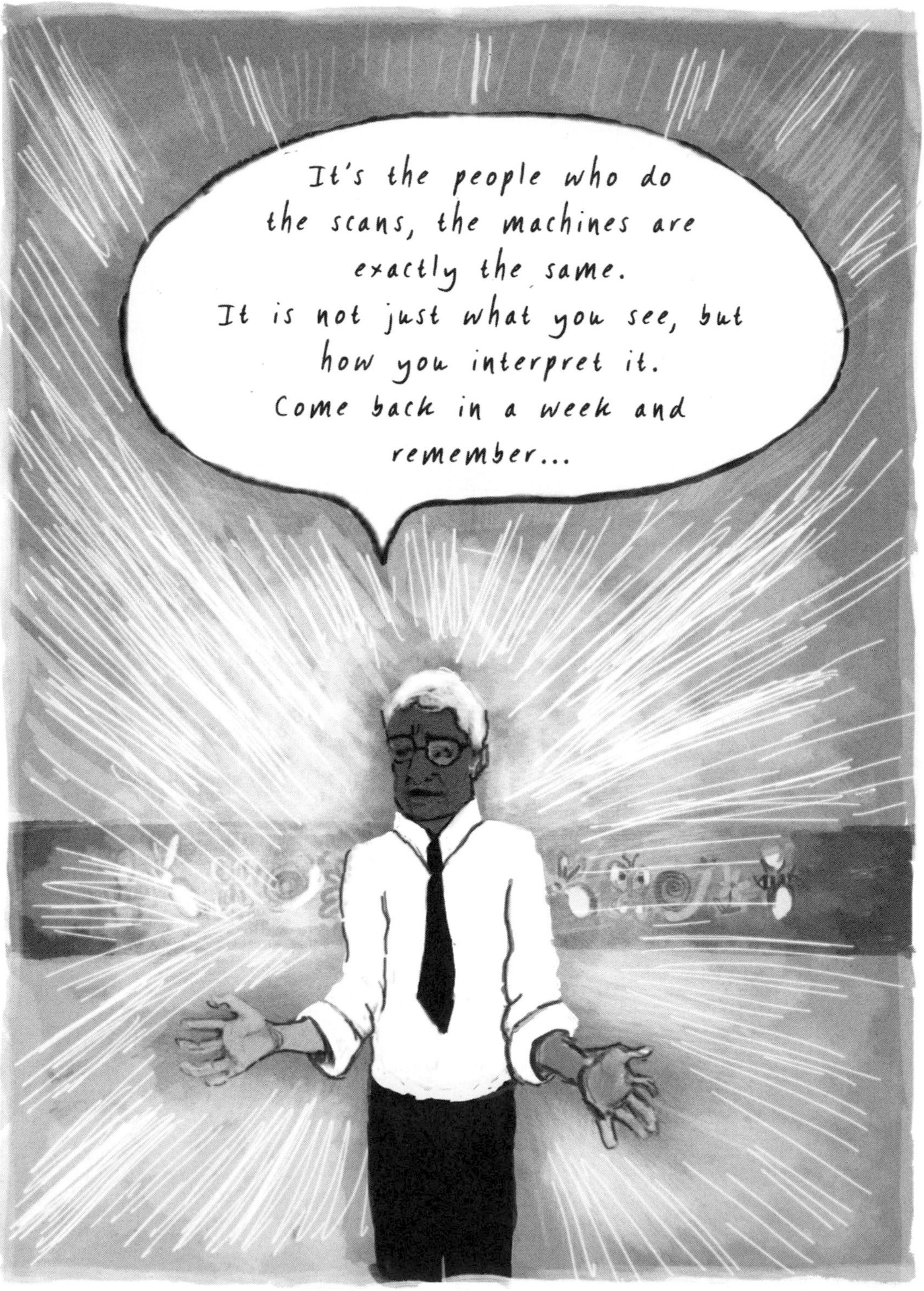
It's the people who do the scans, the machines are exactly the same. It is not just what you see, but how you interpret it. Come back in a week and remember...

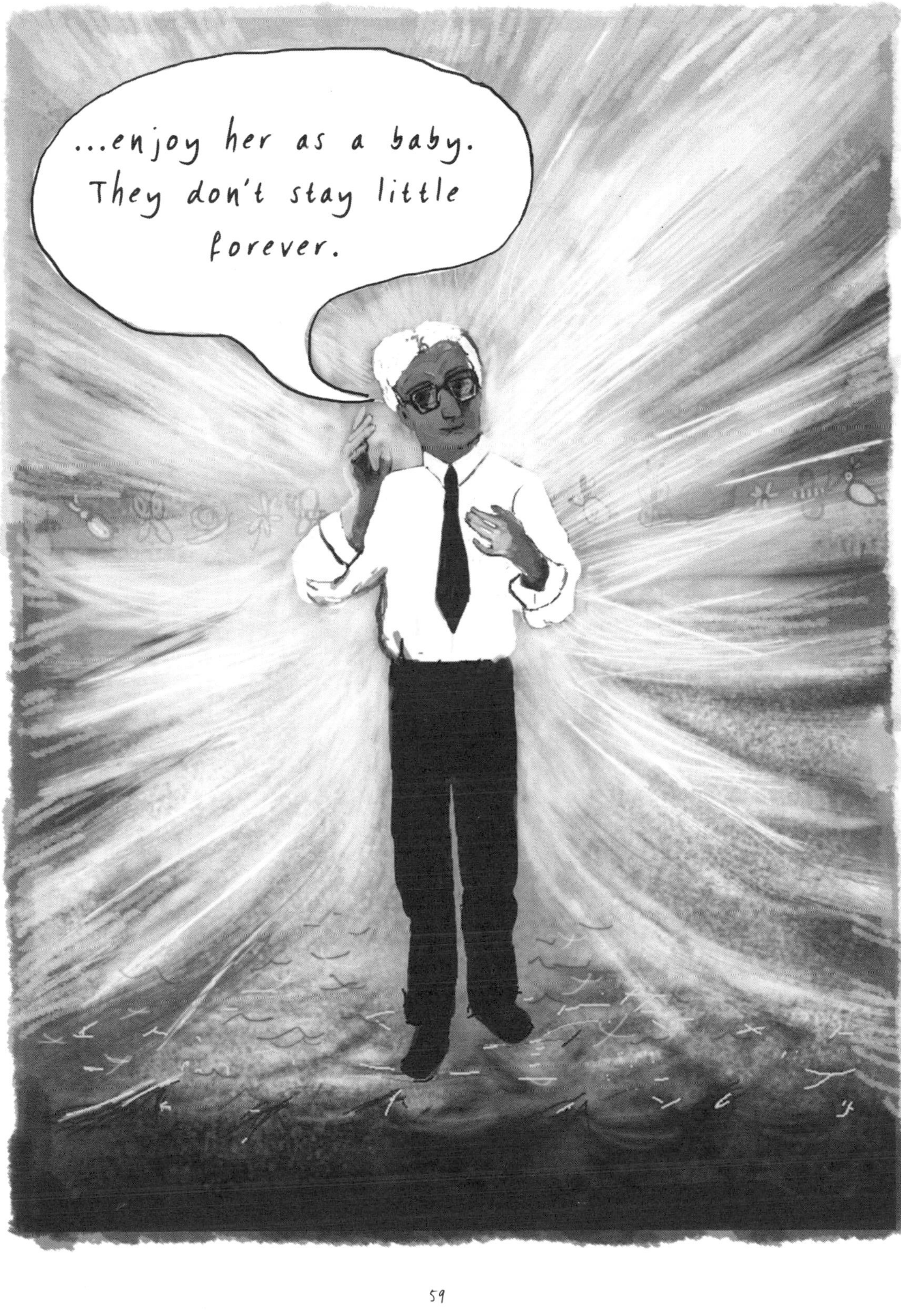
...enjoy her as a baby. They don't stay little forever.

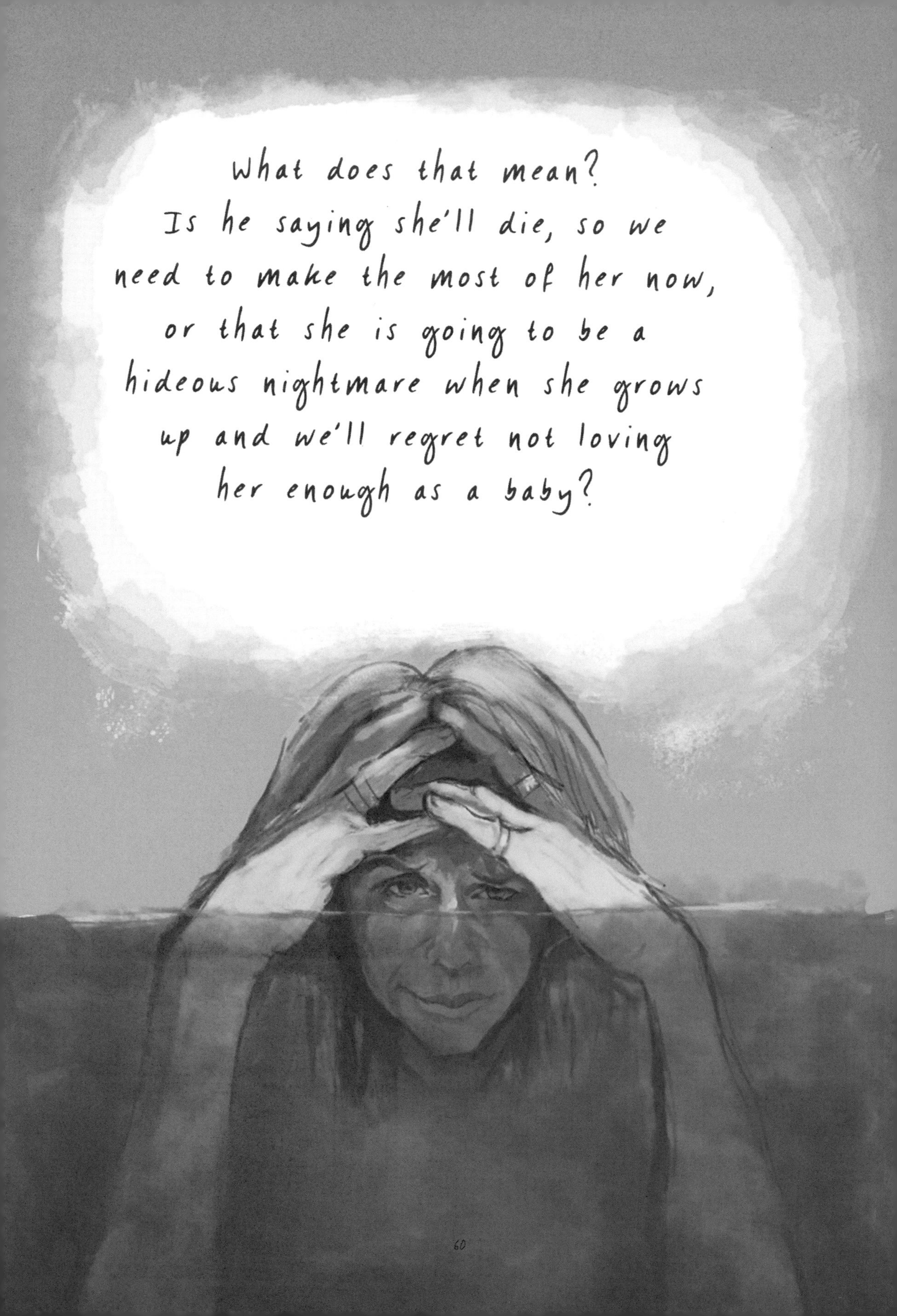
What does that mean? Is he saying she'll die, so we need to make the most of her now, or that she is going to be a hideous nightmare when she grows up and we'll regret not loving her enough as a baby?

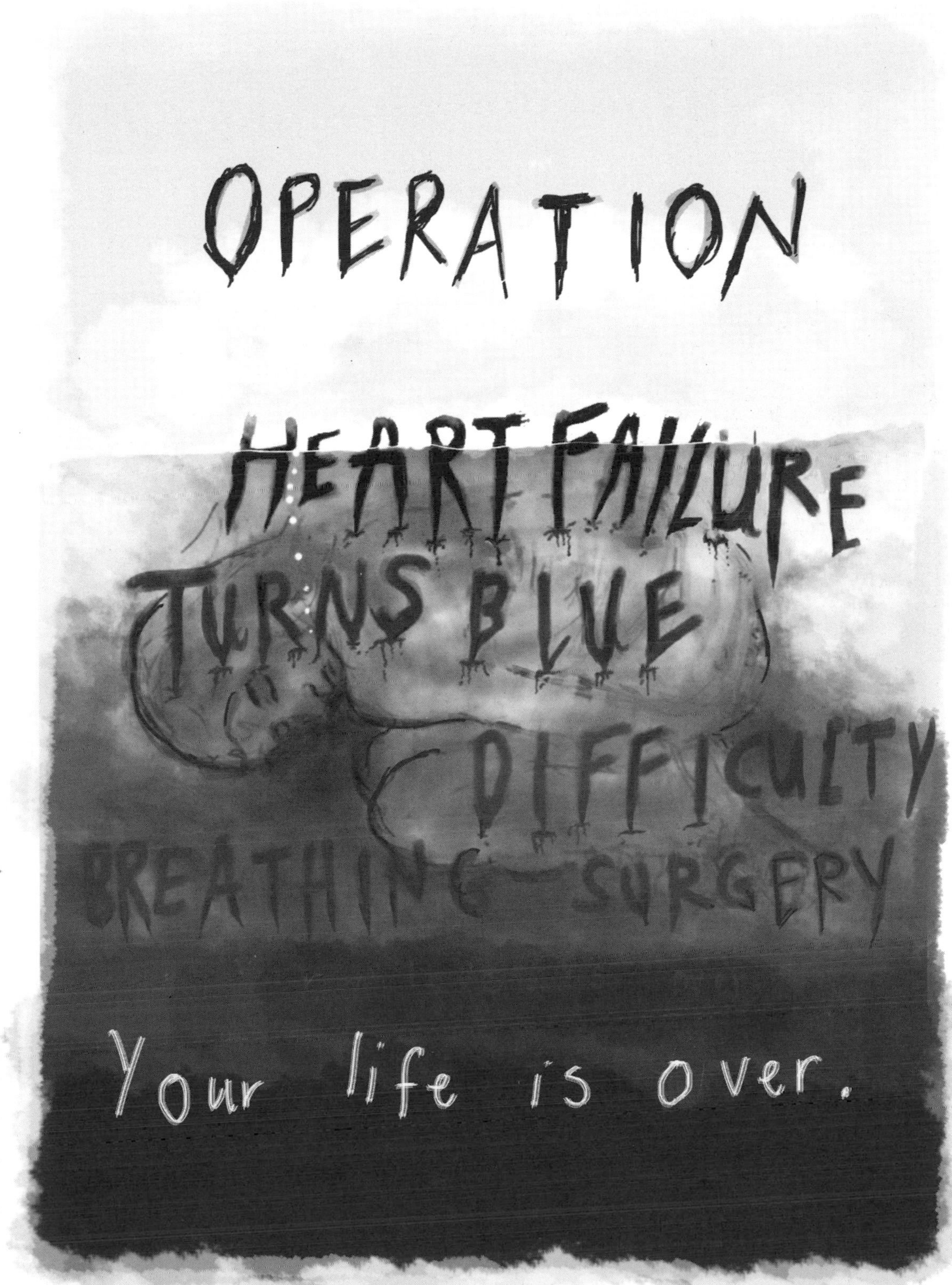
OPERATION
HEART FAILURE
TURNS BLUE
DIFFICULTY
BREATHING
SURGERY
Your life is over.

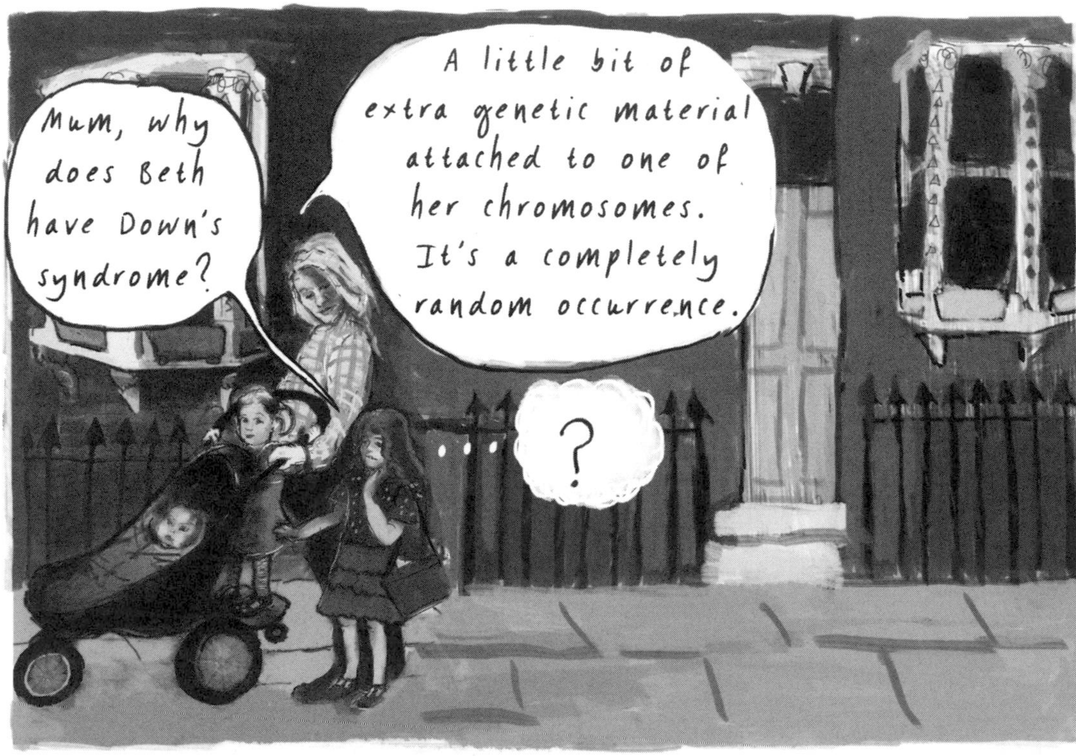
Mum, why does Beth have Down's syndrome?
A little bit of extra genetic material attached to one of her chromosomes. It's a completely random occurrence.
?

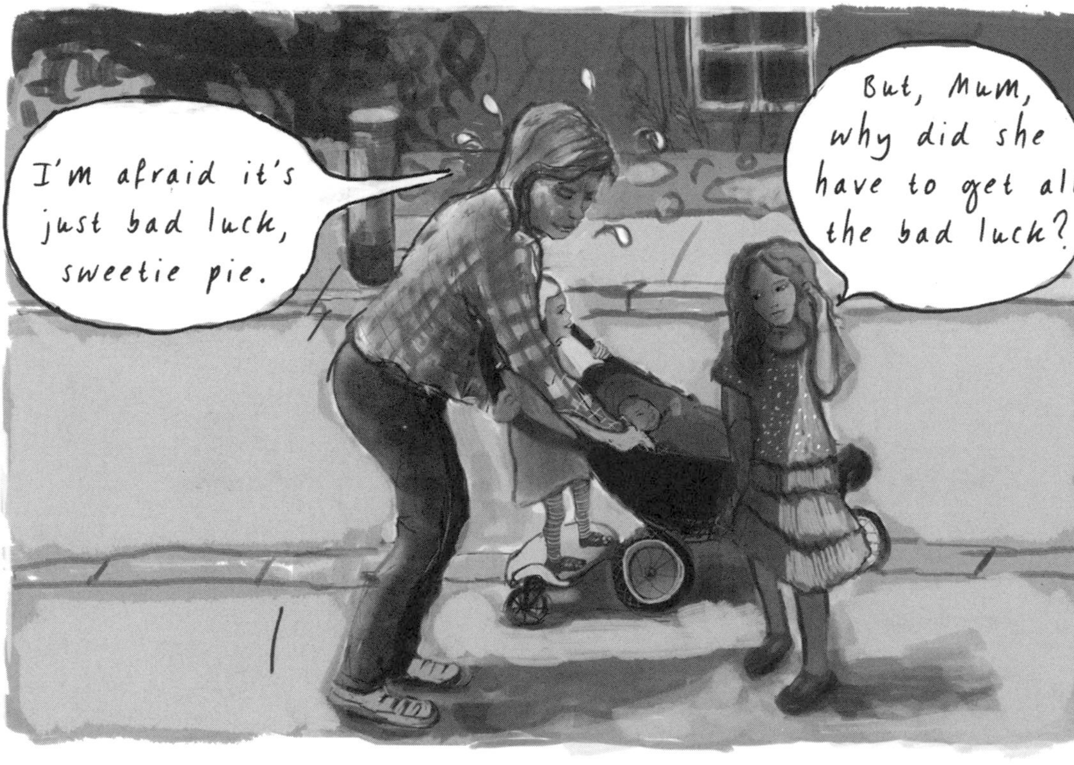
I'm afraid it's just bad luck, sweetie pie.
But, Mum, why did she have to get all the bad luck?

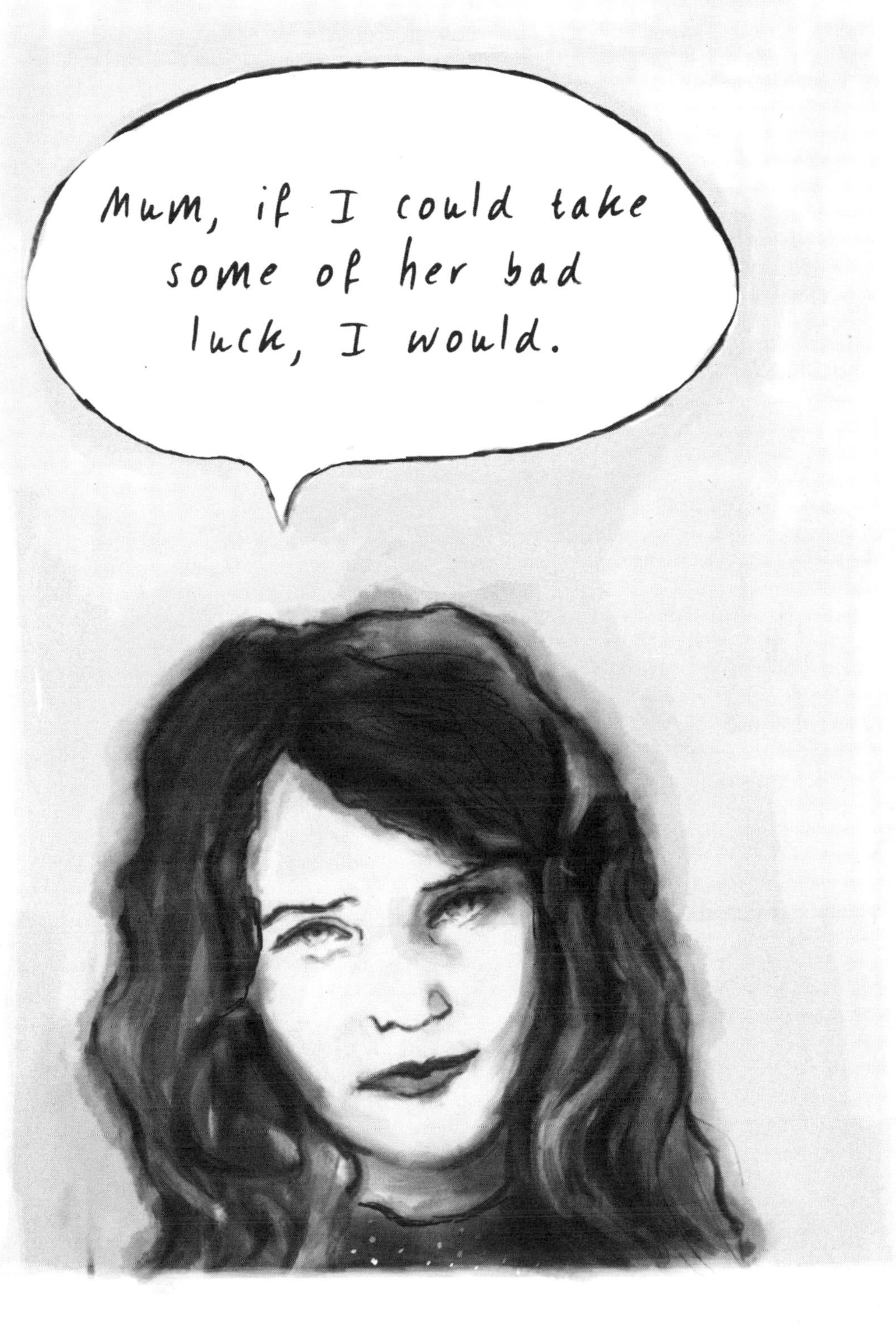
Mum, if I could take some of her bad luck, I would.

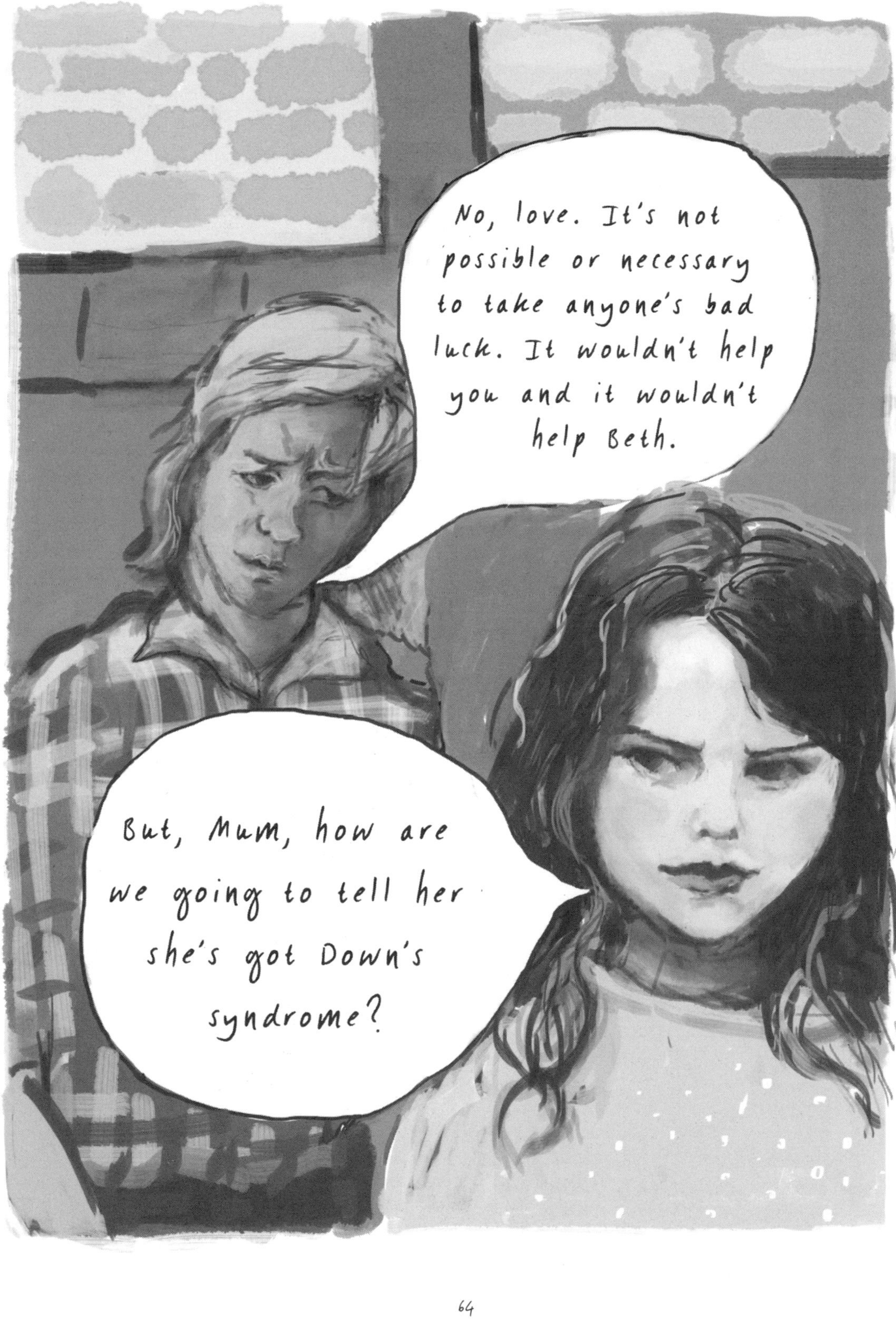
No, love. It's not possible or necessary to take anyone's bad luck. It wouldn't help you and it wouldn't help Beth.
But, Mum, how are we going to tell her she's got Down's syndrome?

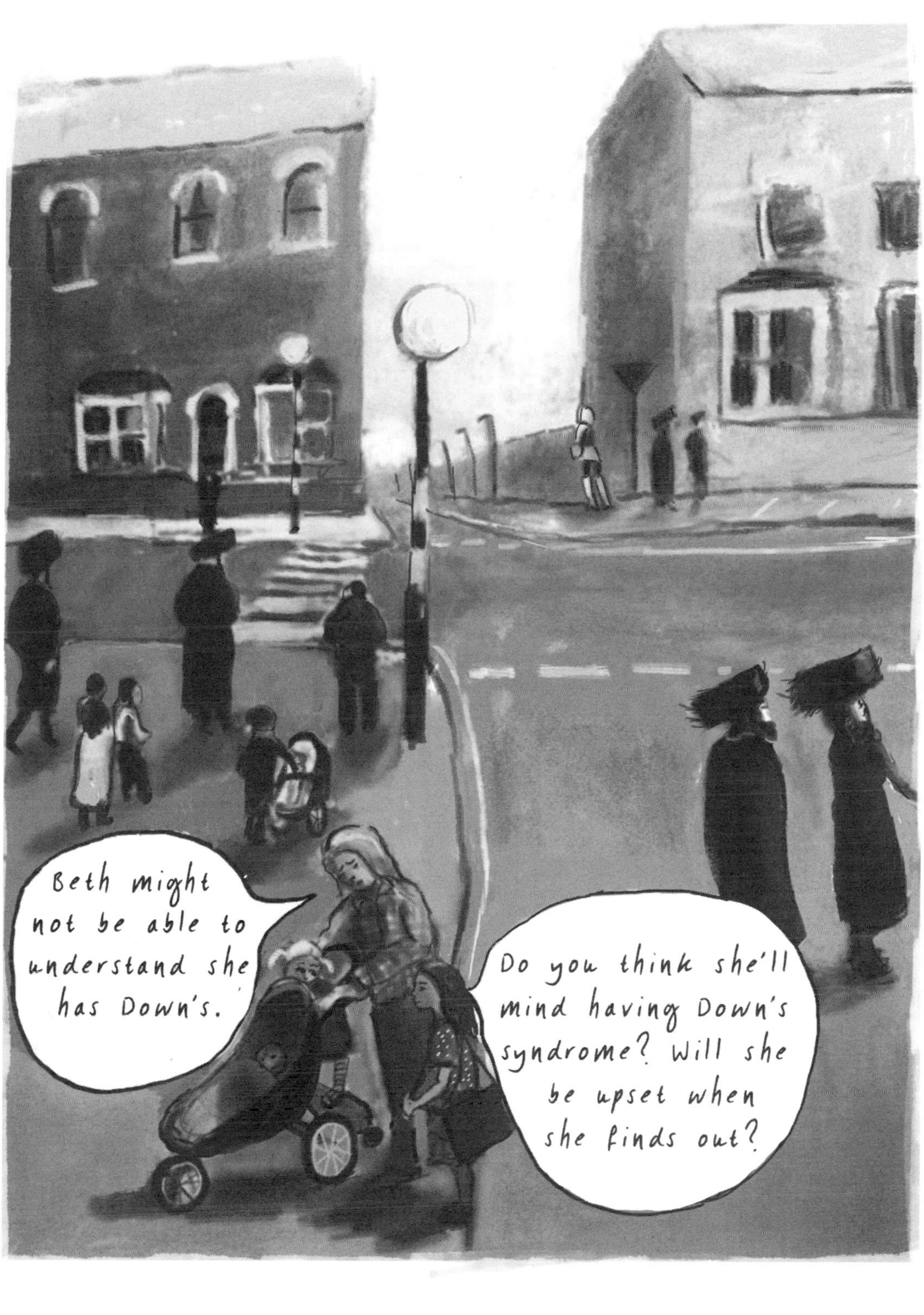
Beth might not be able to understand she has Down's.
Do you think she'll mind having Down's syndrome? Will she be upset when she finds out?

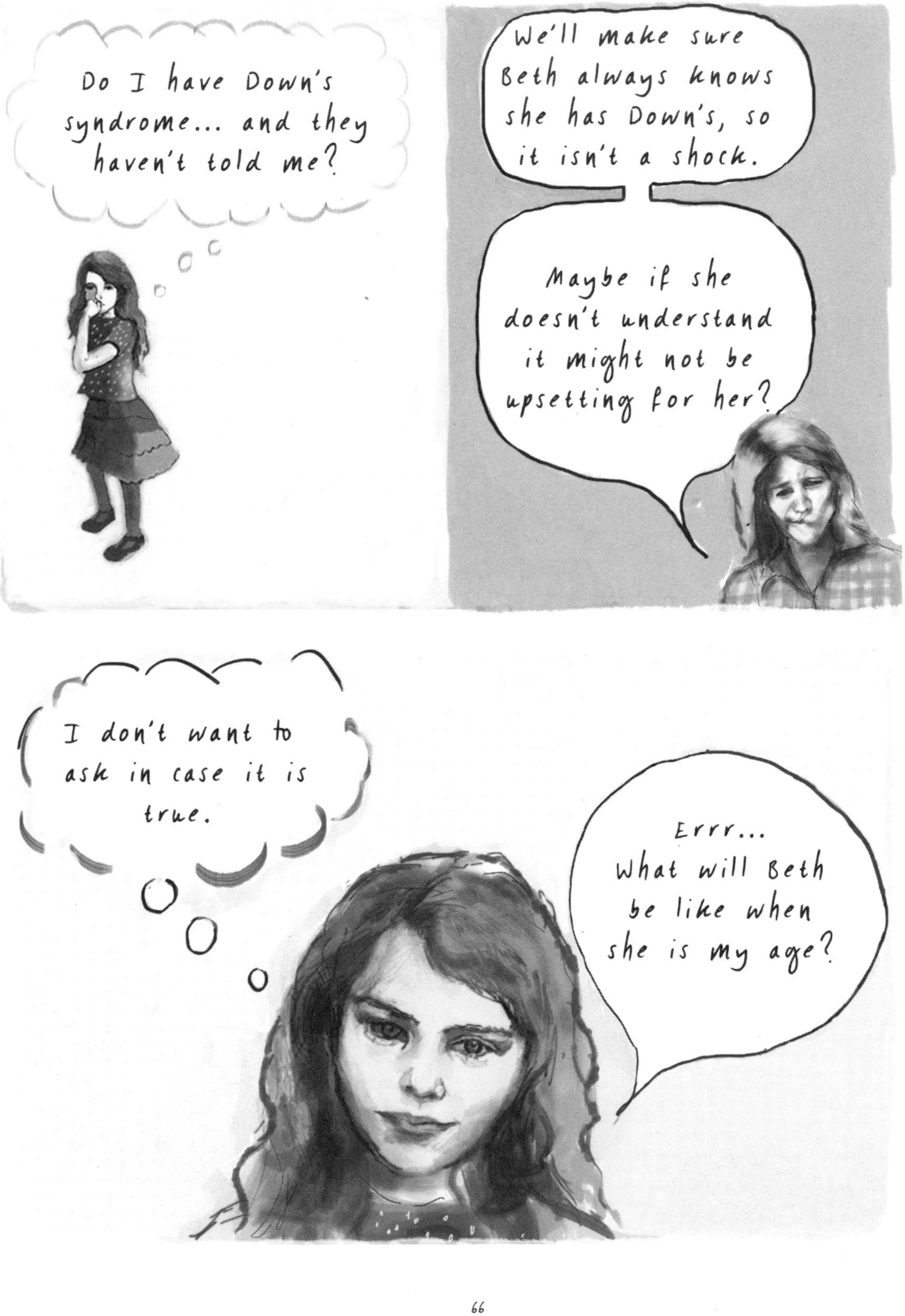
Do I have Down's syndrome... and they haven't told me?
We'll make sure Beth always knows she has Down's, so it isn't a shock.
Maybe if she doesn't understand it might not be upsetting for her?
I don't want to ask in case it is true.
Errr... What will Beth be like when she is my age?

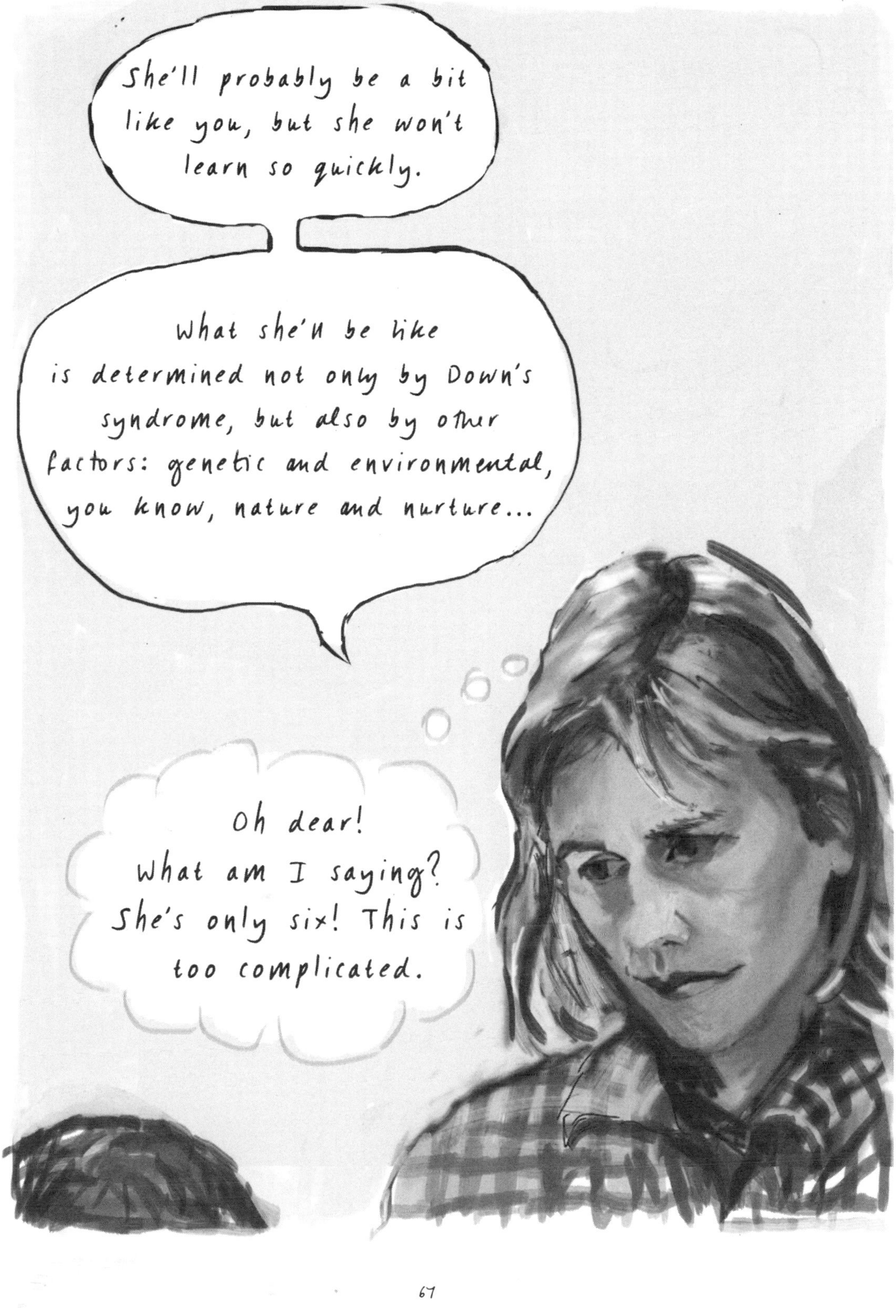
She'll probably be a bit like you, but she won't learn so quickly.
What she'll be like is determined not only by Down's syndrome, but also by other factors: genetic and environmental, you know, nature and nurture...
Oh dear! What am I saying? She's only six! This is too complicated.

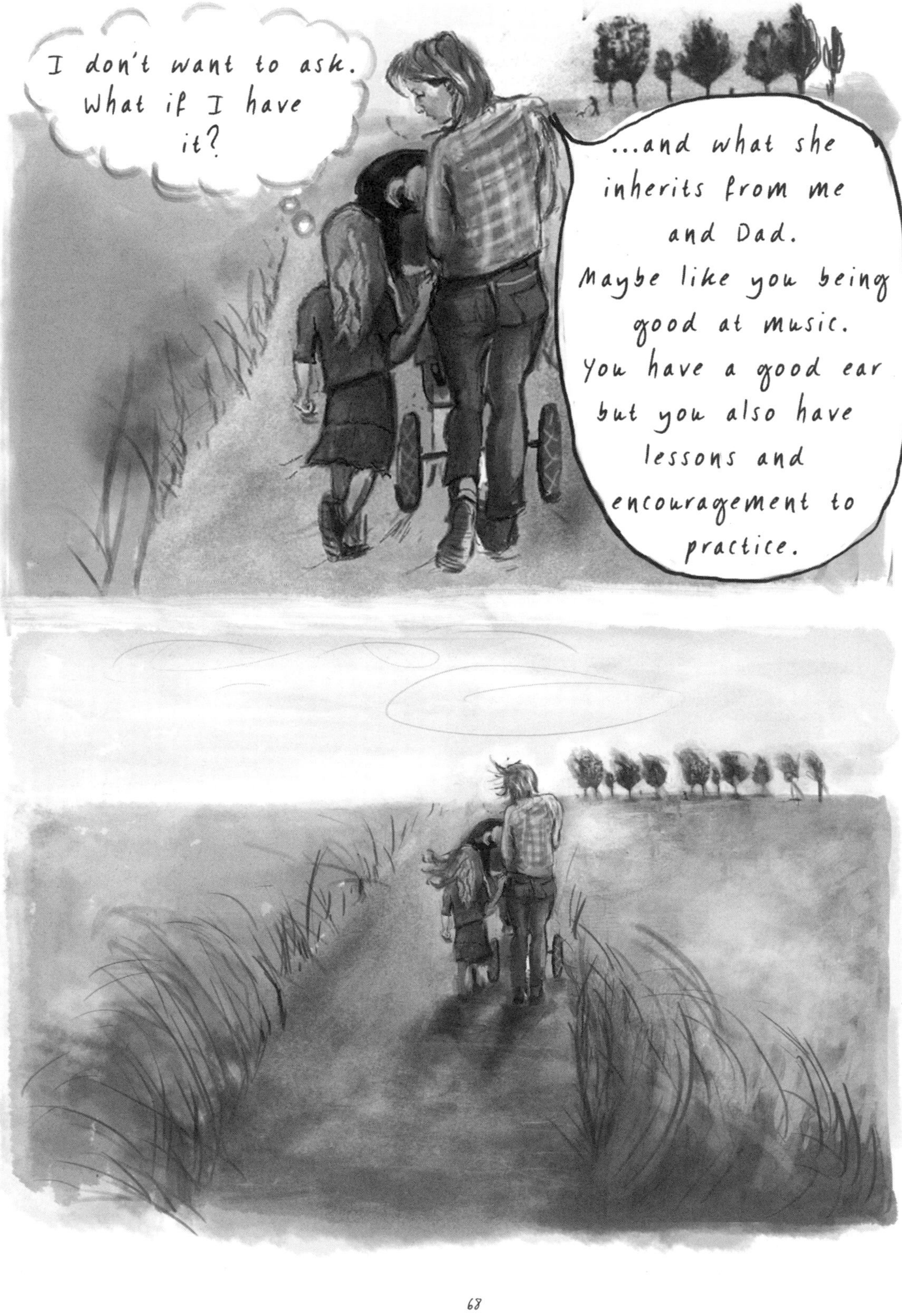
I don't want to ask. What if I have it?
...and what she inherits from me and Dad. Maybe like you being good at music. You have a good ear but you also have lessons and encouragement to practice.

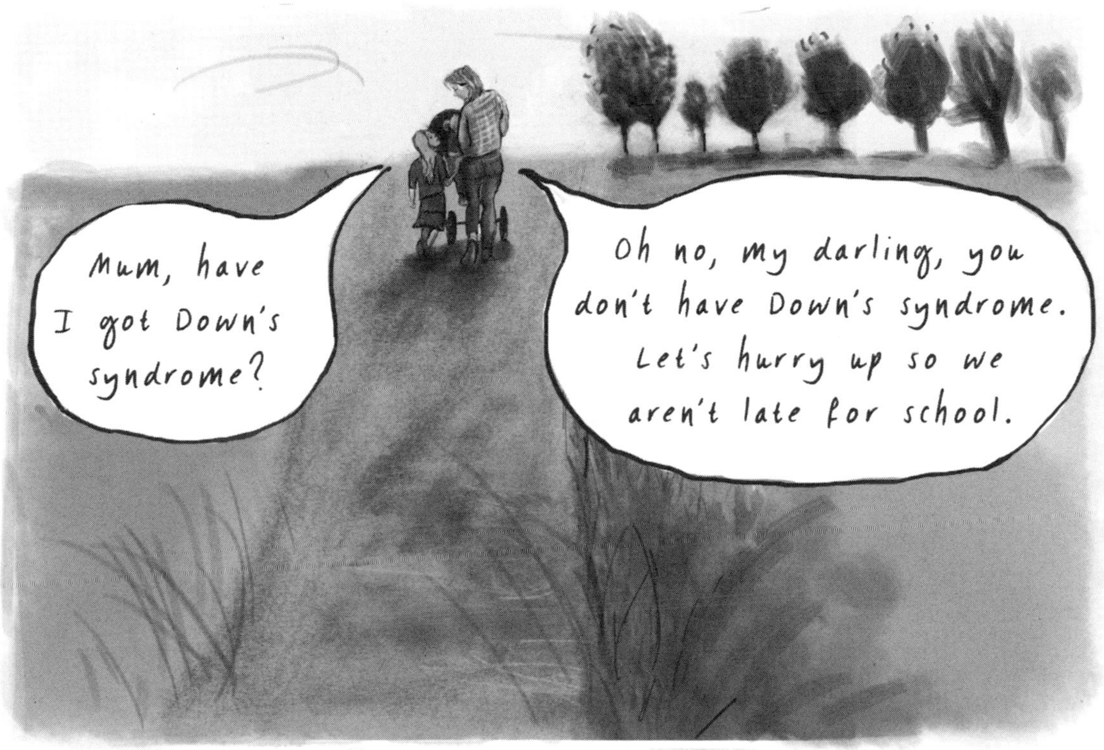
Mum, have I got Down's syndrome?
Oh no, my darling, you don't have Down's syndrome. Let's hurry up so we aren't late for school.

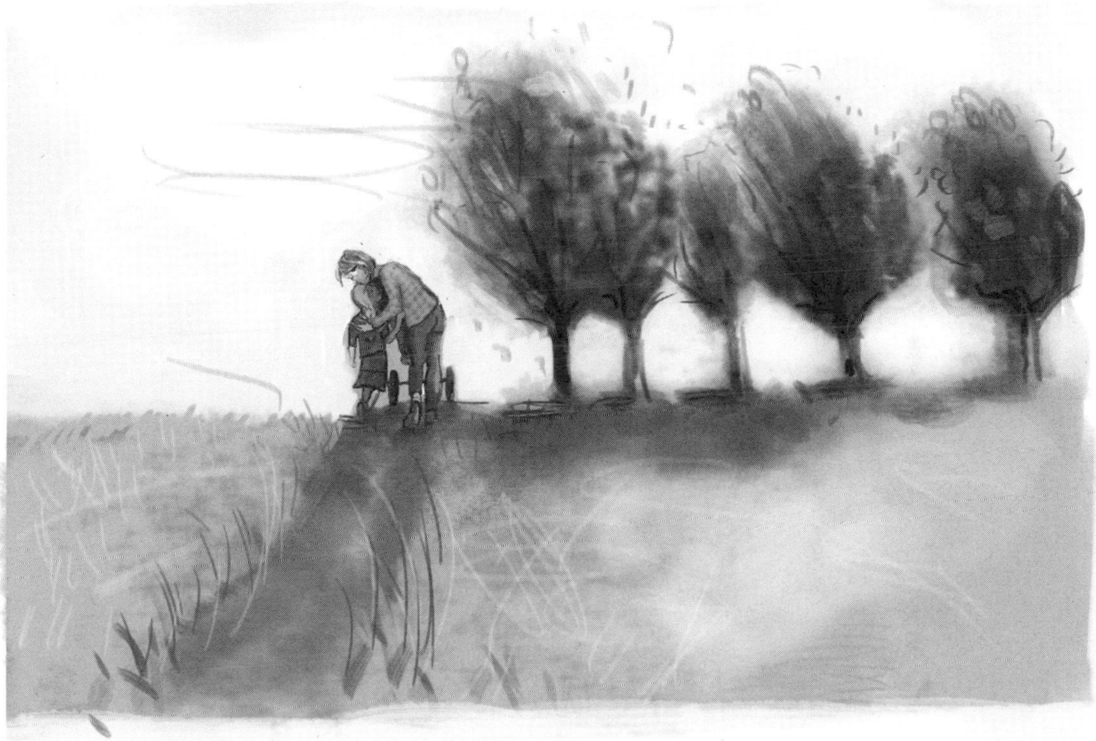

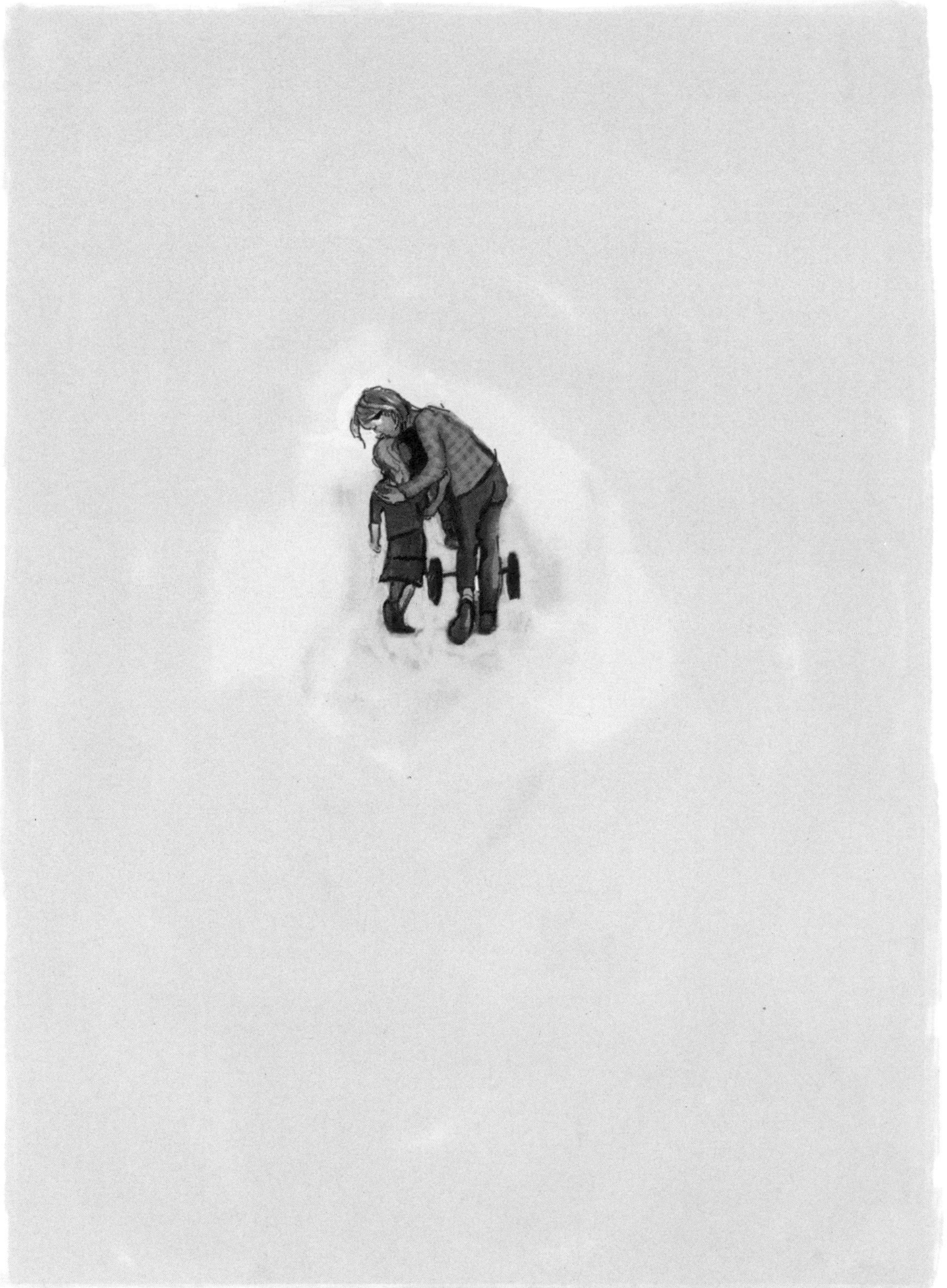

Part Two

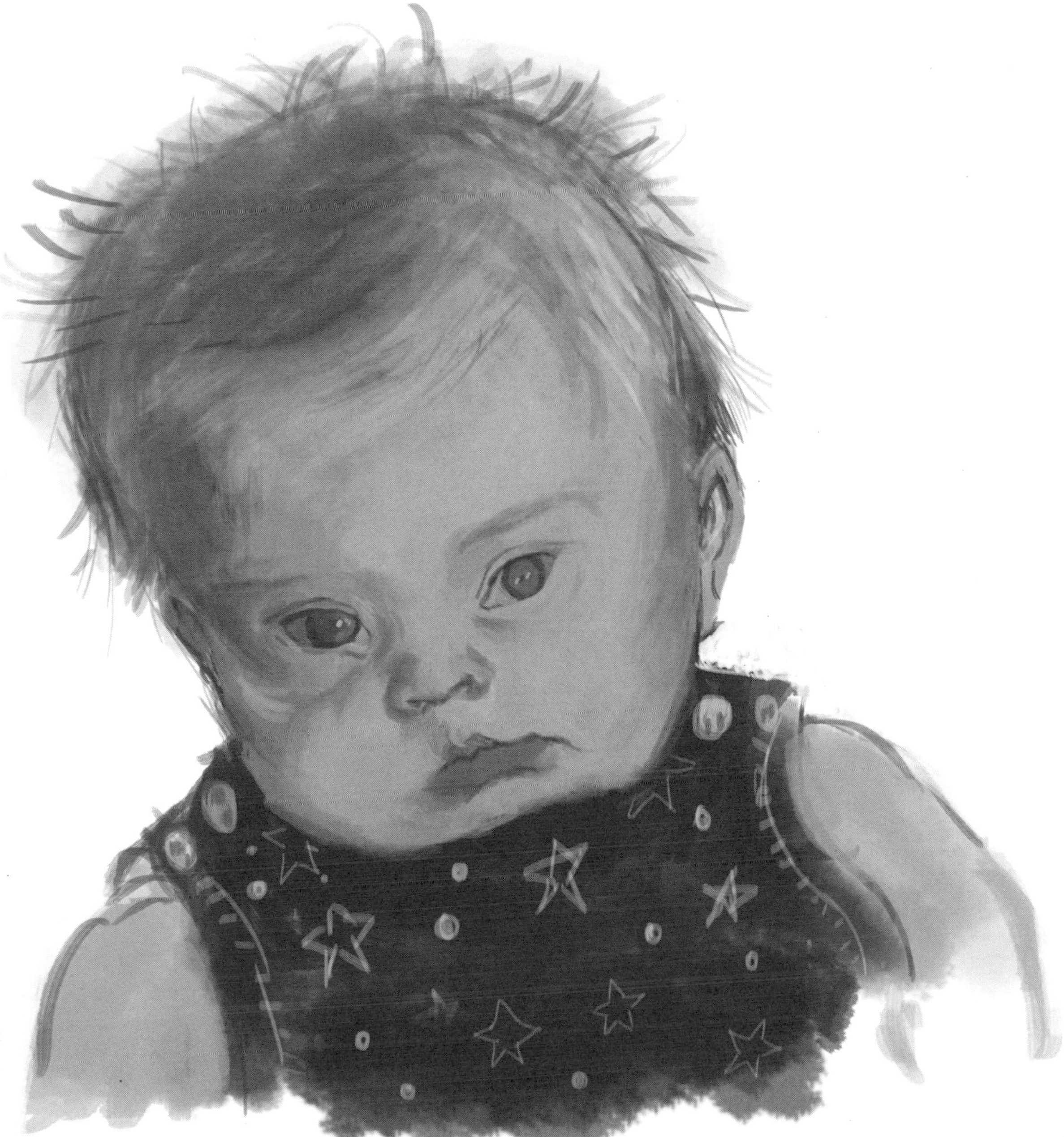

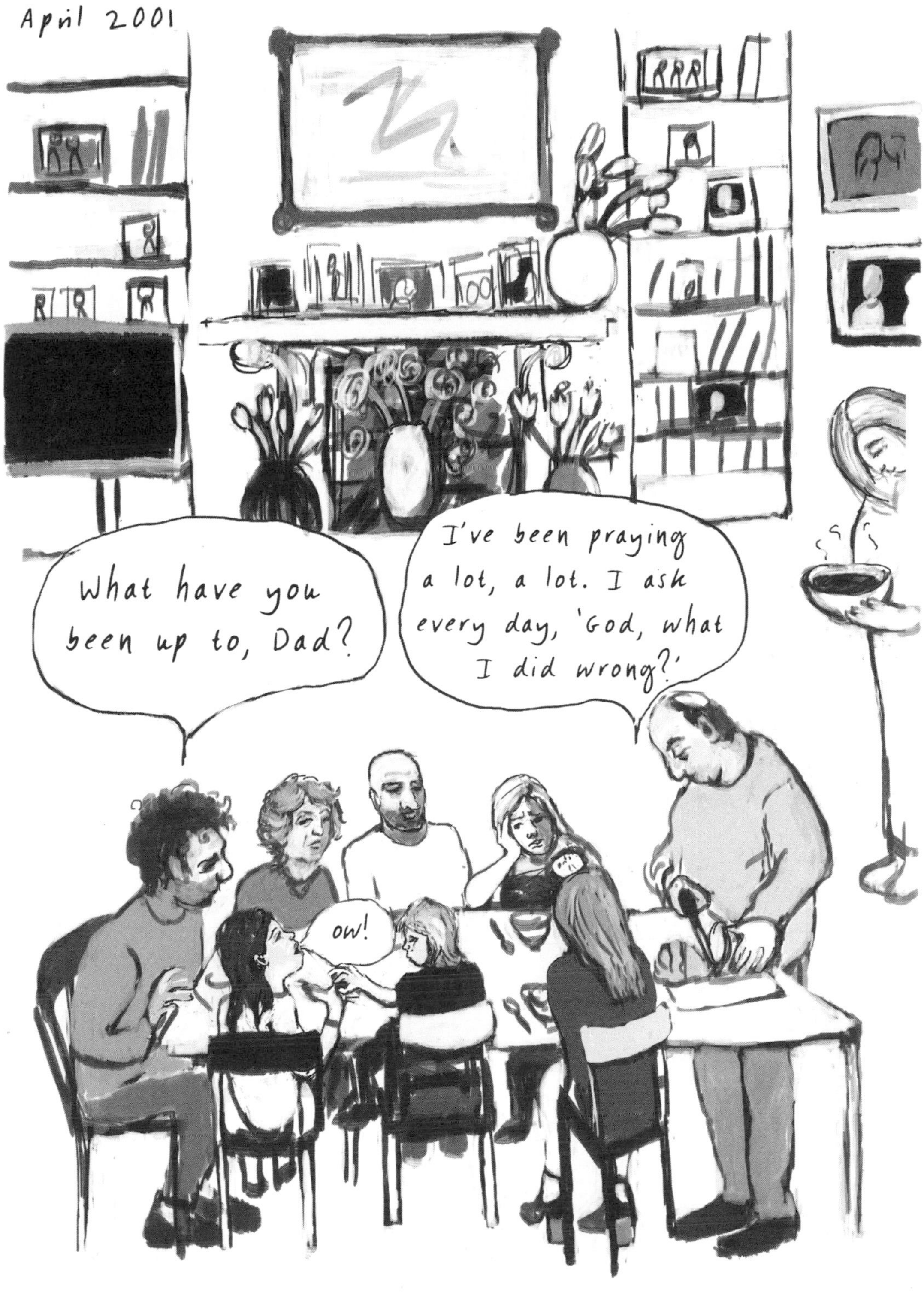
April 2001
What have you been up to, Dad?
I've been praying a lot, a lot. I ask every day, 'God, what I did wrong?'
ow!

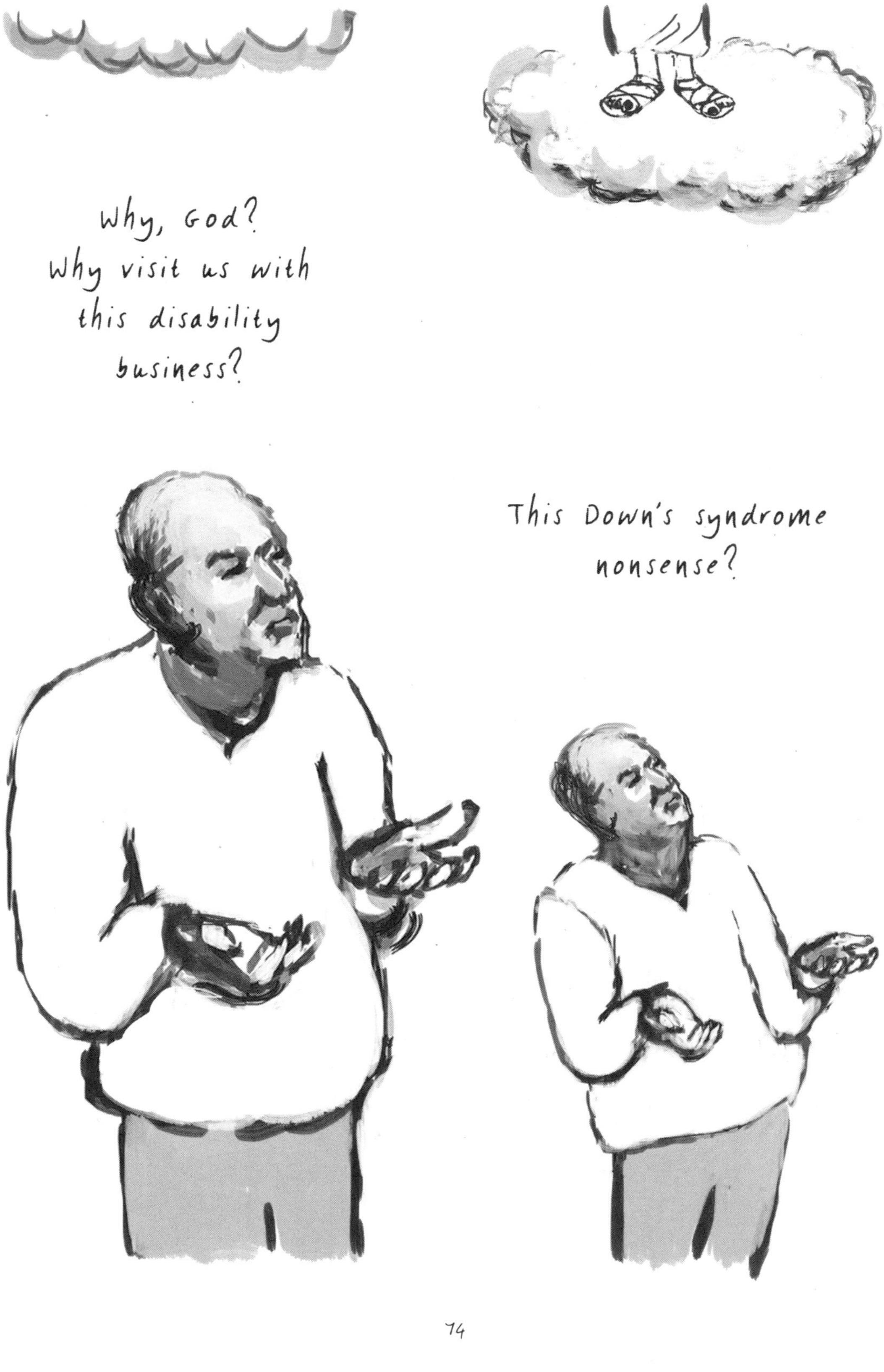
Why, God?
Why visit us with
this disability
business?
This Down's syndrome
nonsense?

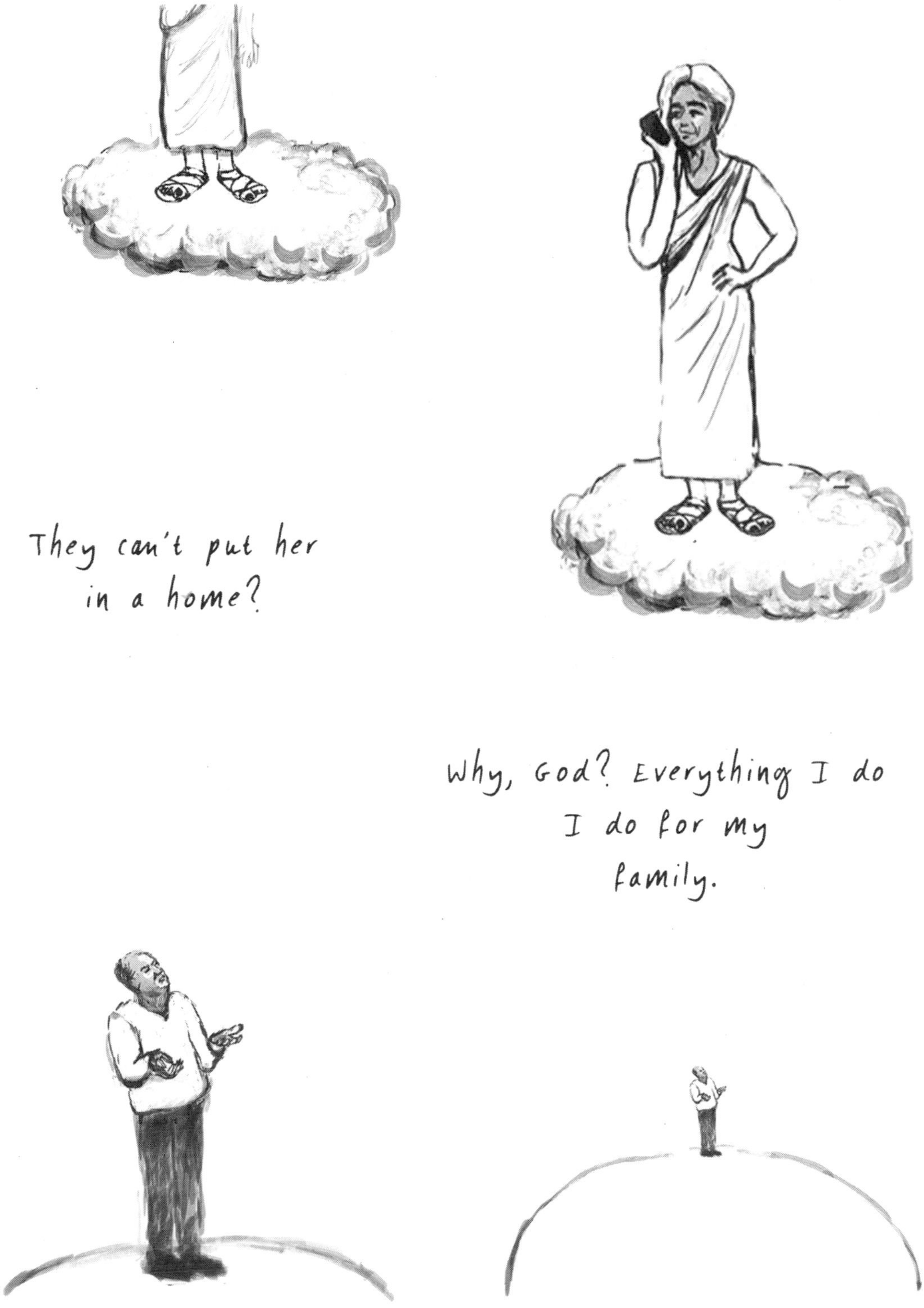
They can't put her in a home?
Why, God? Everything I do I do for my family.

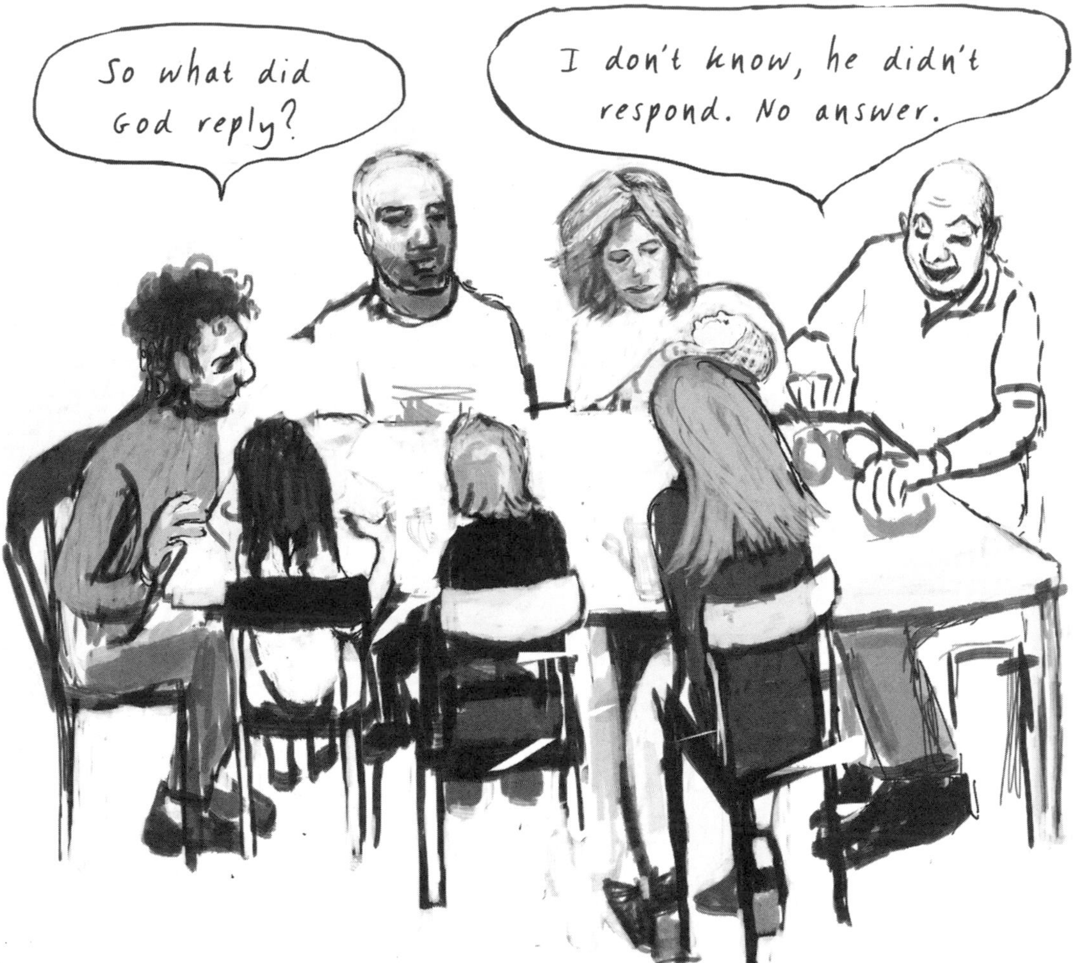
So what did God reply?
I don't know, he didn't respond. No answer.

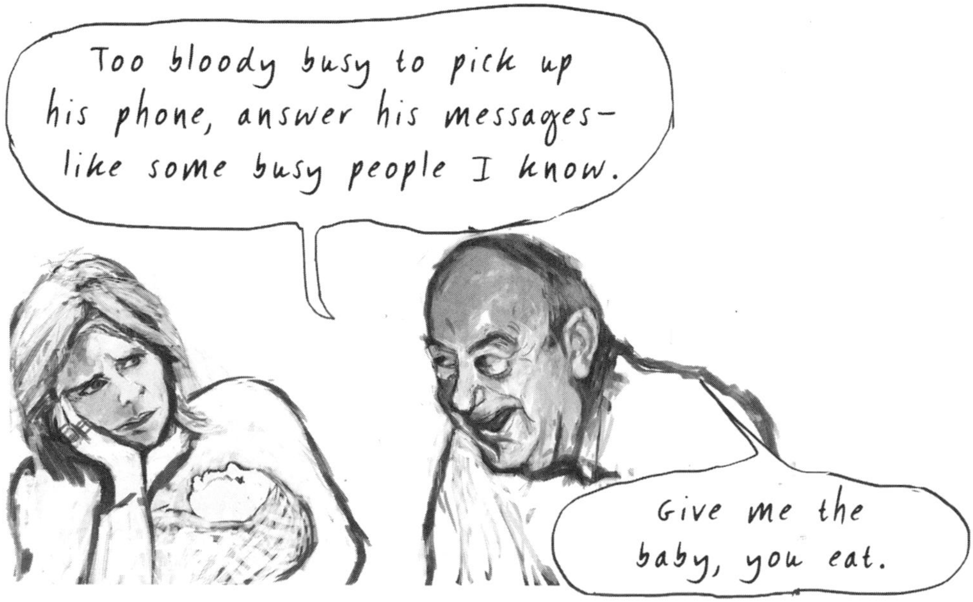
Too bloody busy to pick up his phone, answer his messages- like some busy people I know.
Give me the baby, you eat.

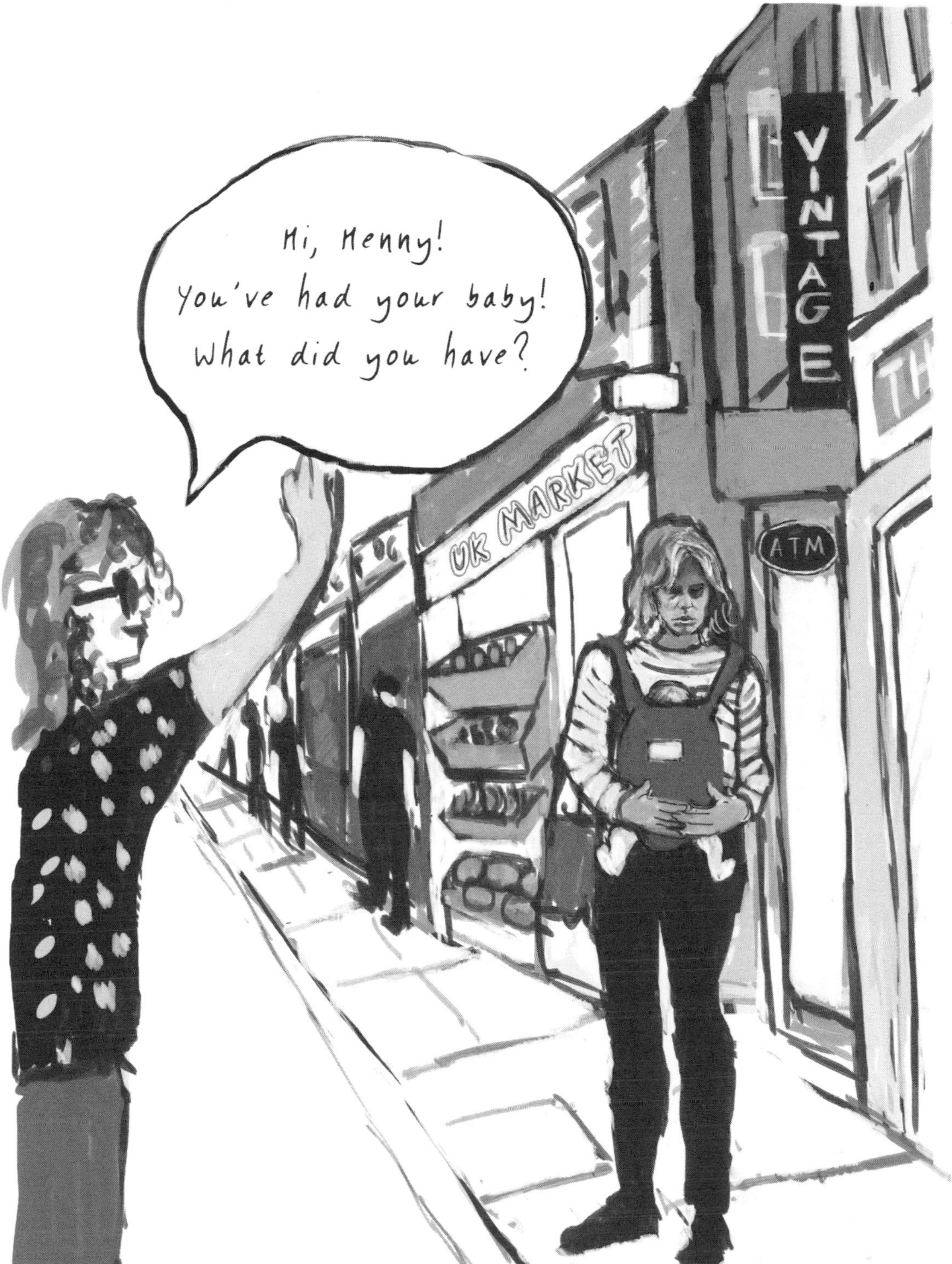
Hi, Henny! You've had your baby! What did you have?
VINTAGE
UK MARKET
ATM

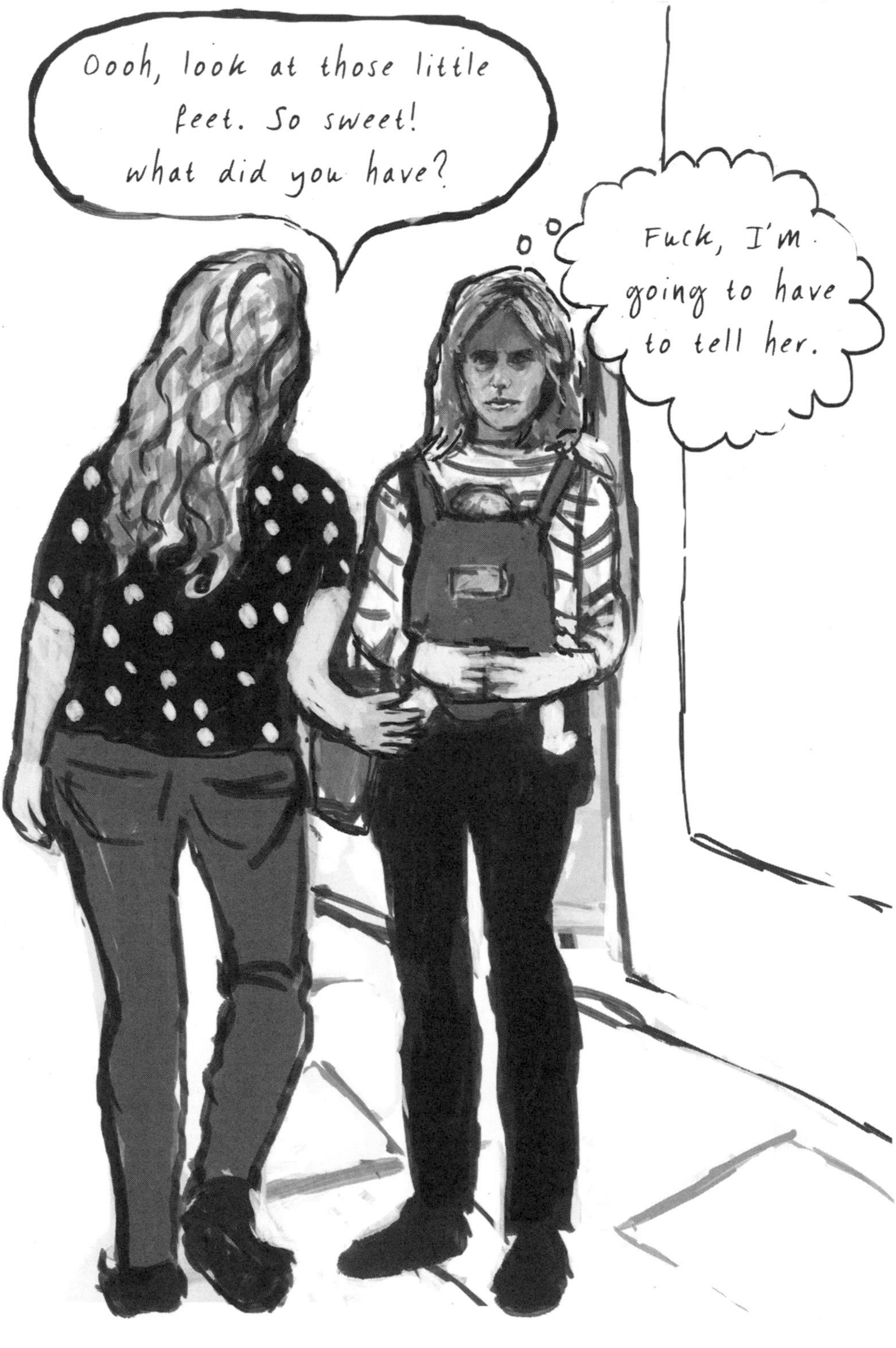
Oooh, look at those little feet. So sweet! what did you have?
Fuck, I'm going to have to tell her.

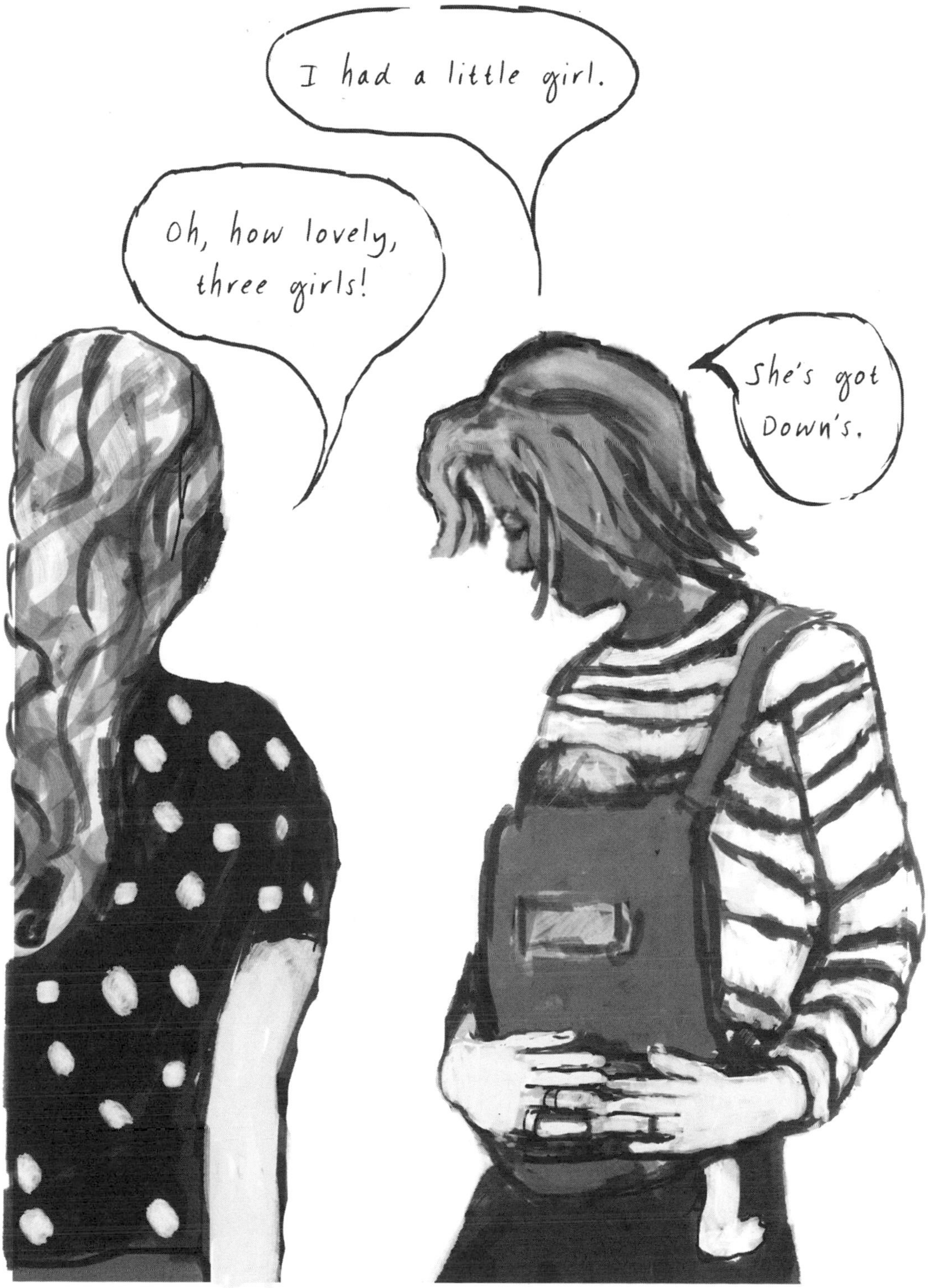
I had a little girl.
Oh, how lovely, three girls!
She's got Down's.

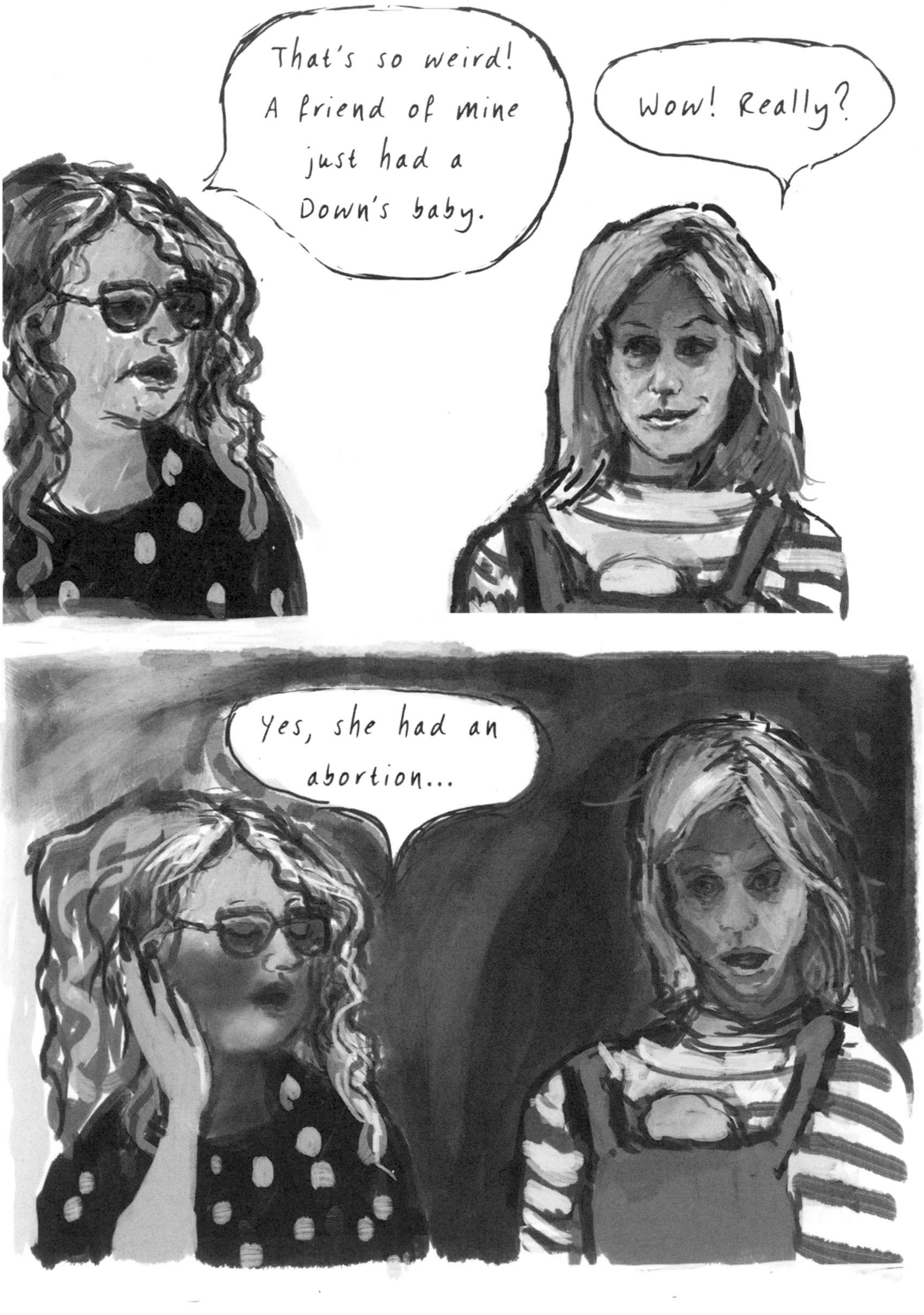
That's so weird! A friend of mine just had a Down's baby.
Wow! Really?
Yes, she had an abortion...

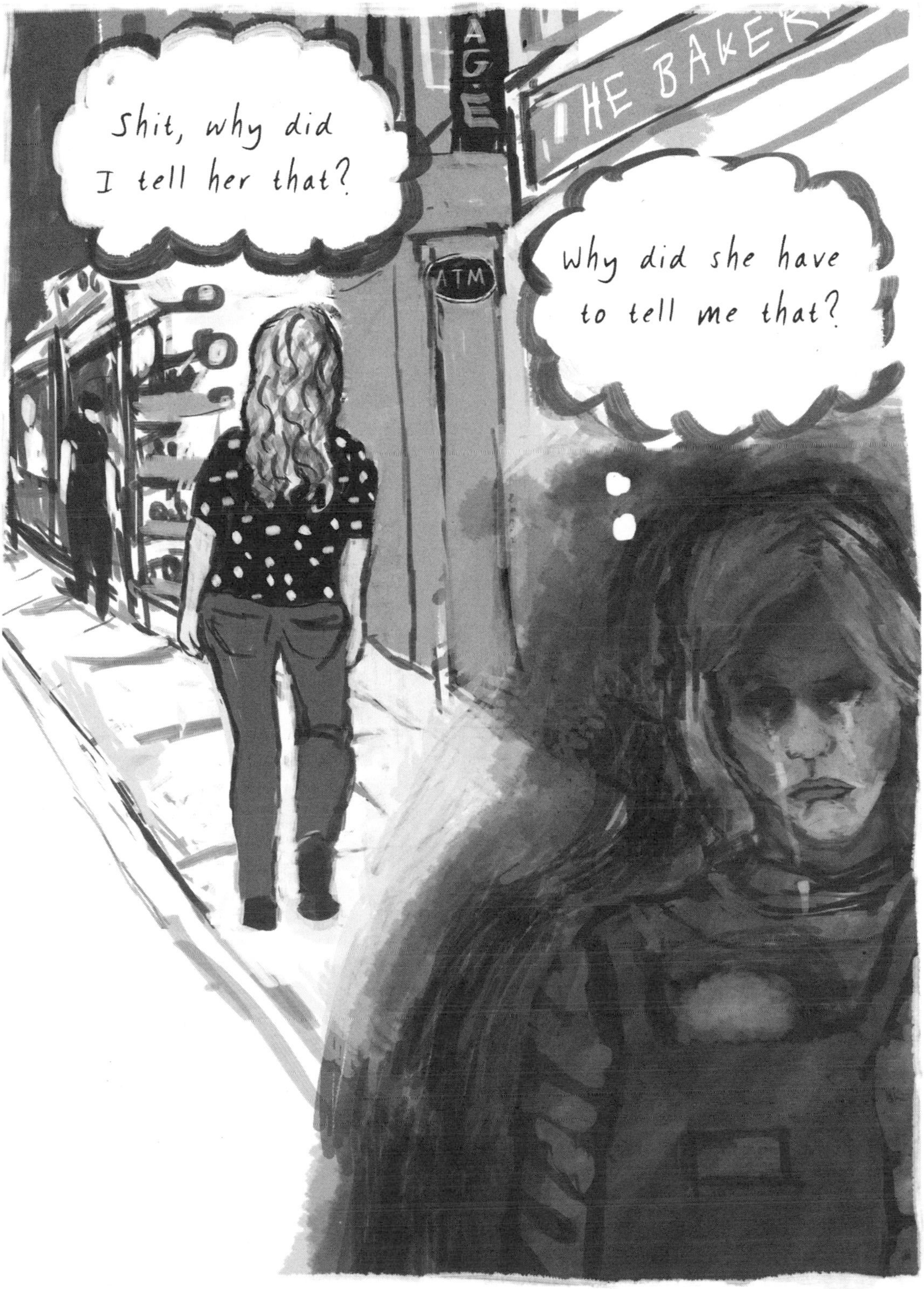
Shit, why did I tell her that?
Why did she have to tell me that?
THE BAKER
AGE
ATM

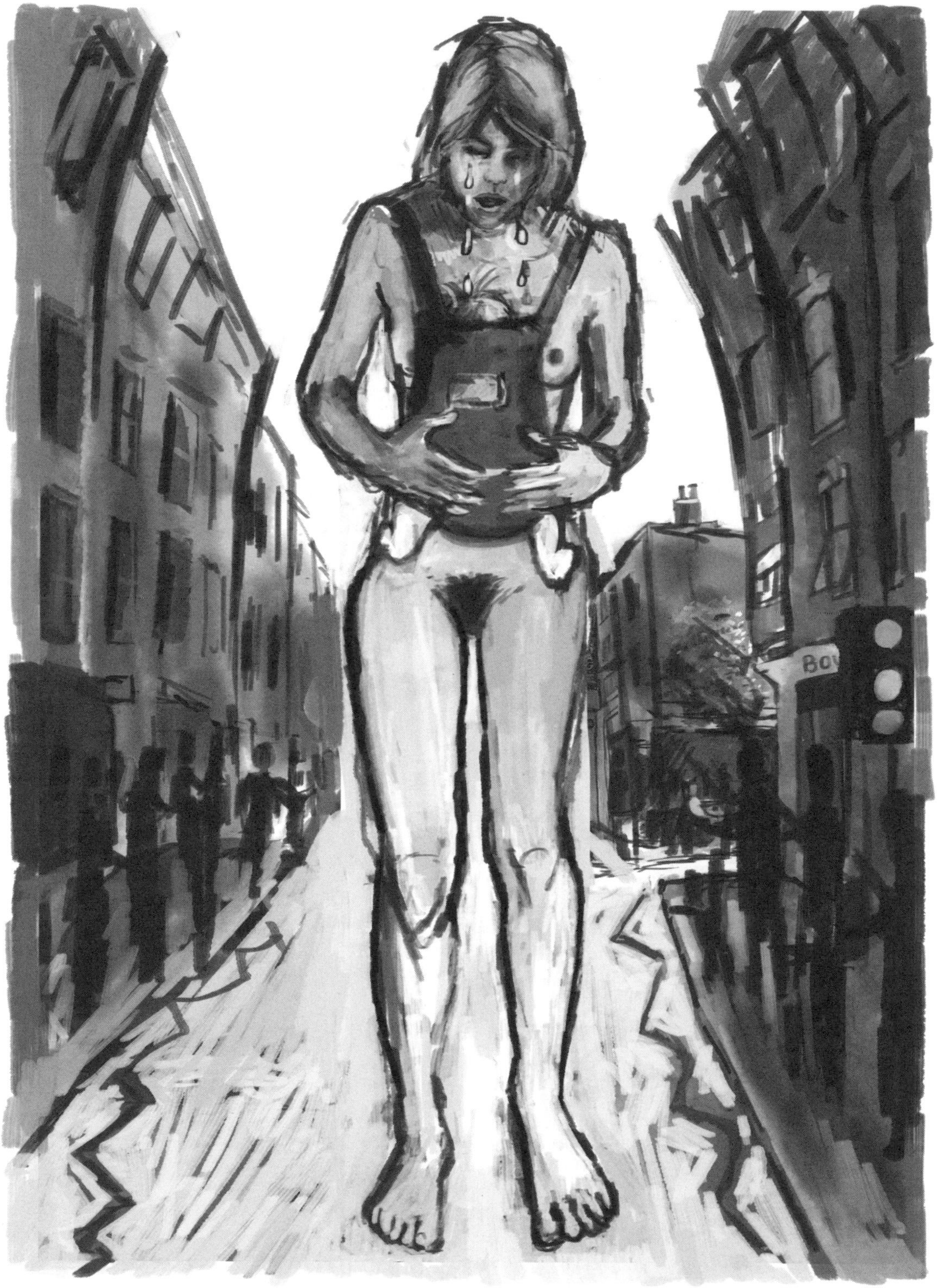

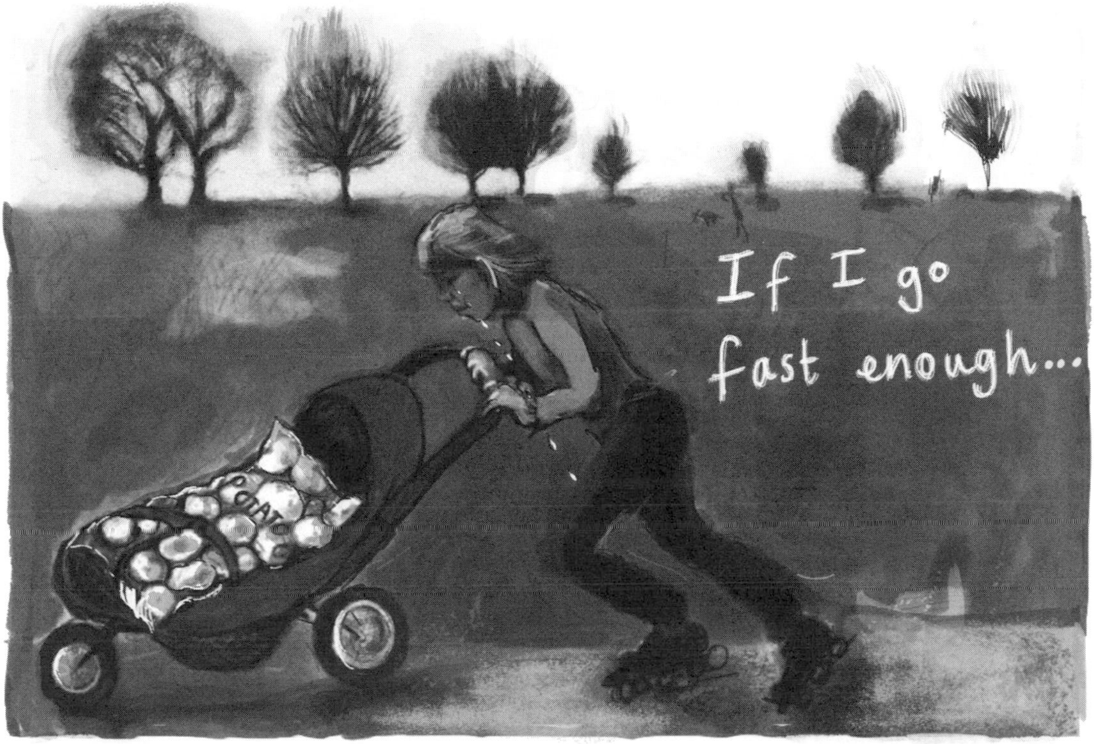
If I go fast enough...
POTATO

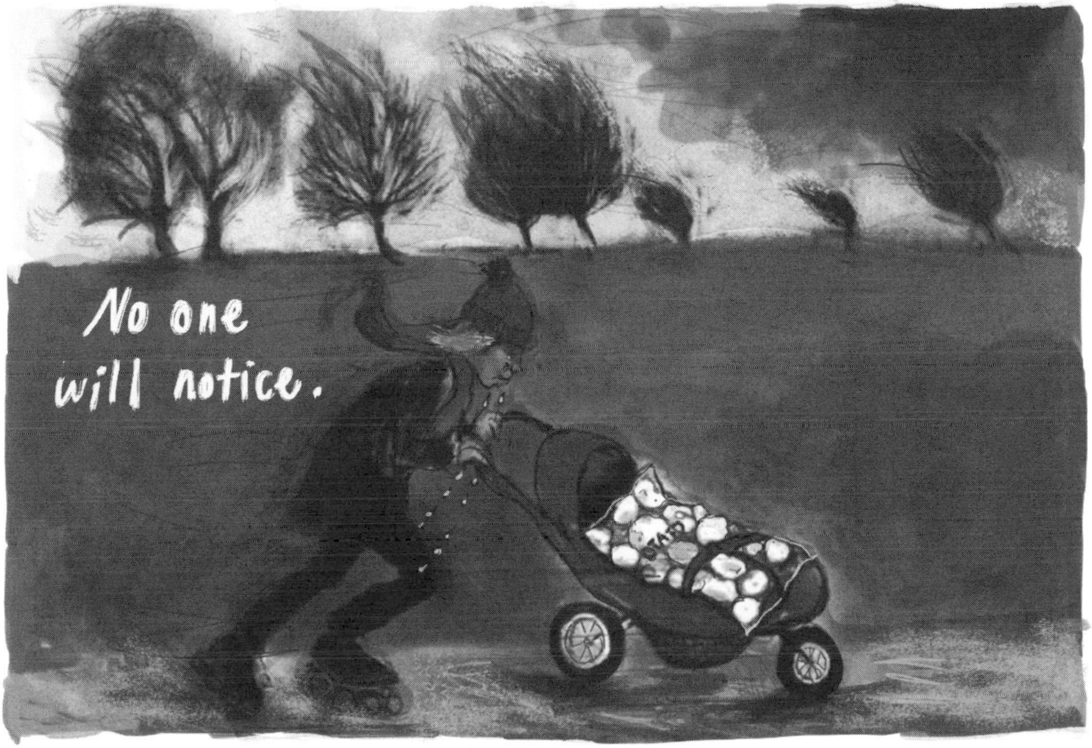
No one will notice.

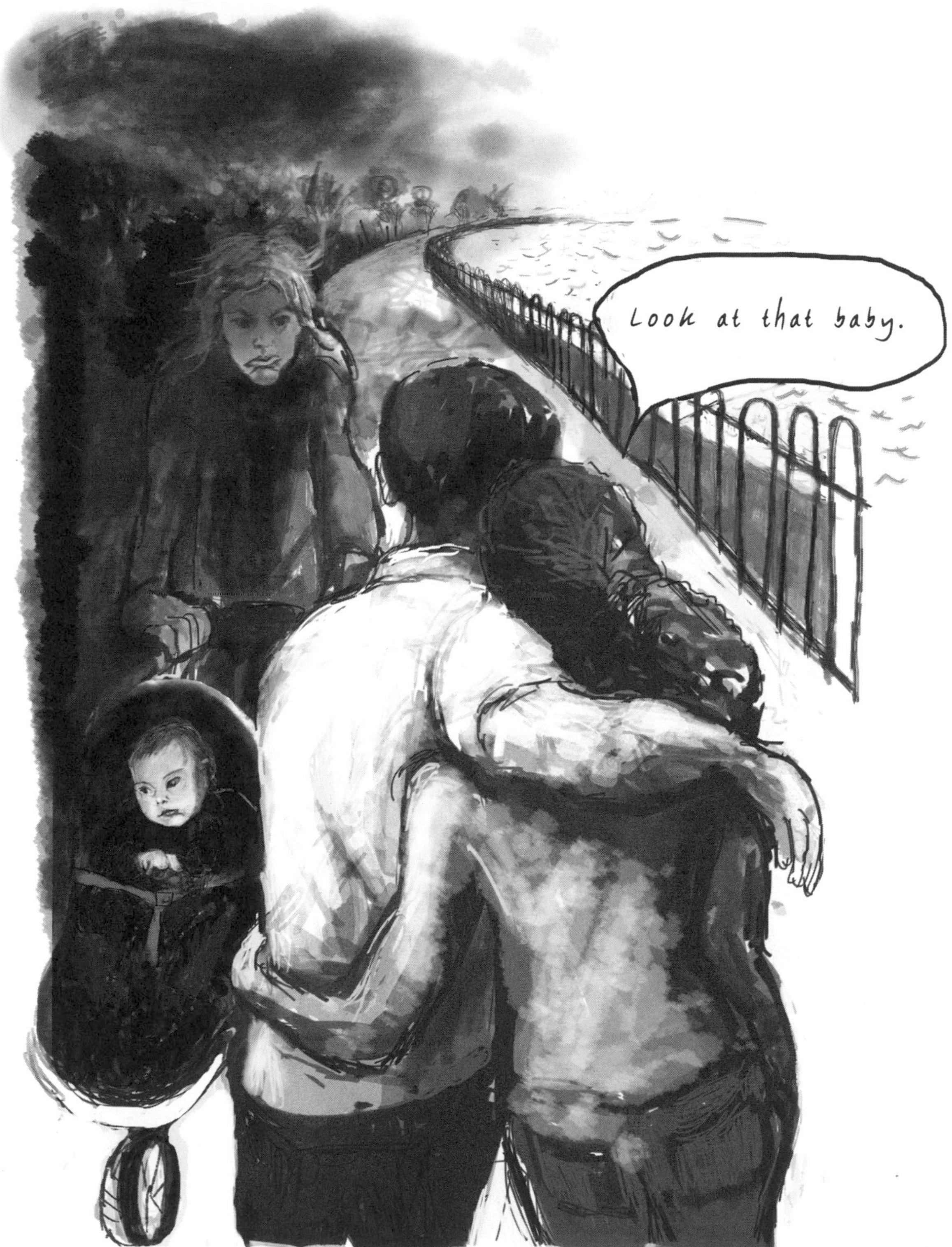
Look at that baby.

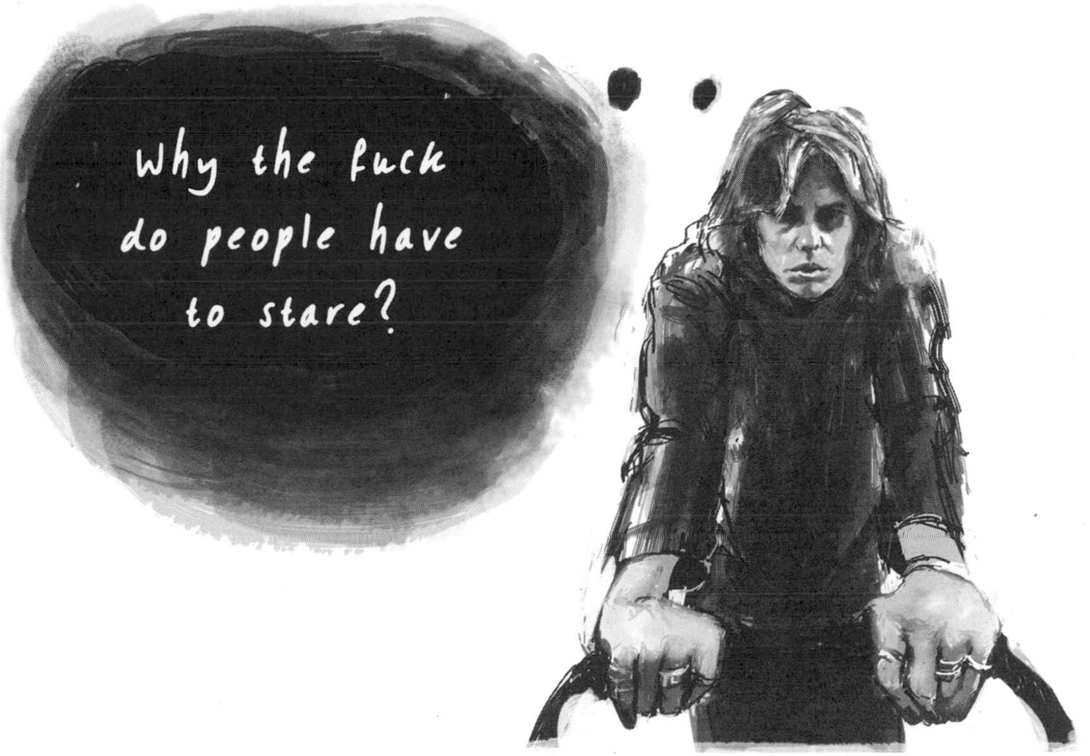
Why the fuck do people have to stare?

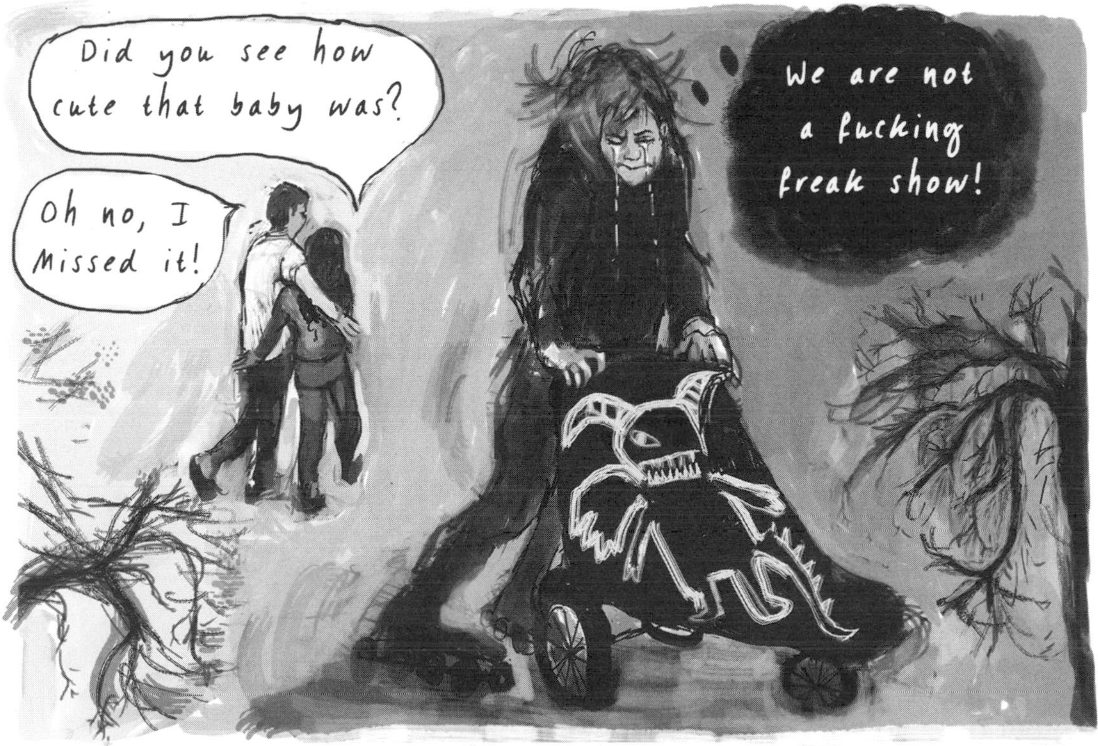
Did you see how cute that baby was?
Oh no, I missed it!
We are not a fucking freak show!

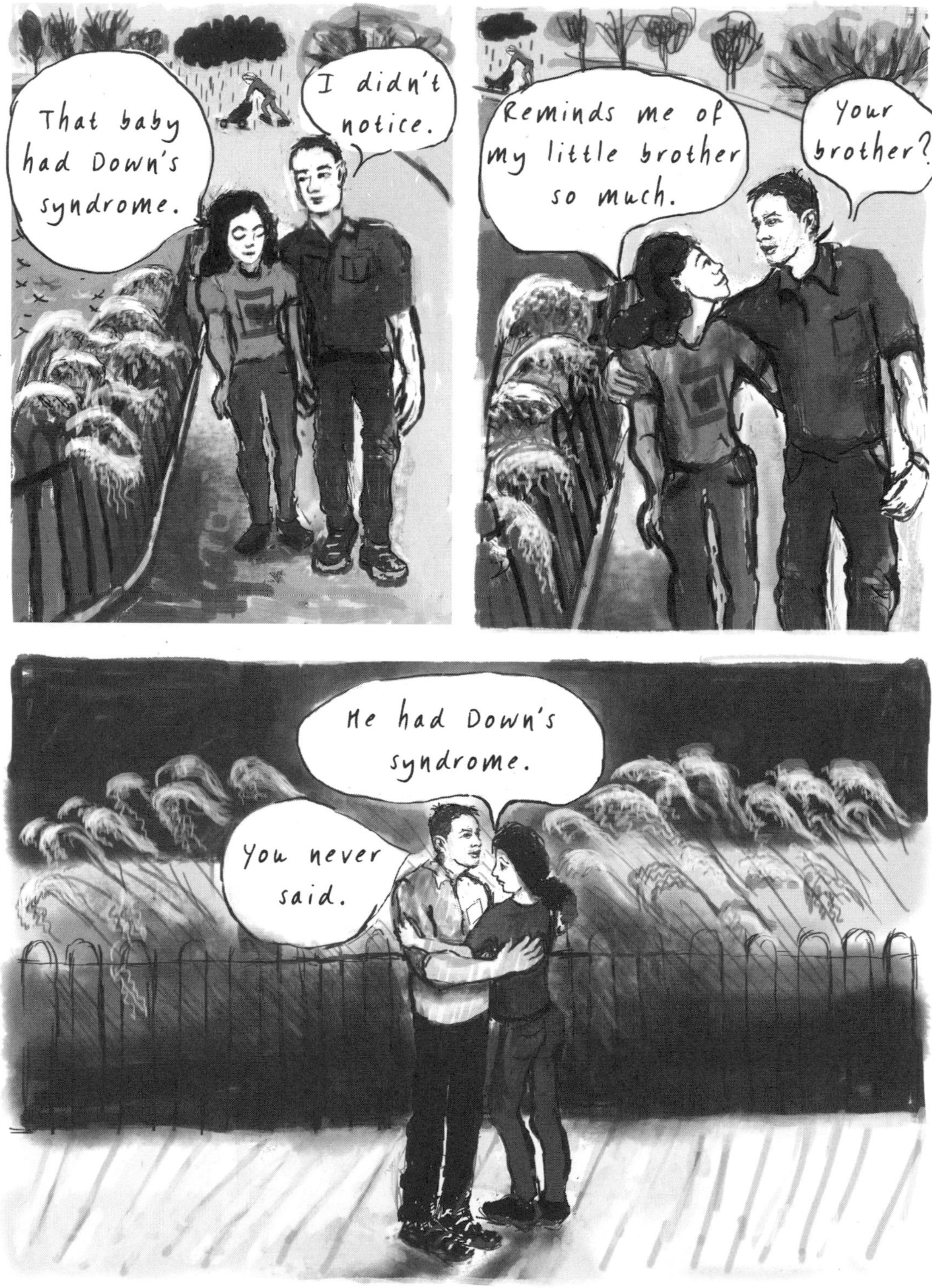
That baby had Down's syndrome.
I didn't notice.
Reminds me of my little brother so much.
Your brother?
He had Down's syndrome.
You never said.

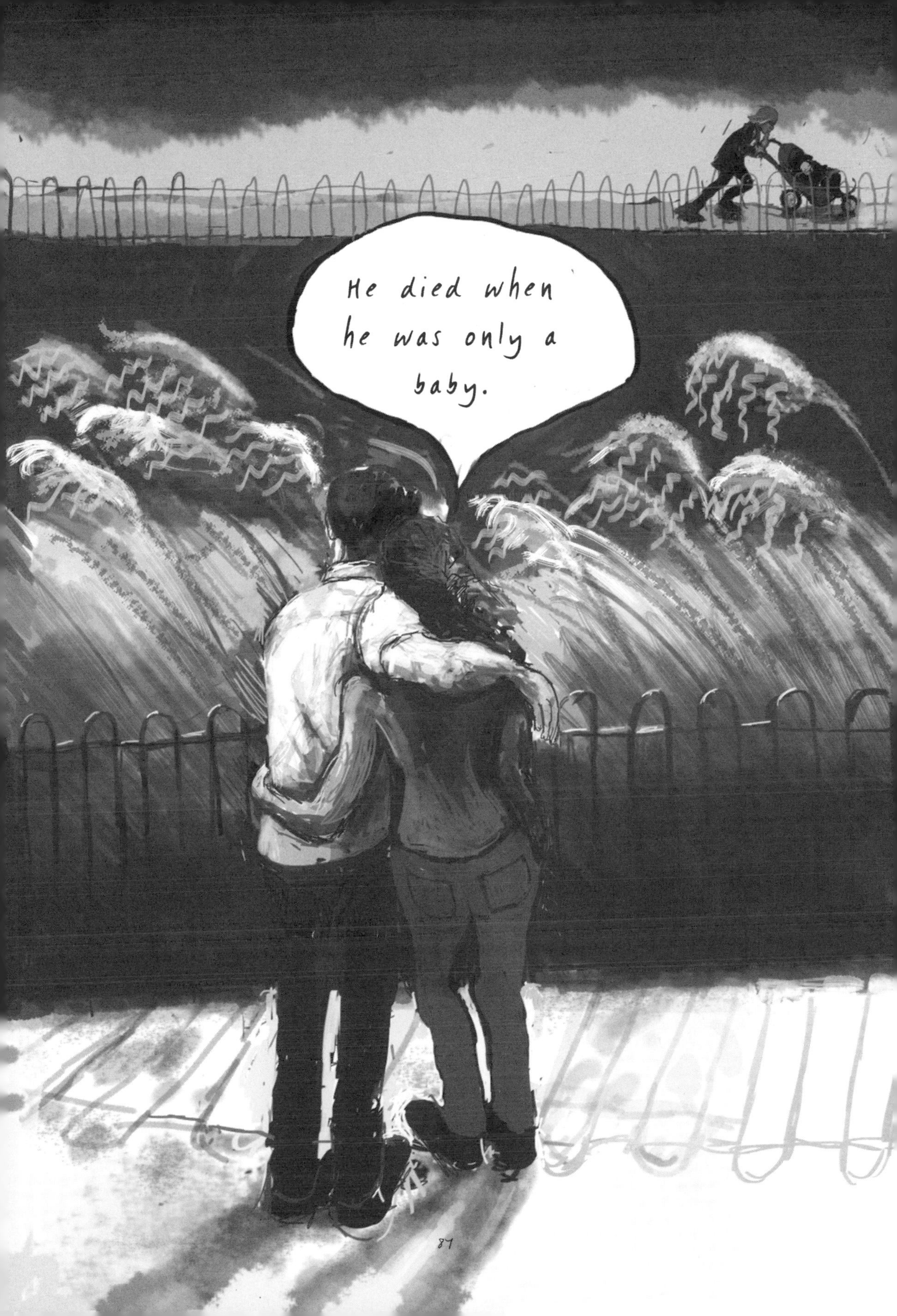
He died when he was only a baby.

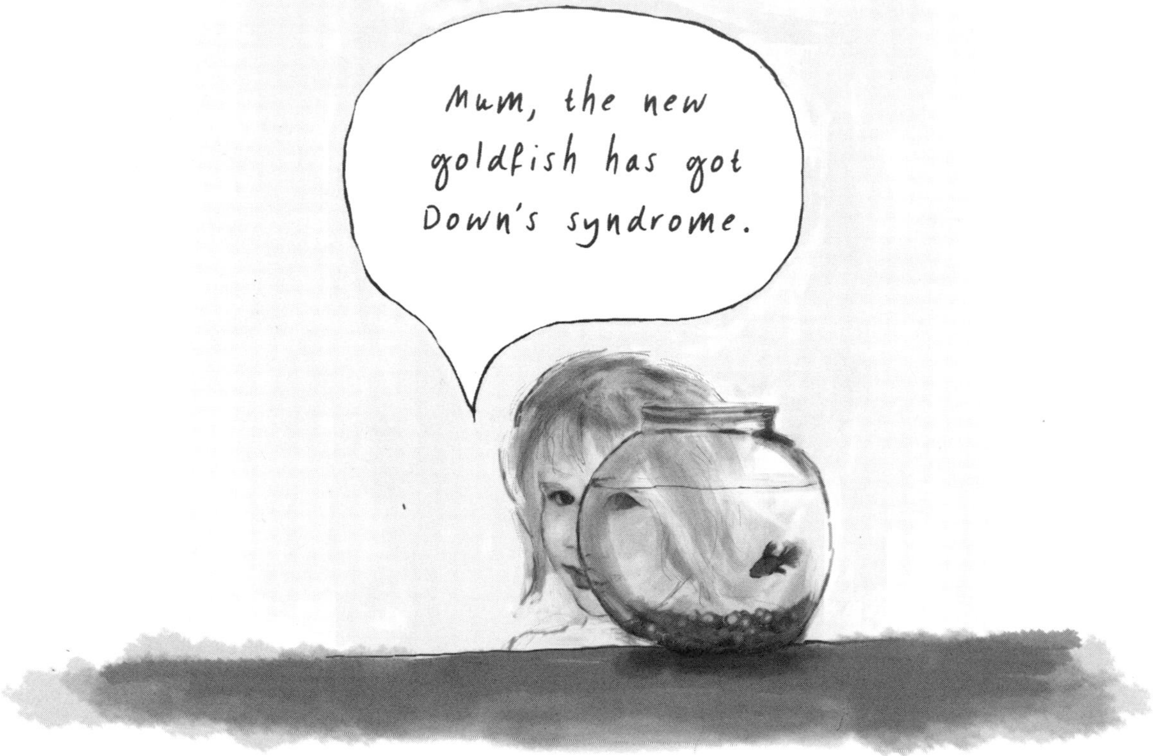
Mum, the new goldfish has got Down's syndrome.

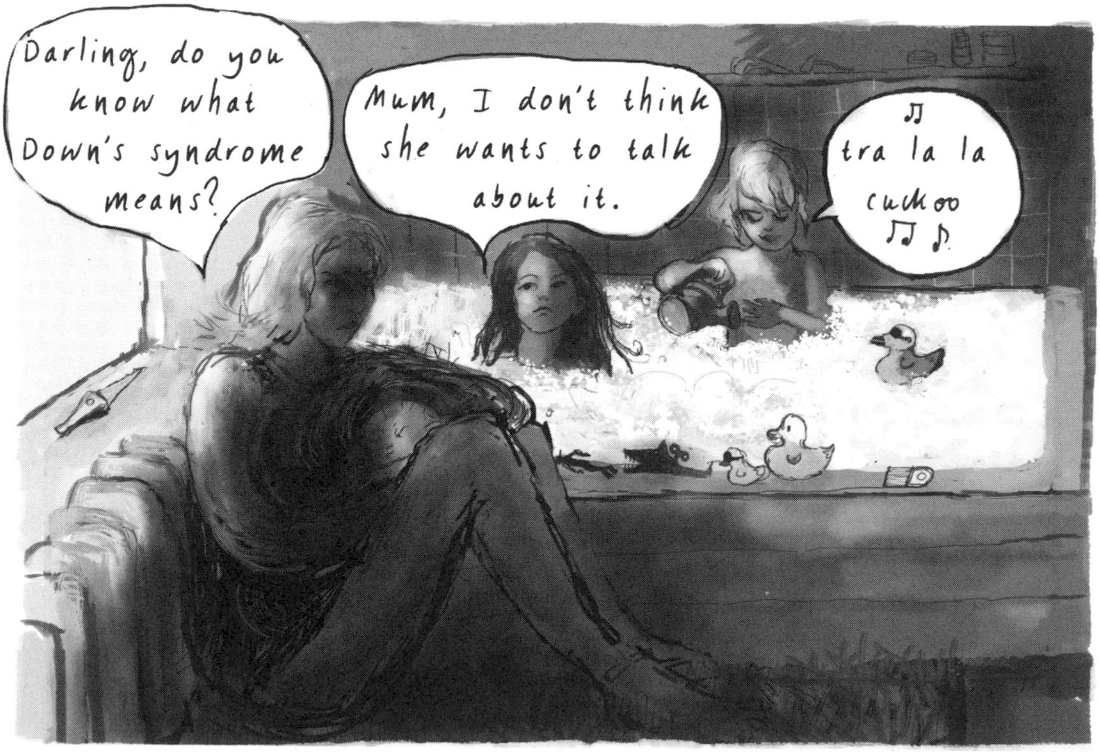
Darling, do you know what Down's syndrome means?
Mum, I don't think she wants to talk about it.
♫ tra la la cuckoo ♫ ♪

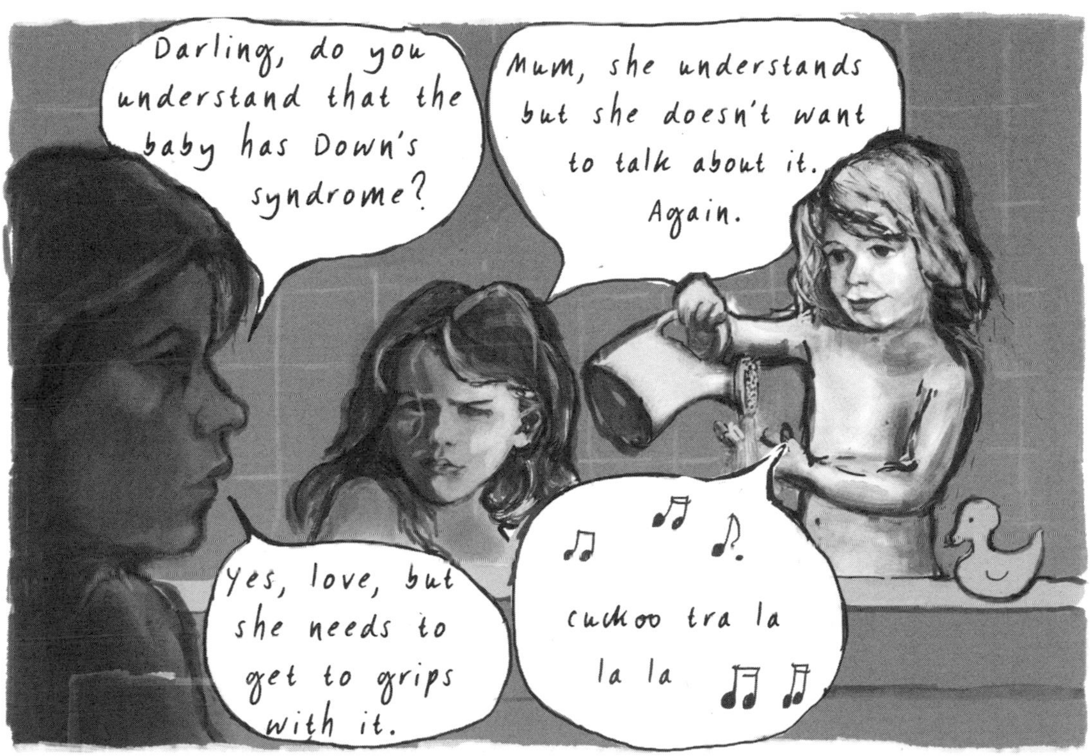
Darling, do you understand that the baby has Down's syndrome?
Mum, she understands but she doesn't want to talk about it. Again.
Yes, love, but she needs to get to grips with it.
cuckoo tra la la la

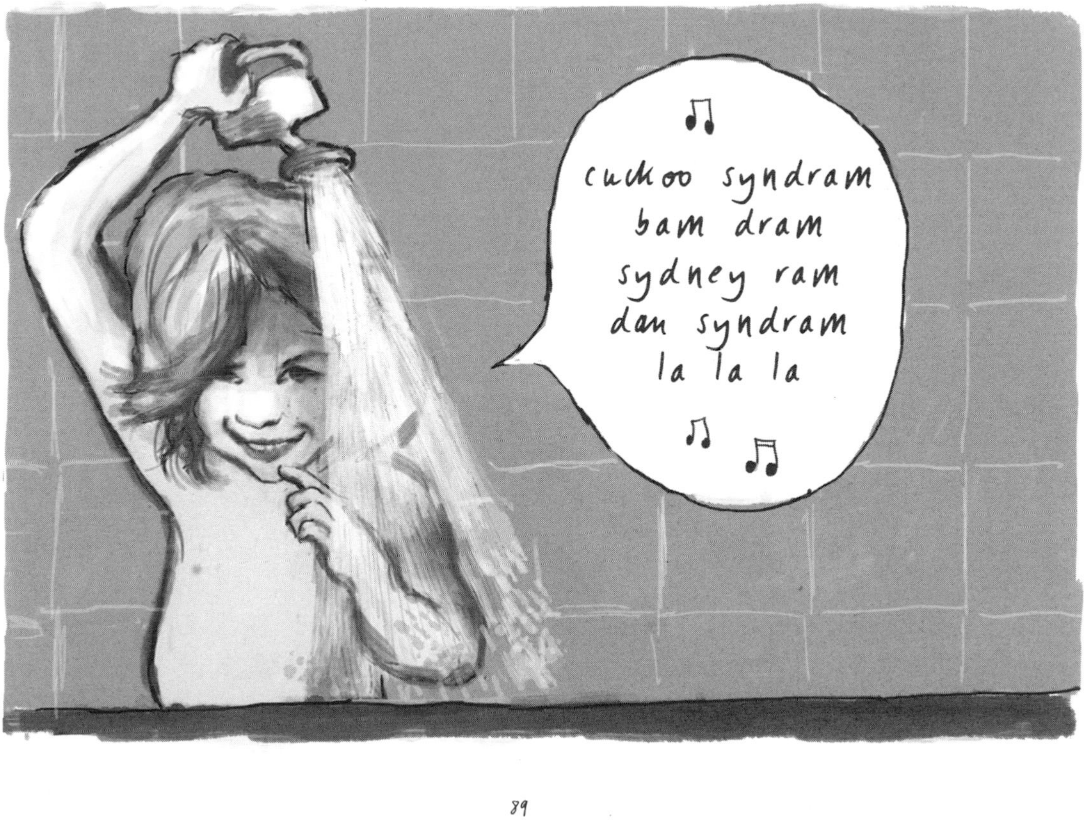
cuckoo syndram bam dram sydney ram dan syndram la la la

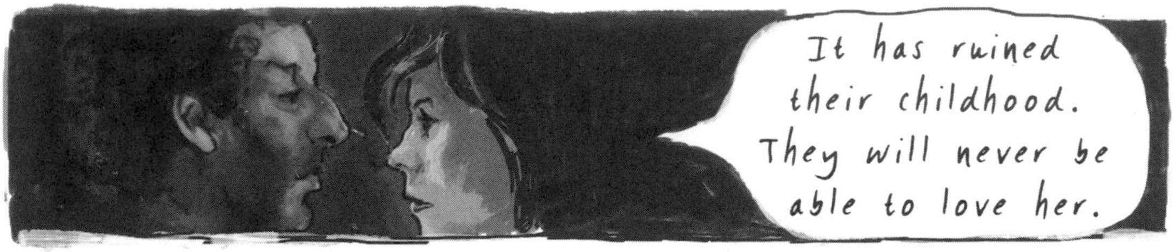
It has ruined their childhood. They will never be able to love her.

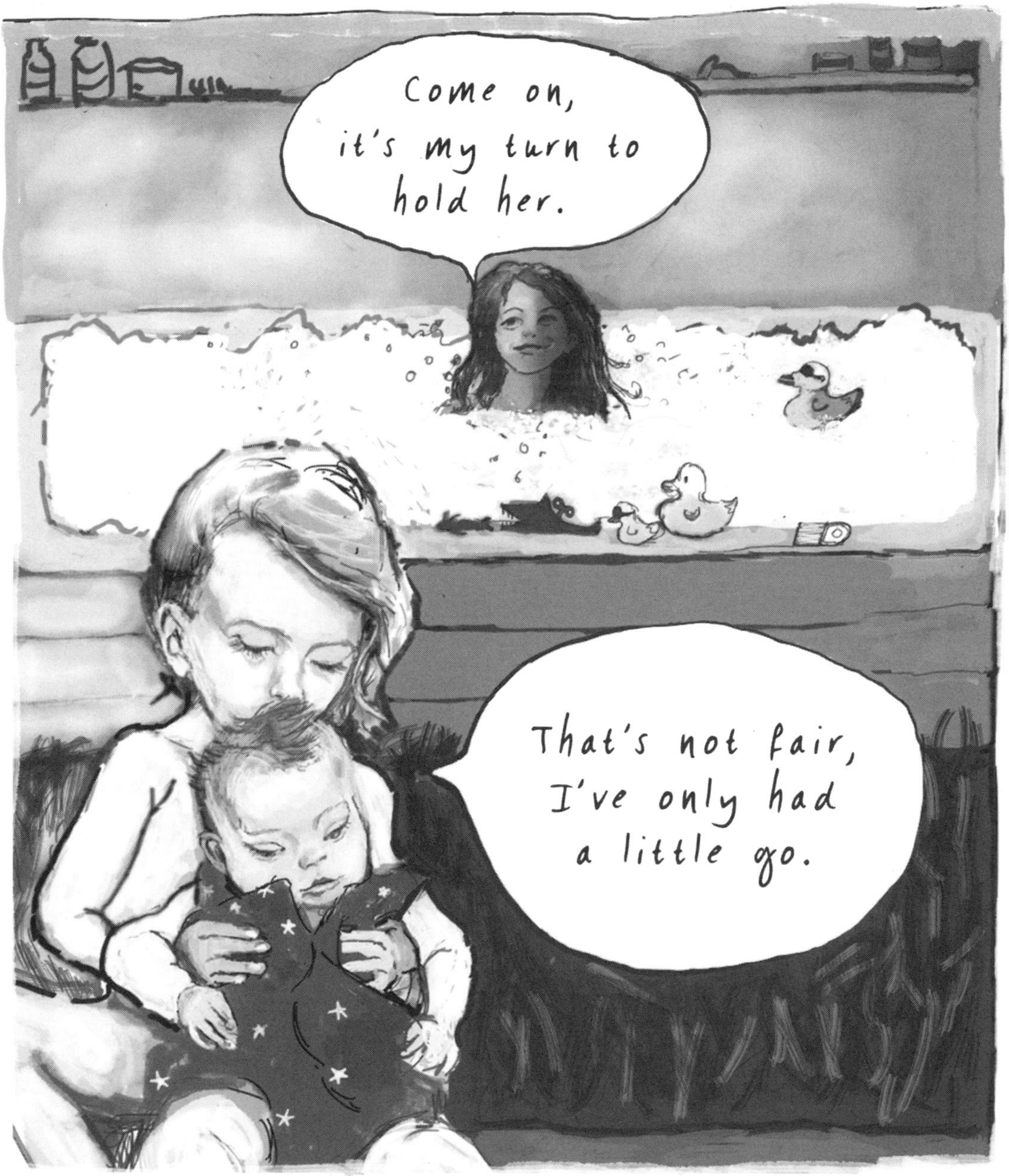
Come on, it's my turn to hold her.
That's not fair, I've only had a little go.

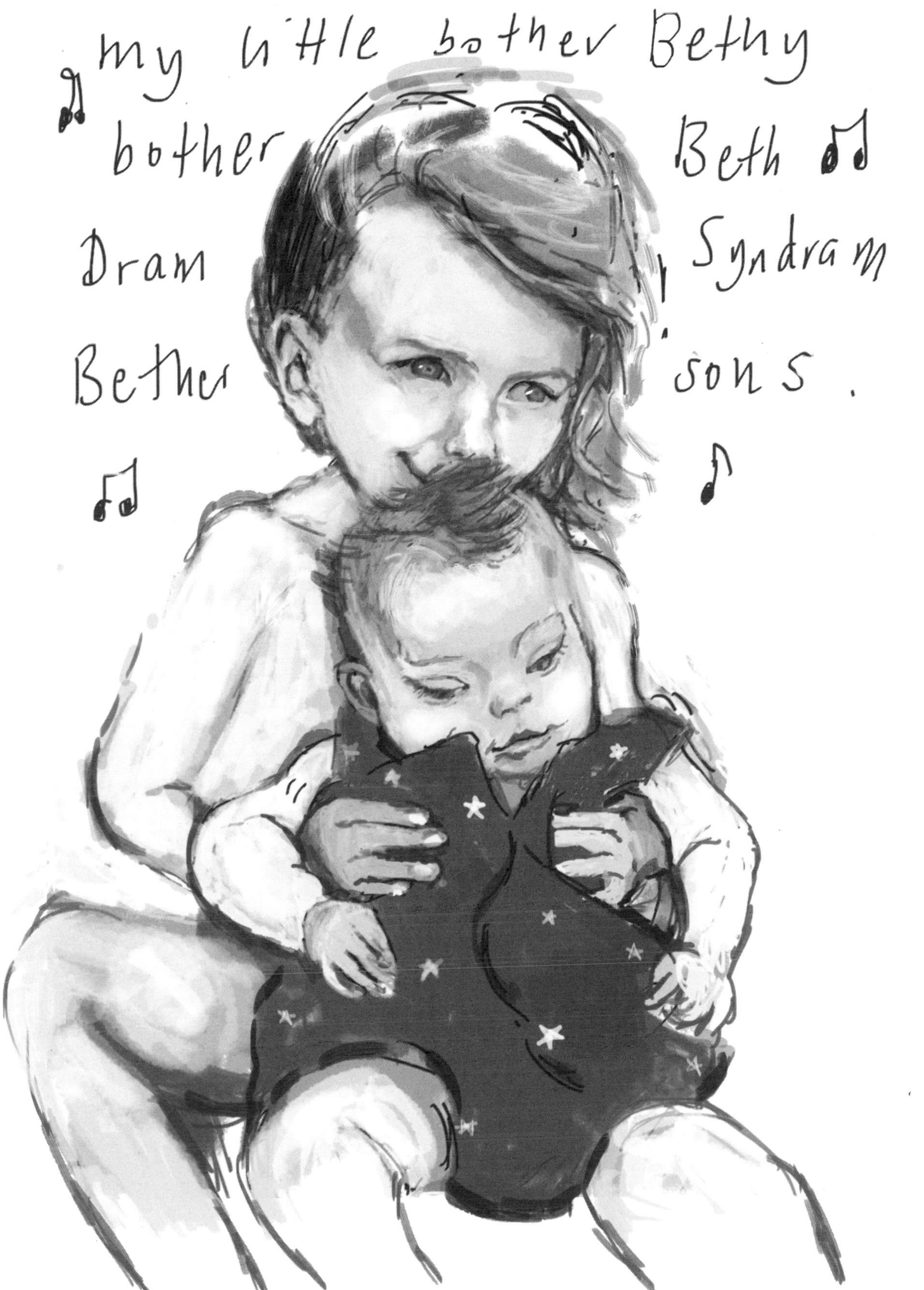
my little bother Bethy
bother Beth
Dram Syndram
Bether sons.

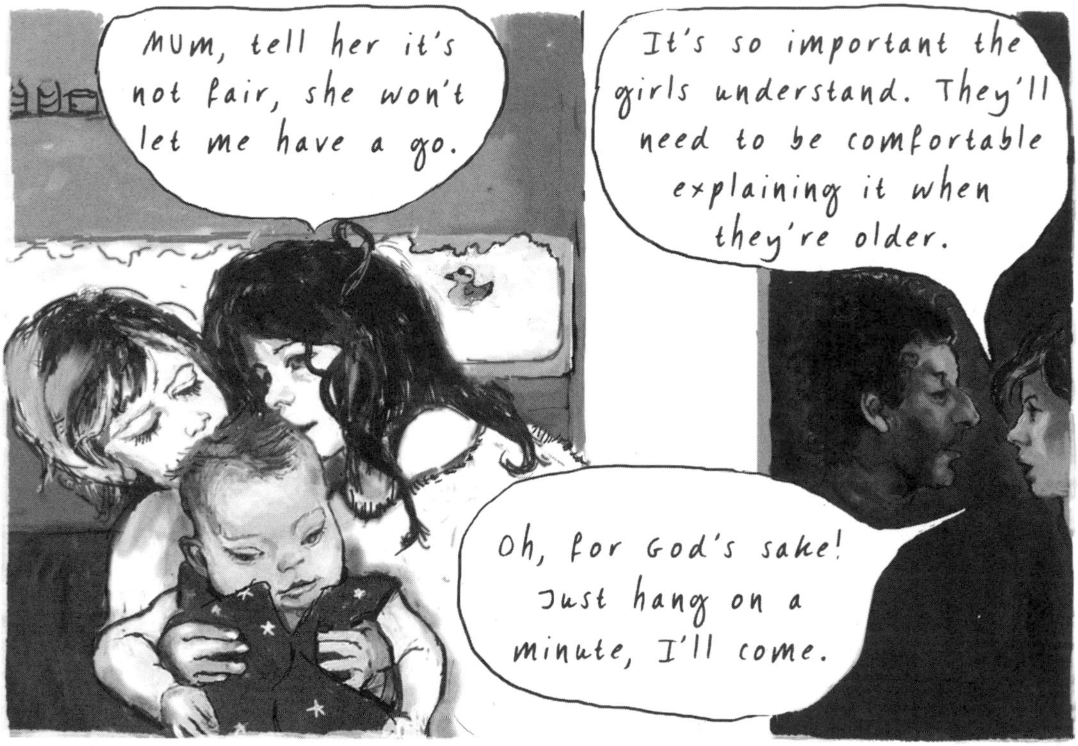
MUM, tell her it's not fair, she won't let me have a go.
It's so important the girls understand. They'll need to be comfortable explaining it when they're older.
Oh, for God's sake! Just hang on a minute, I'll come.

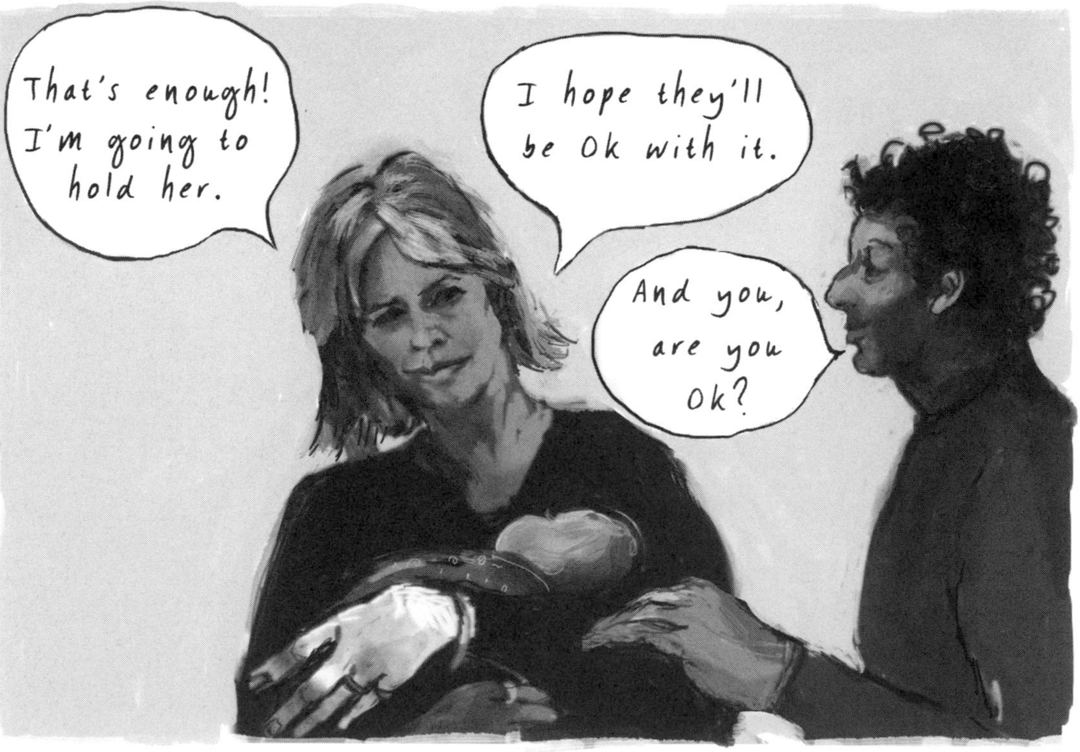
That's enough! I'm going to hold her.
I hope they'll be Ok with it.
And you, are you Ok?

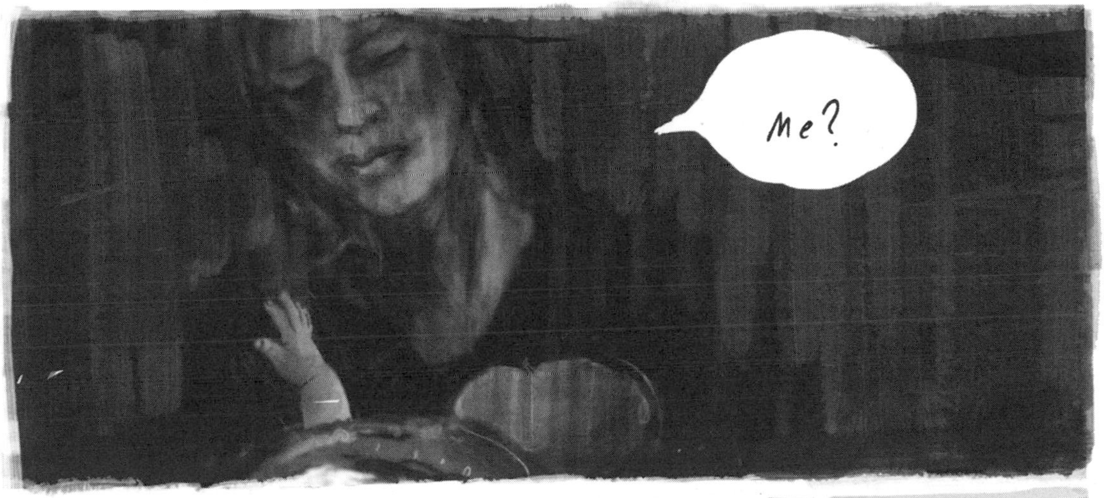
Me?

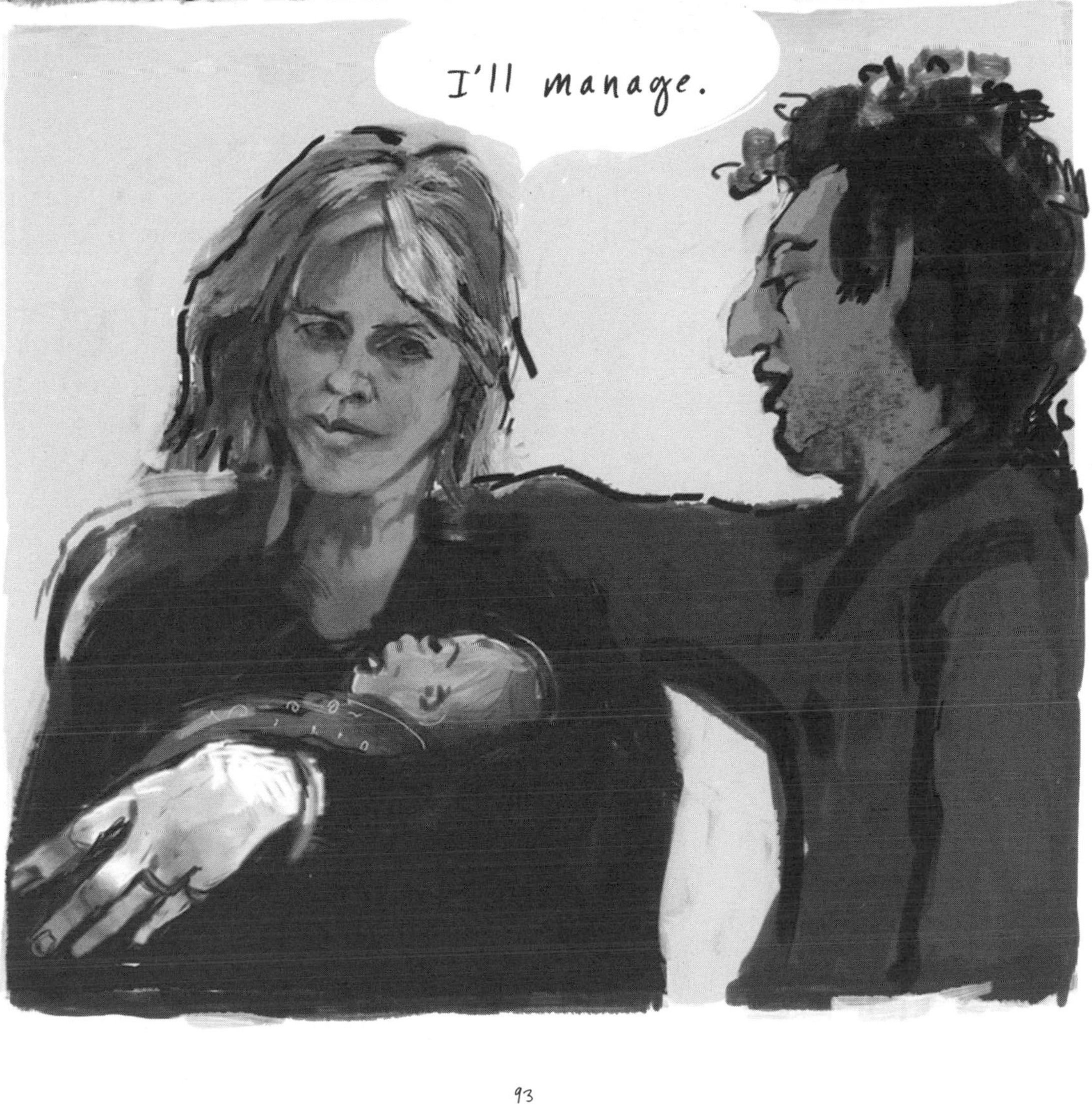
I'll manage.

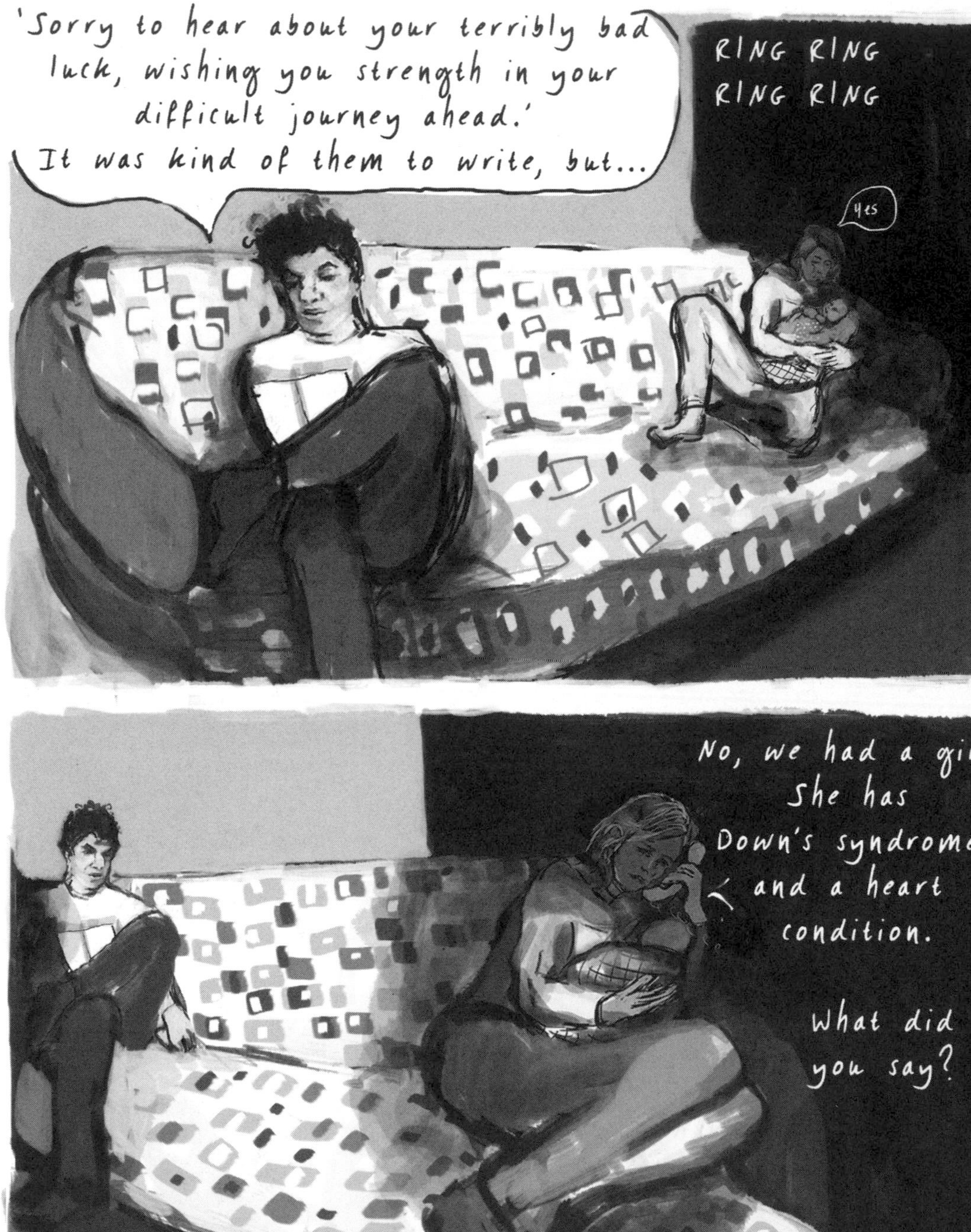
'Sorry to hear about your terribly bad luck, wishing you strength in your difficult journey ahead.' It was kind of them to write, but...
RING RING RING RING
yes
No, we had a girl. She has Down's syndrome and a heart condition.
What did you say?

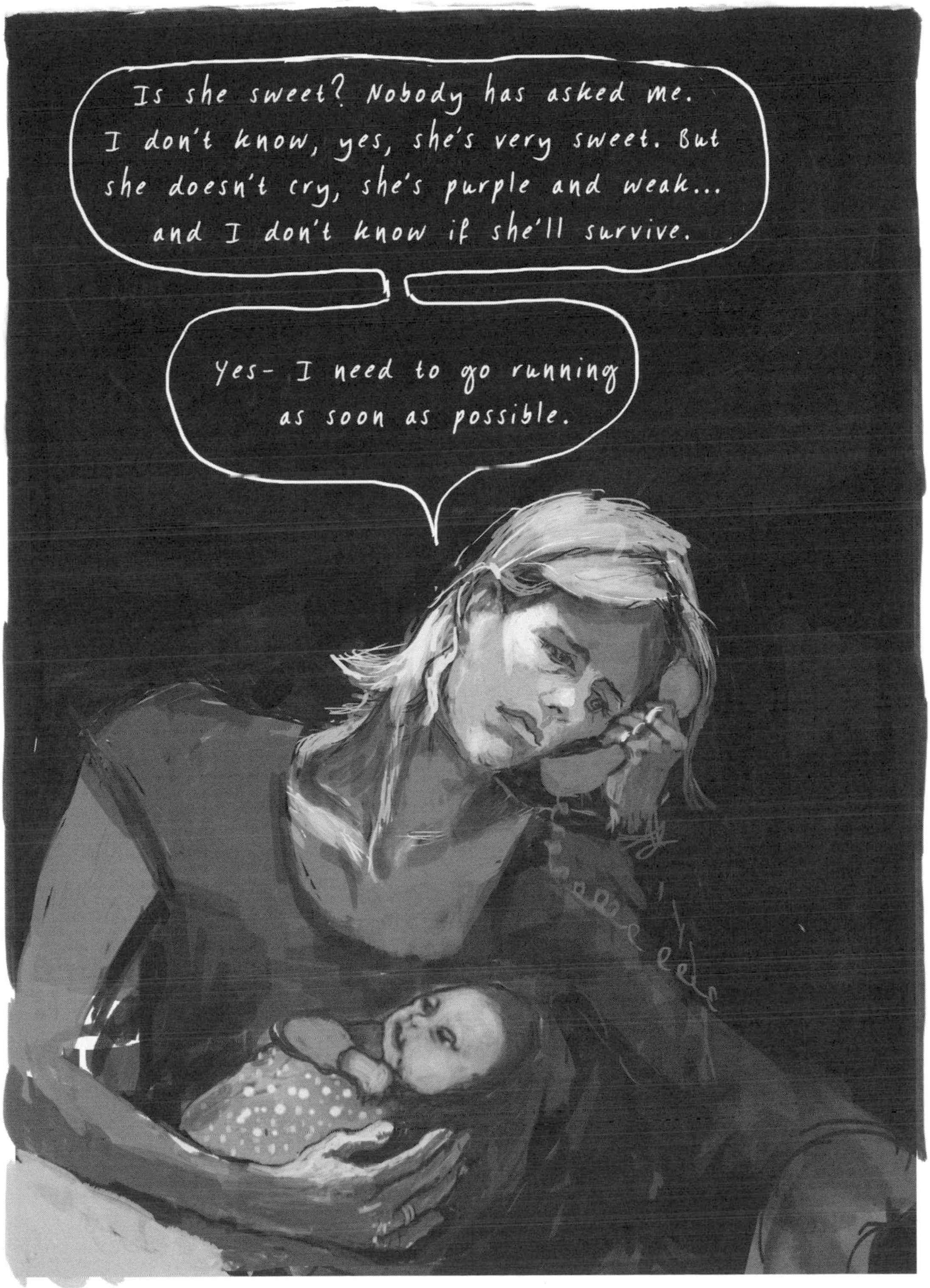
Is she sweet? Nobody has asked me. I don't know, yes, she's very sweet. But she doesn't cry, she's purple and weak... and I don't know if she'll survive.
Yes- I need to go running as soon as possible.

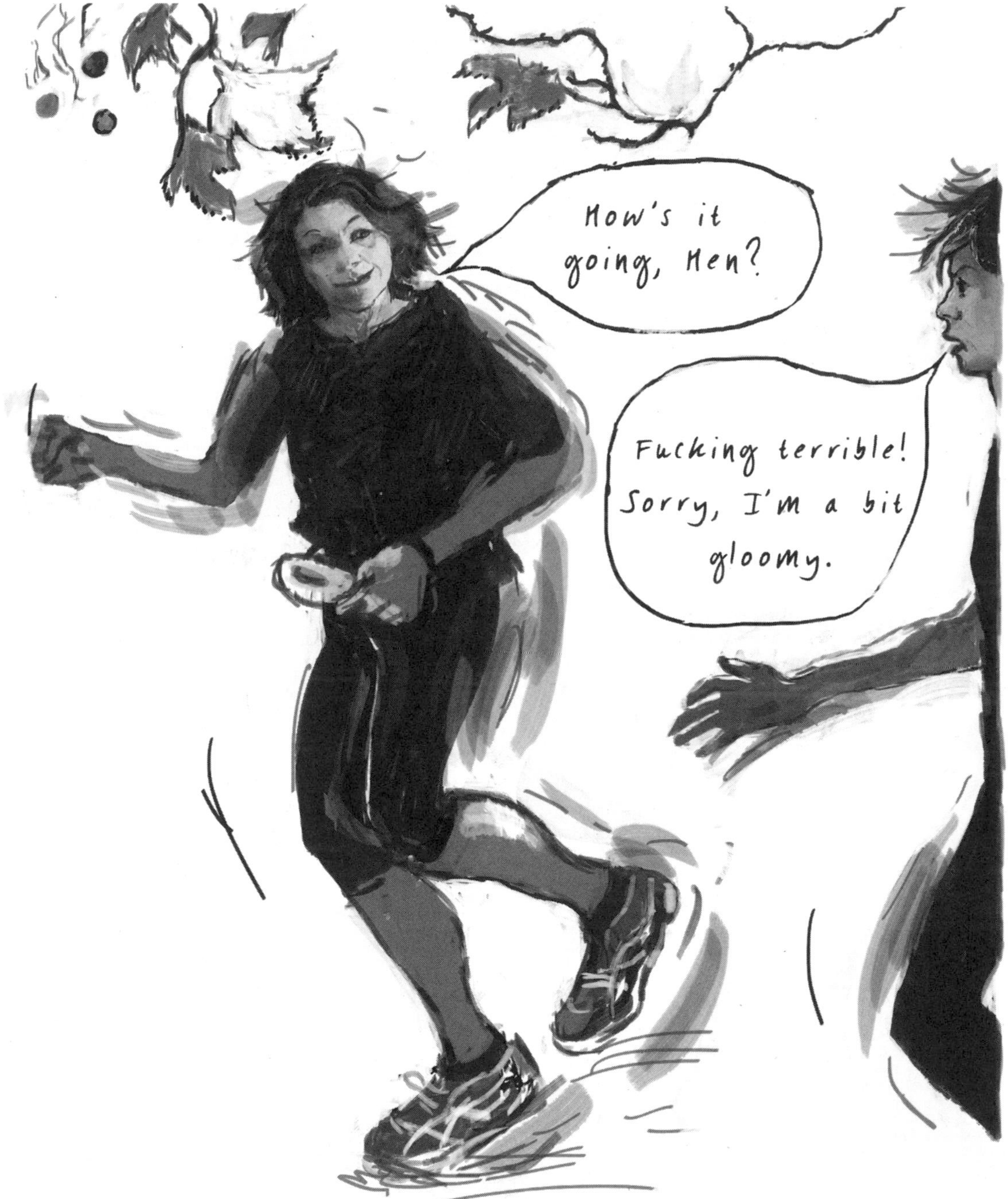
How's it going, Hen?
Fucking terrible! Sorry, I'm a bit gloomy.

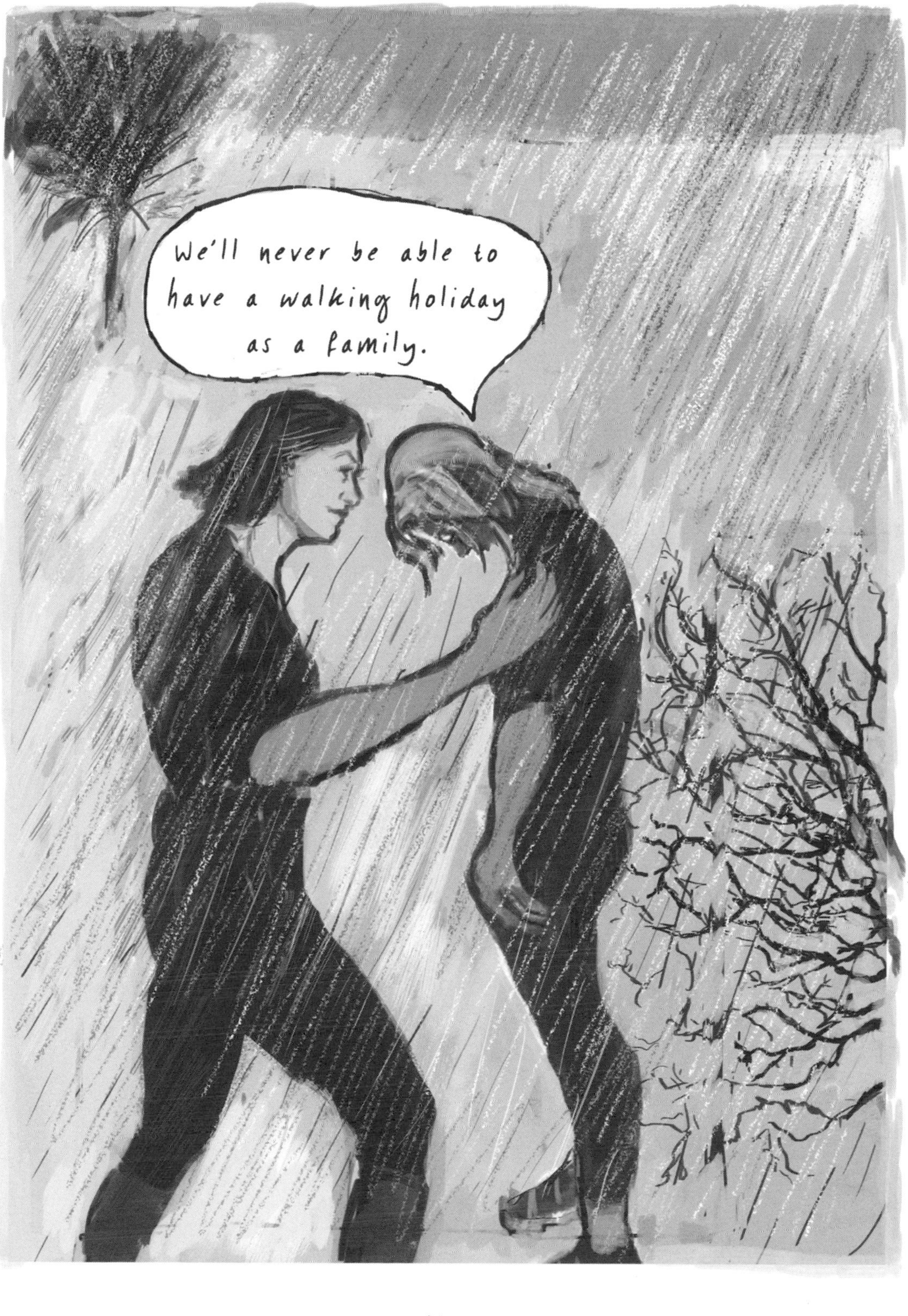
We'll never be able to have a walking holiday as a family.

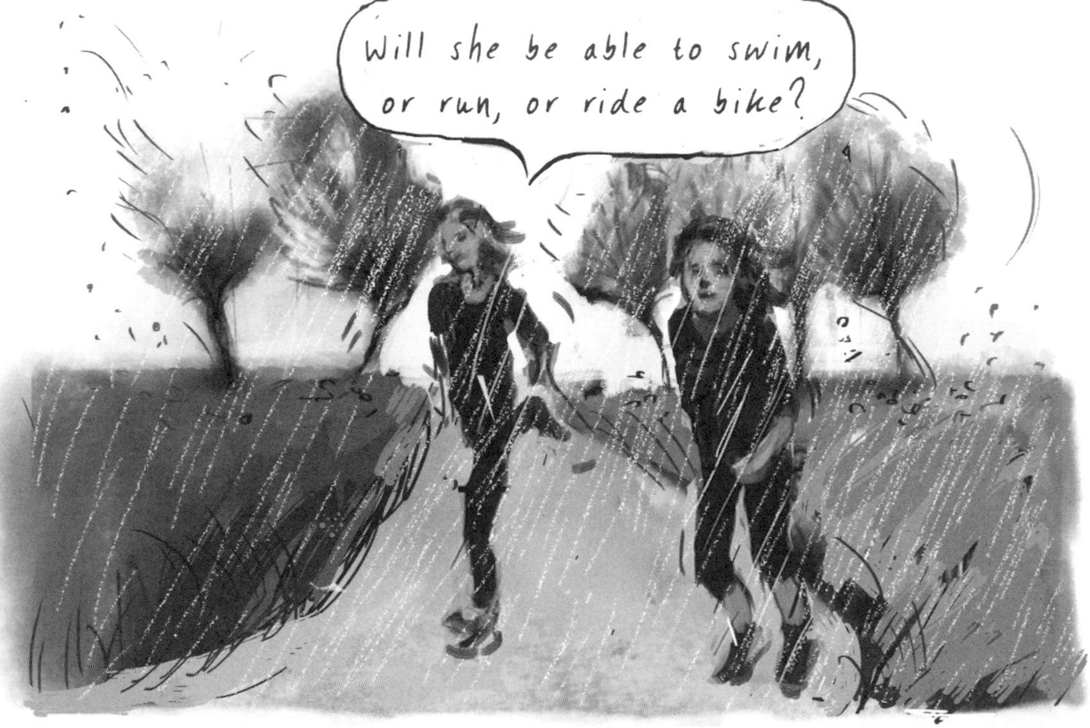
Will she be able to swim, or run, or ride a bike?

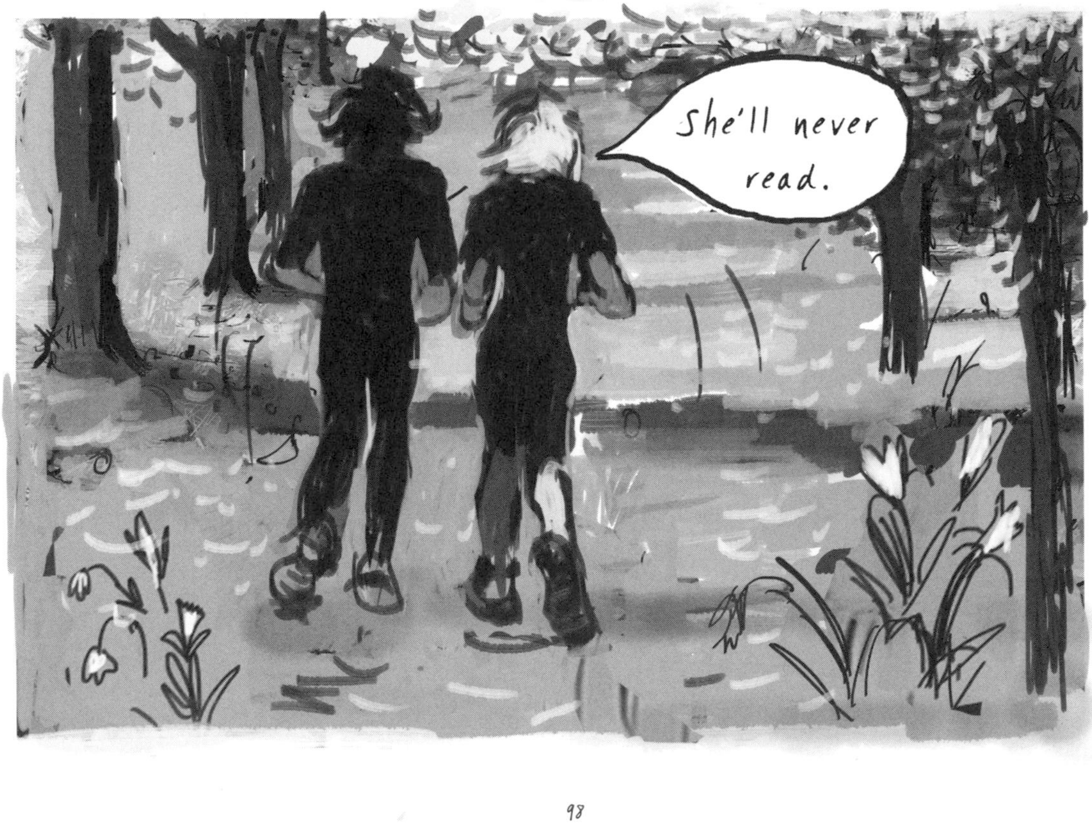
She'll never read.

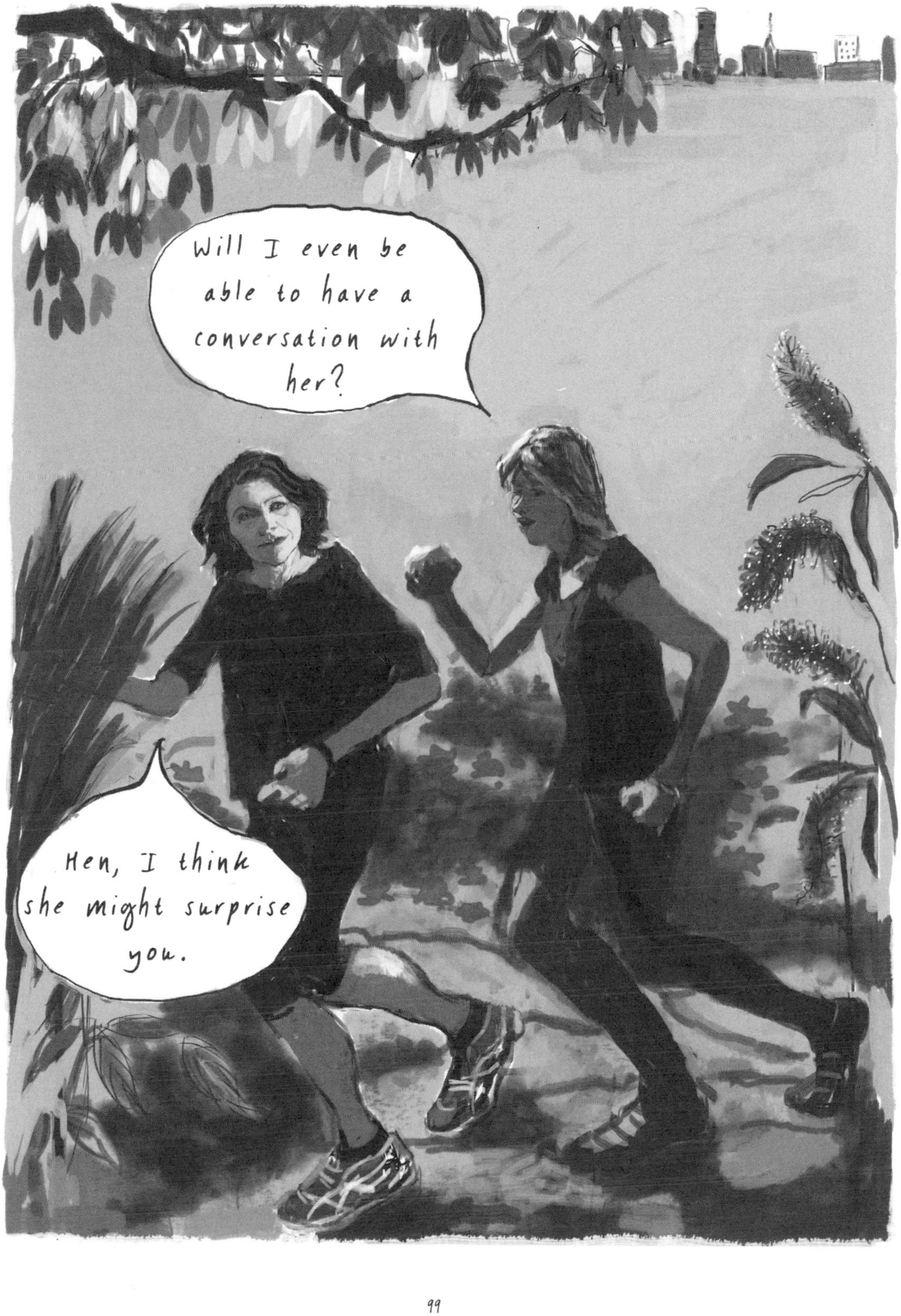
Will I even be able to have a conversation with her?
Hen, I think she might surprise you.

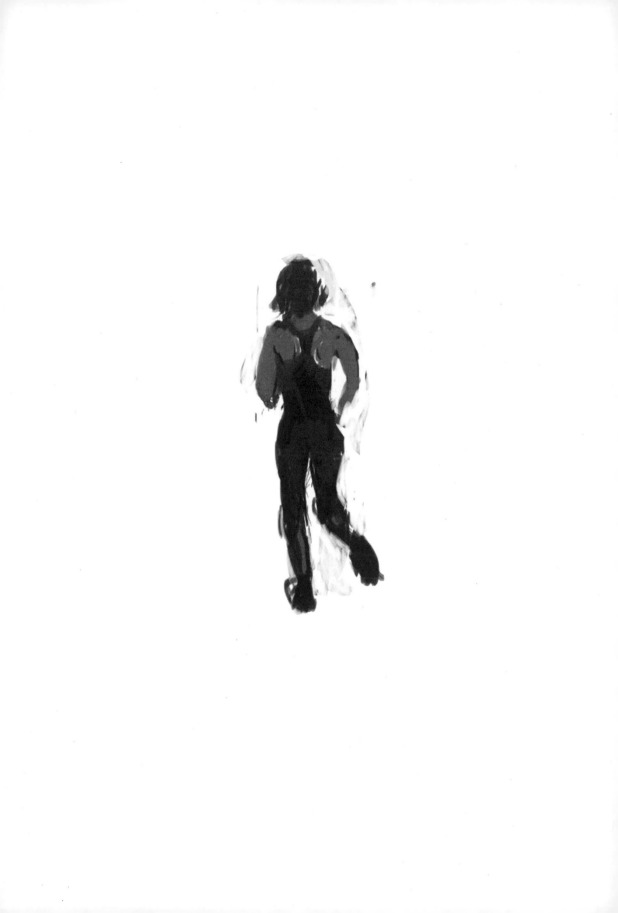

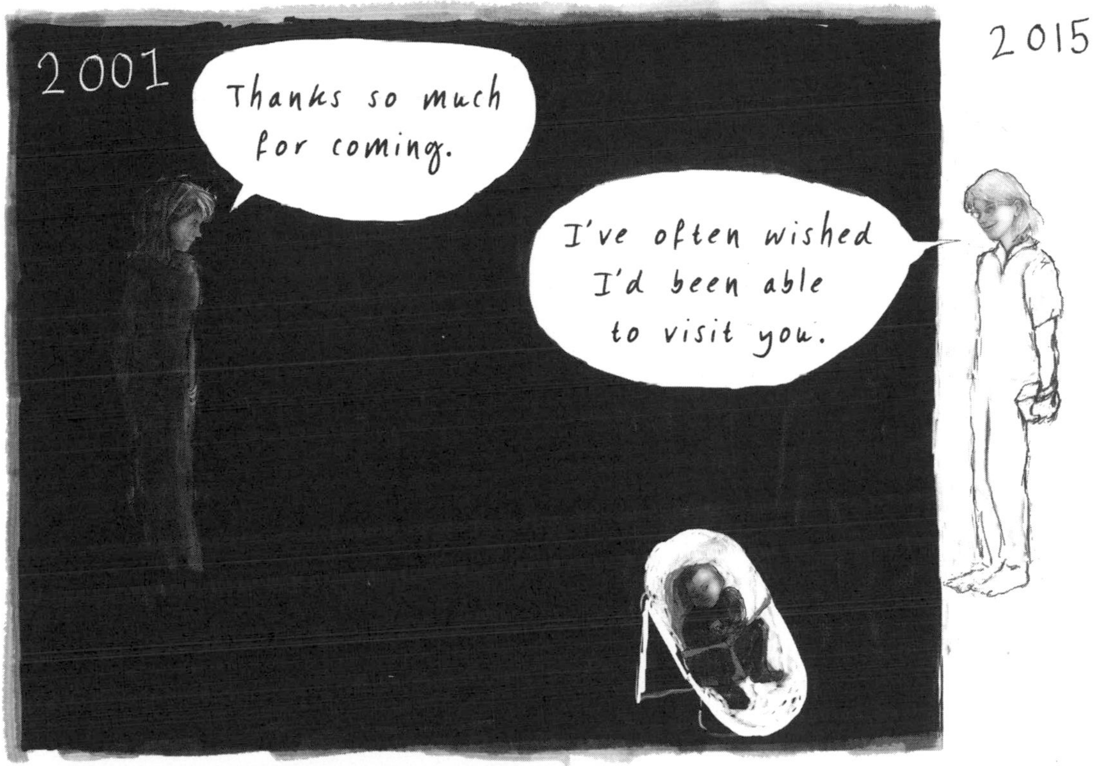
2001
2015
Thanks so much for coming.
I've often wished I'd been able to visit you.

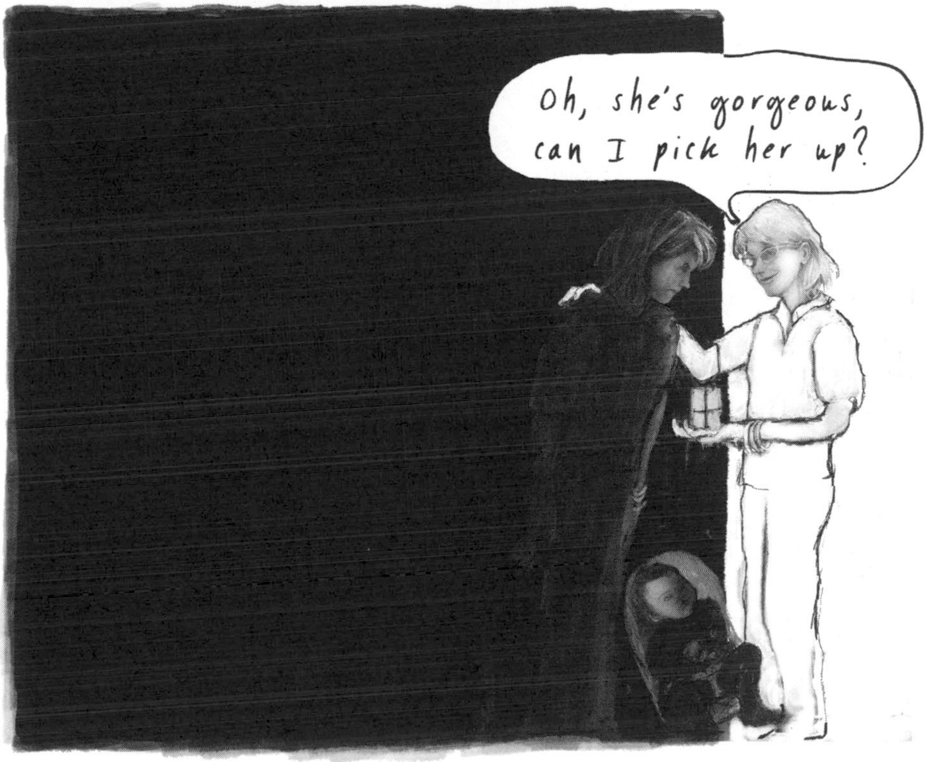
Oh, she's gorgeous, can I pick her up?

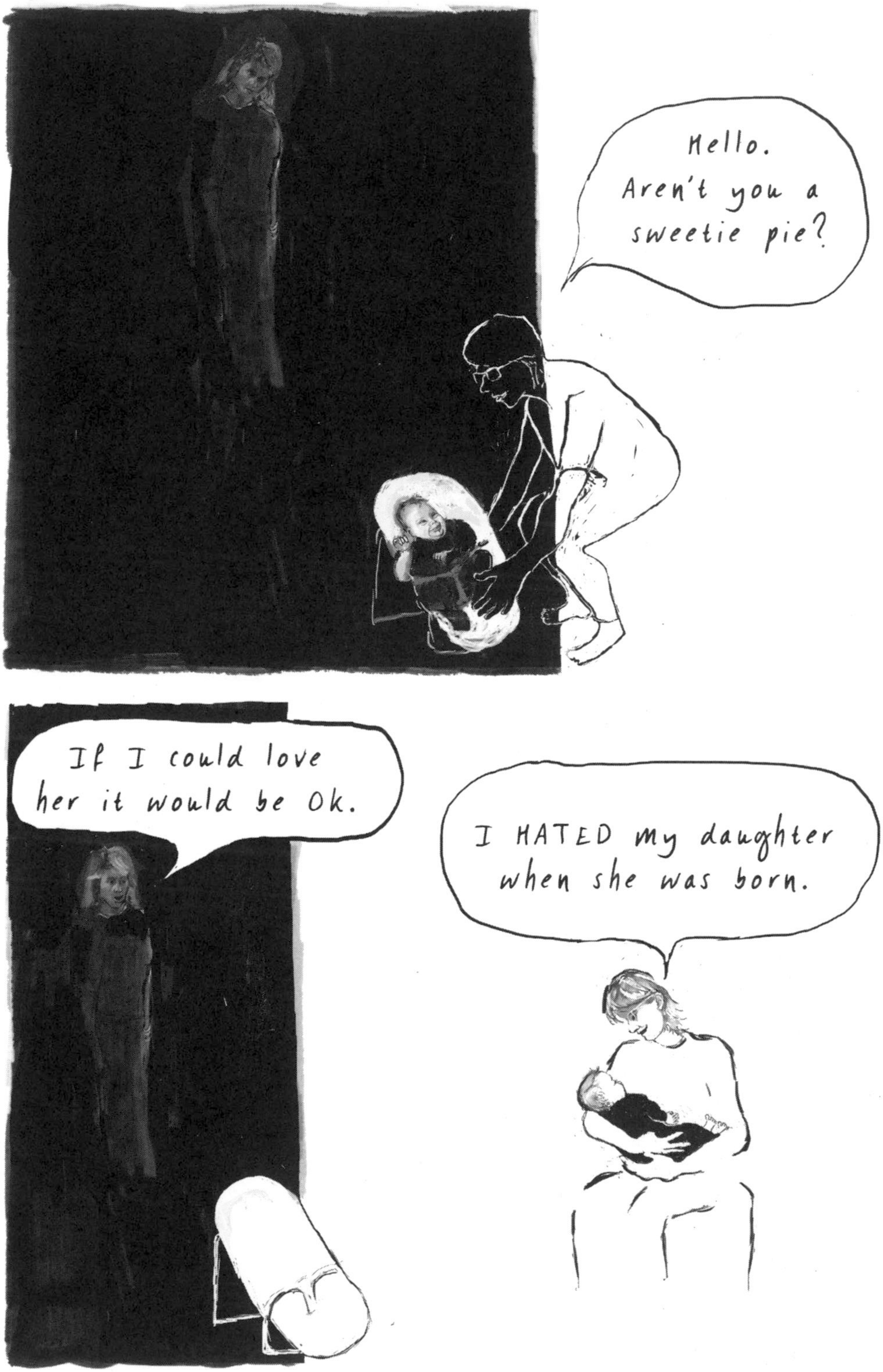
Hello.
Aren't you a sweetie pie?
If I could love her it would be Ok.
I HATED my daughter when she was born.

When she was tiny, I used to go into her bedroom and hope that she had died of cot death.

She's so vulnerable and needs me more, but I hate her for it. I can't stand the way she looks. I can't love her.

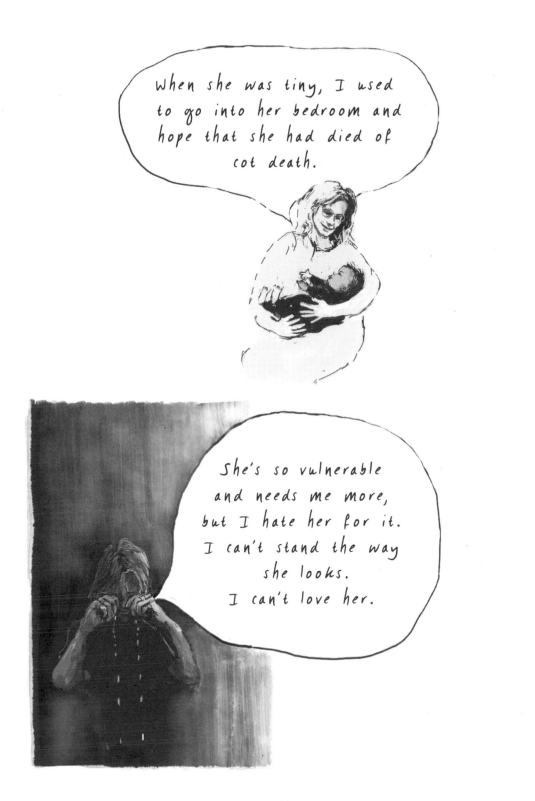

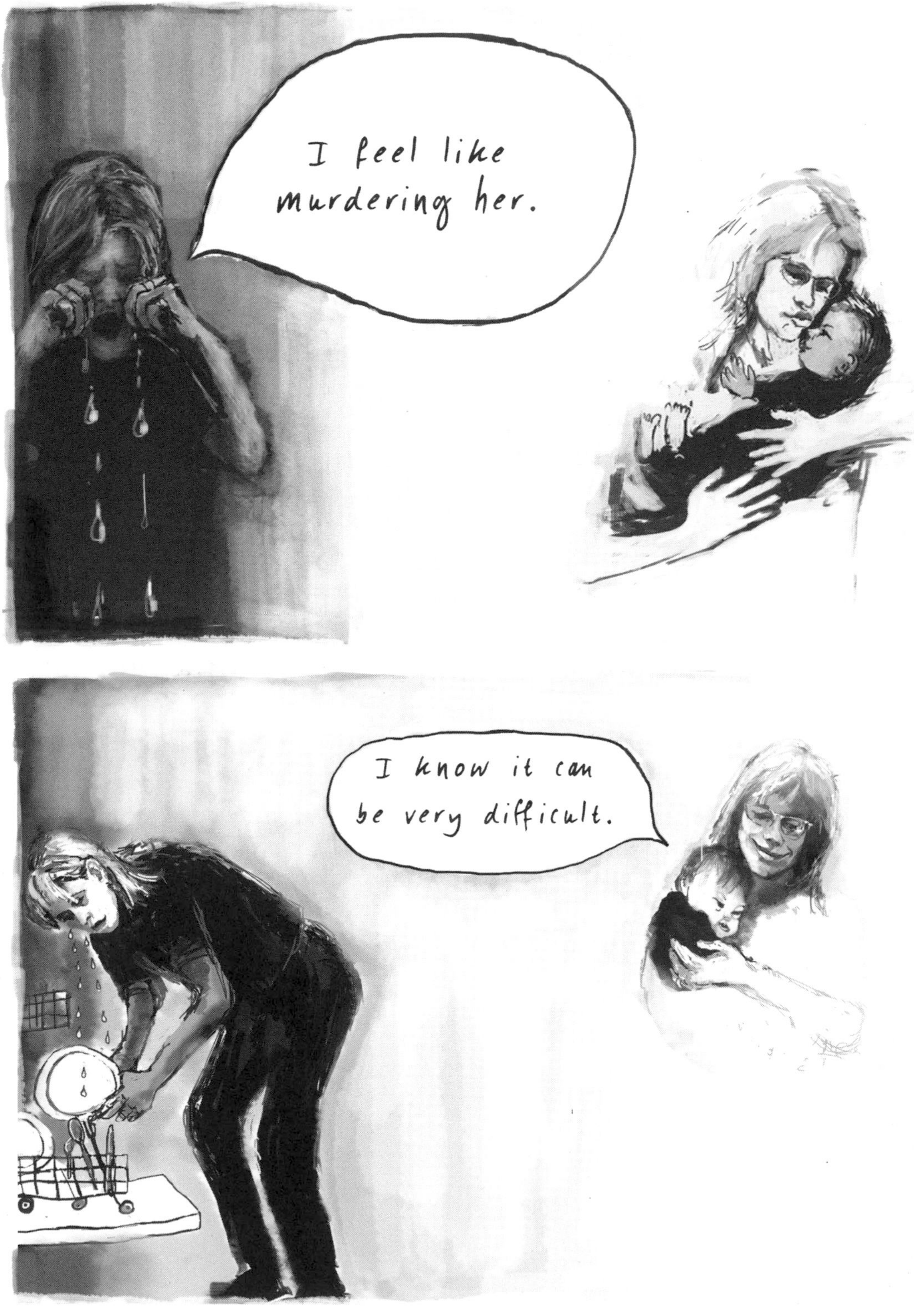
I feel like murdering her.
I know it can be very difficult.

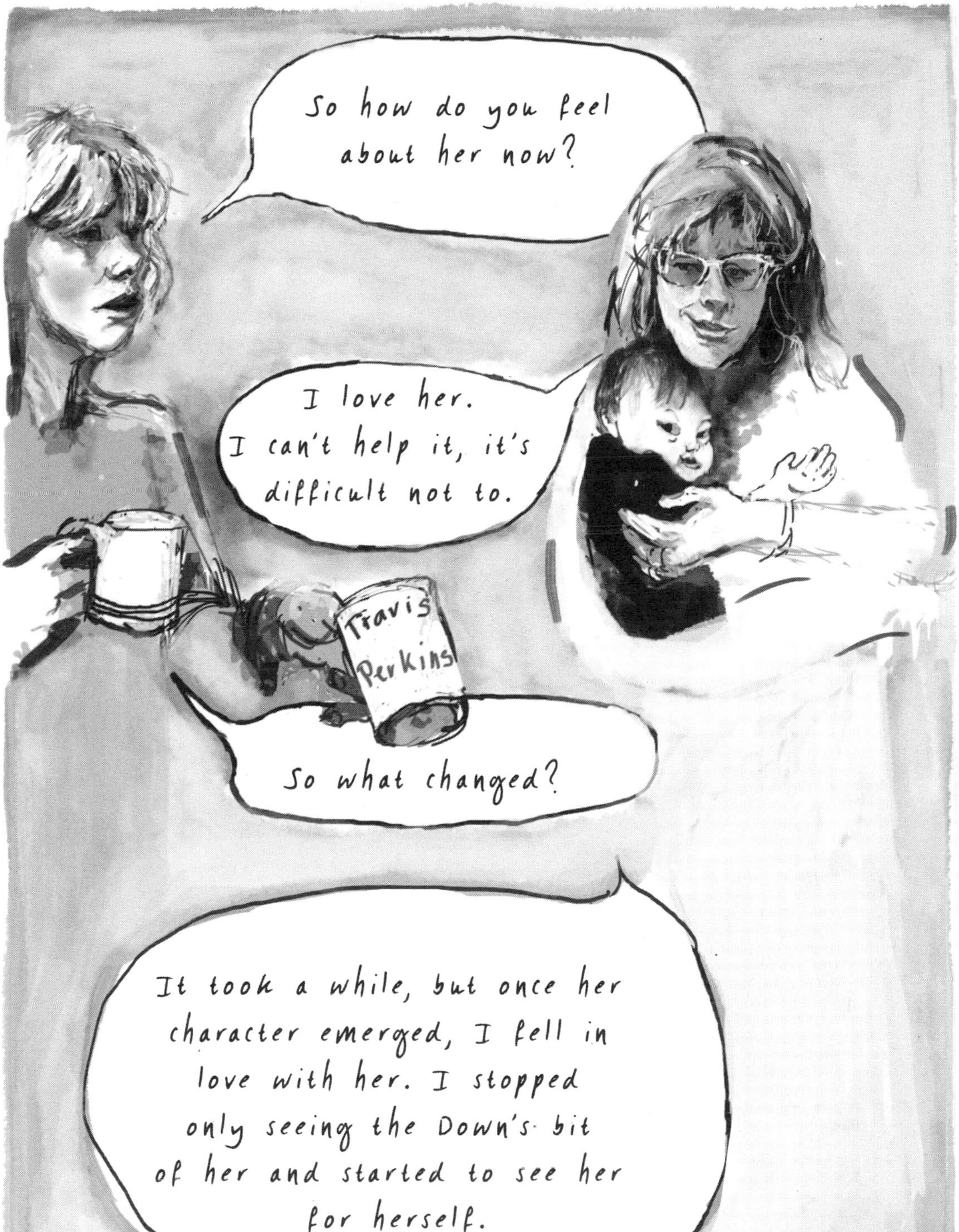
So how do you feel about her now?
I love her. I can't help it, it's difficult not to.
Travis Perkins
So what changed?
It took a while, but once her character emerged, I fell in love with her. I stopped only seeing the Down's bit of her and started to see her for herself.

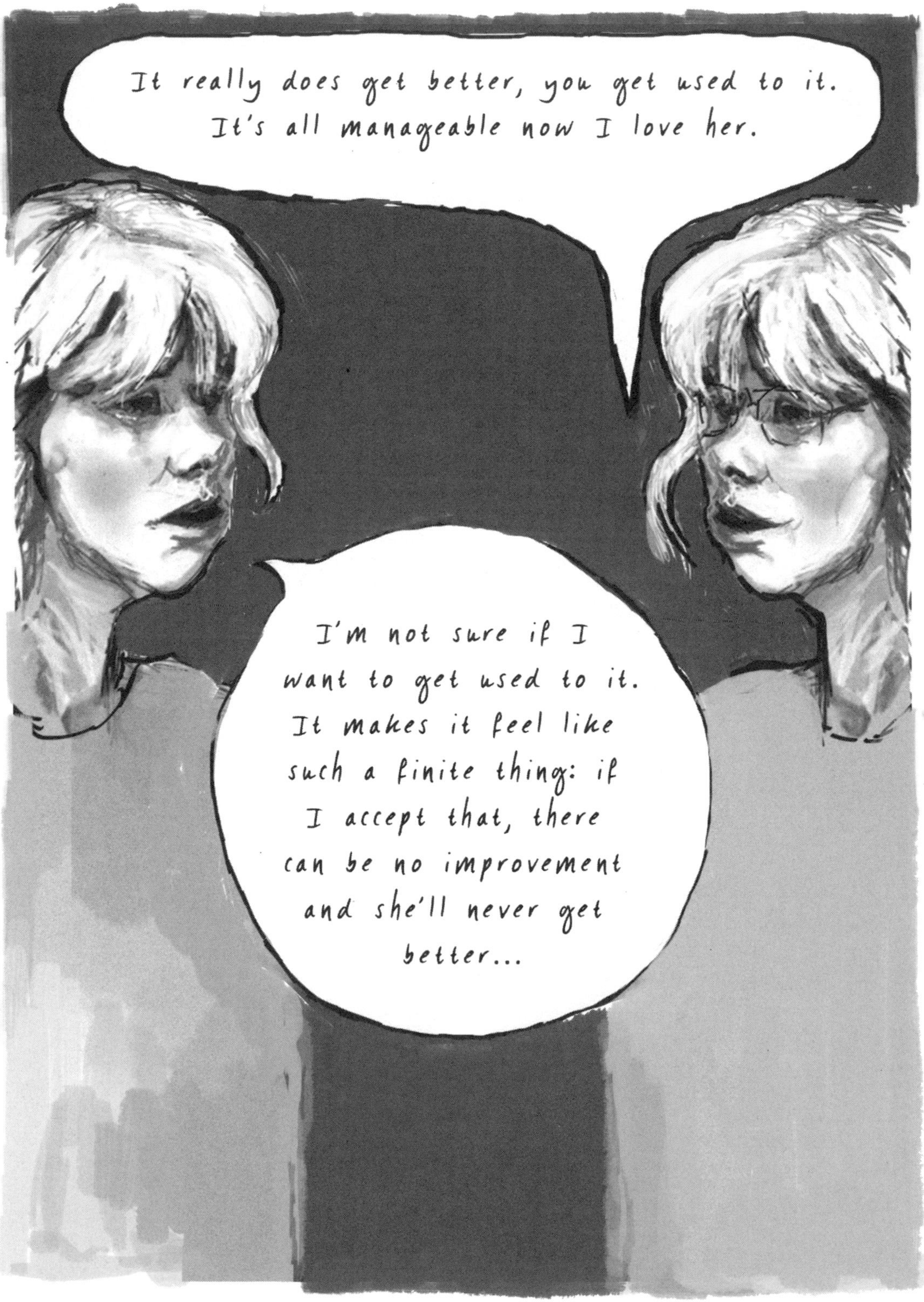
It really does get better, you get used to it. It's all manageable now I love her.
I'm not sure if I want to get used to it. It makes it feel like such a finite thing: if I accept that, there can be no improvement and she'll never get better...

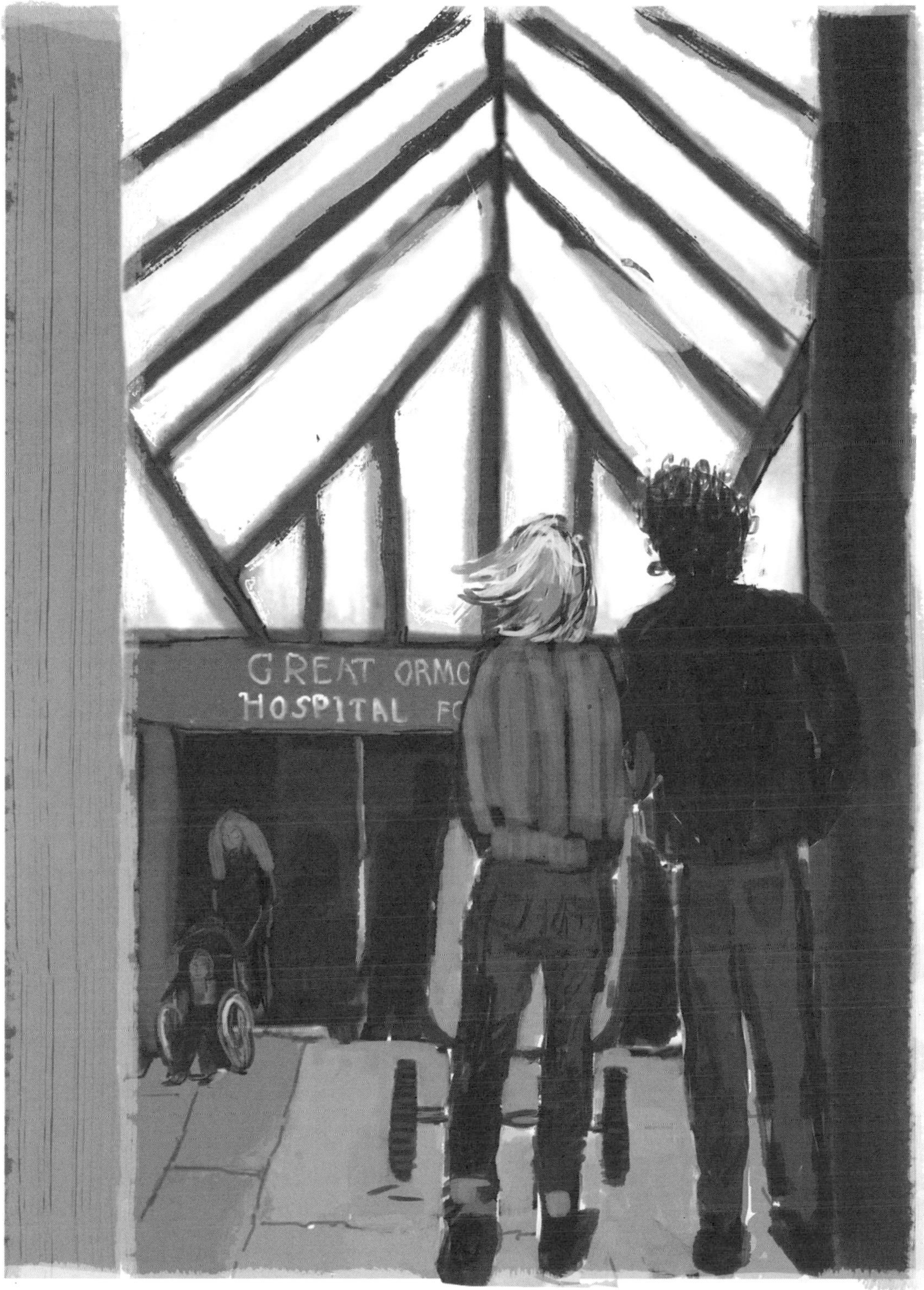
GREAT ORMO
HOSPITAL FO

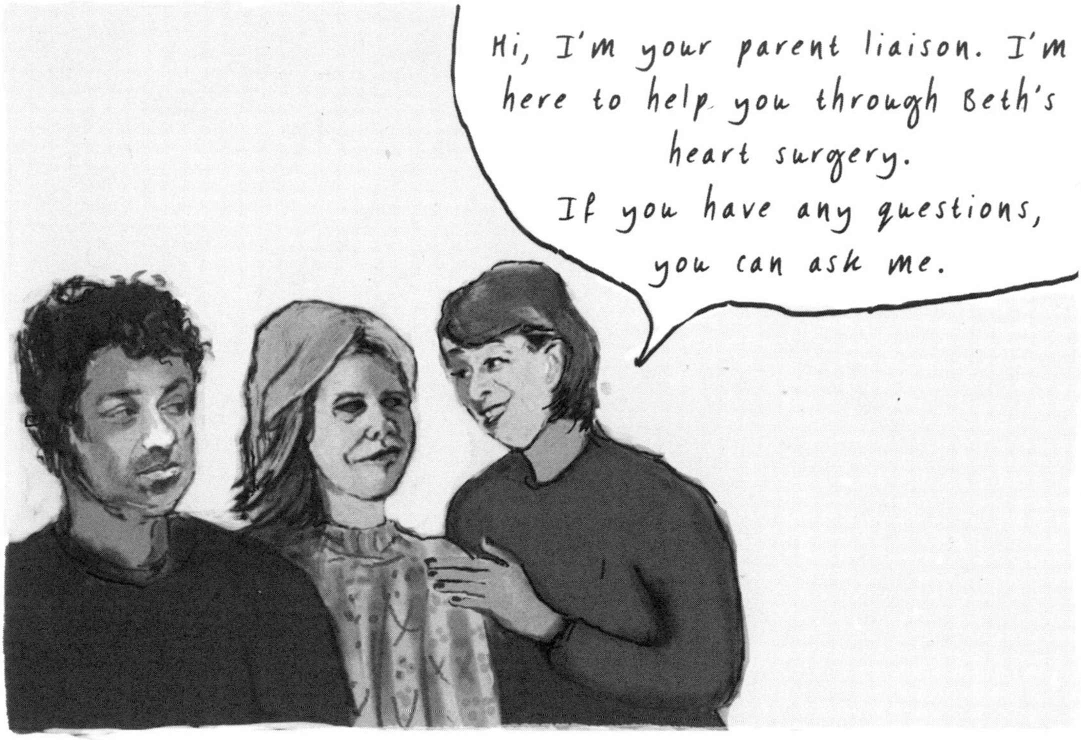
Hi, I'm your parent liaison. I'm here to help you through Beth's heart surgery. If you have any questions, you can ask me.

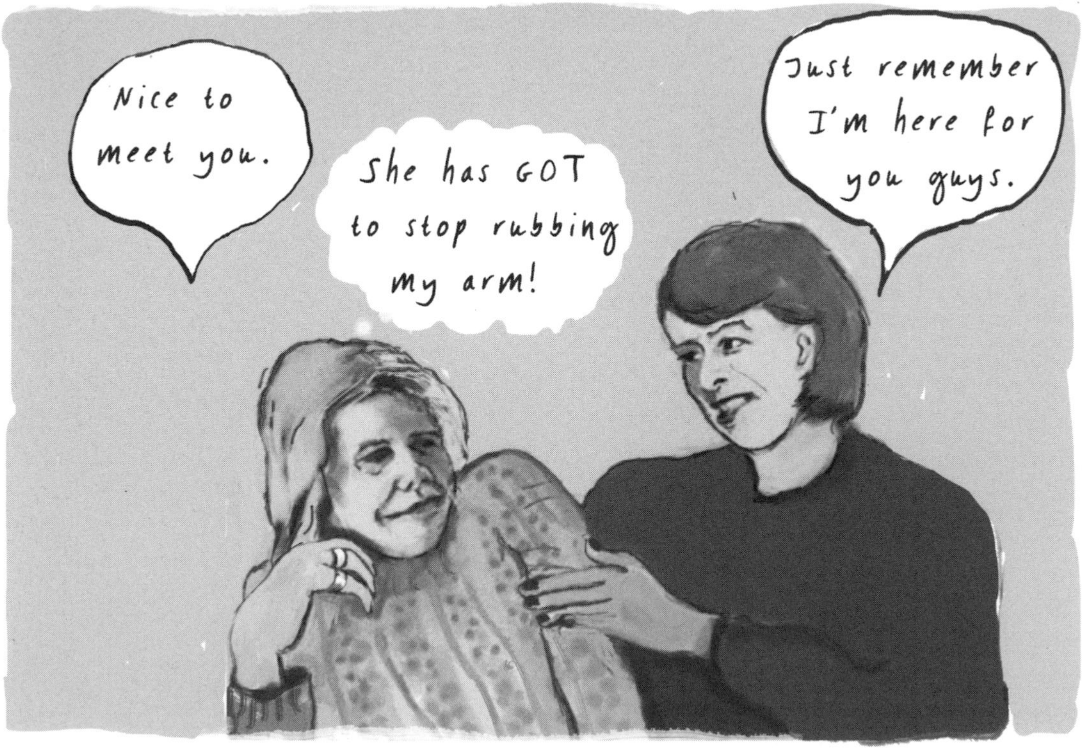
Nice to meet you.
She has GOT to stop rubbing my arm!
Just remember I'm here for you guys.

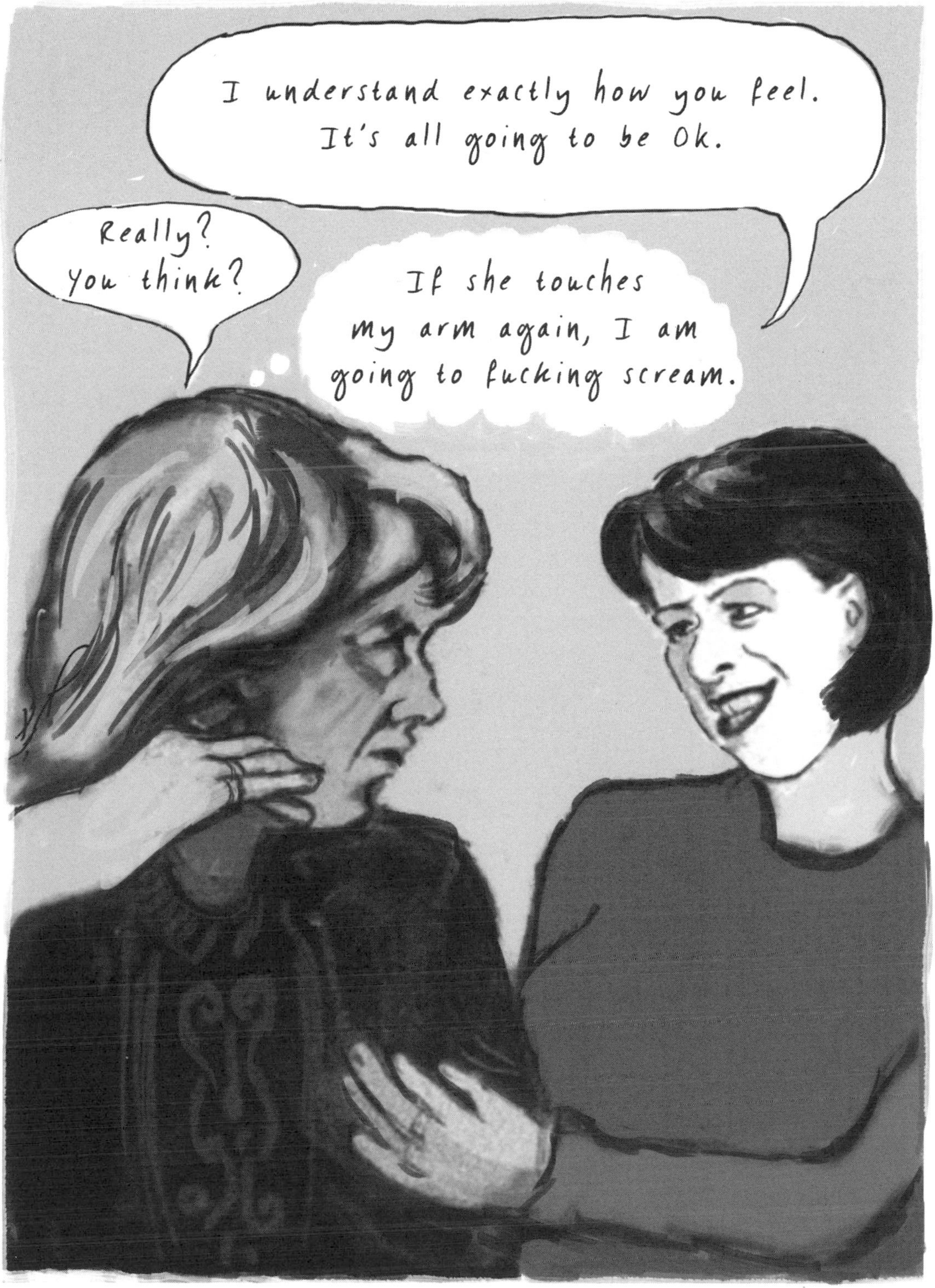
I understand exactly how you feel. It's all going to be Ok.
Really? you think?
If she touches my arm again, I am going to fucking scream.

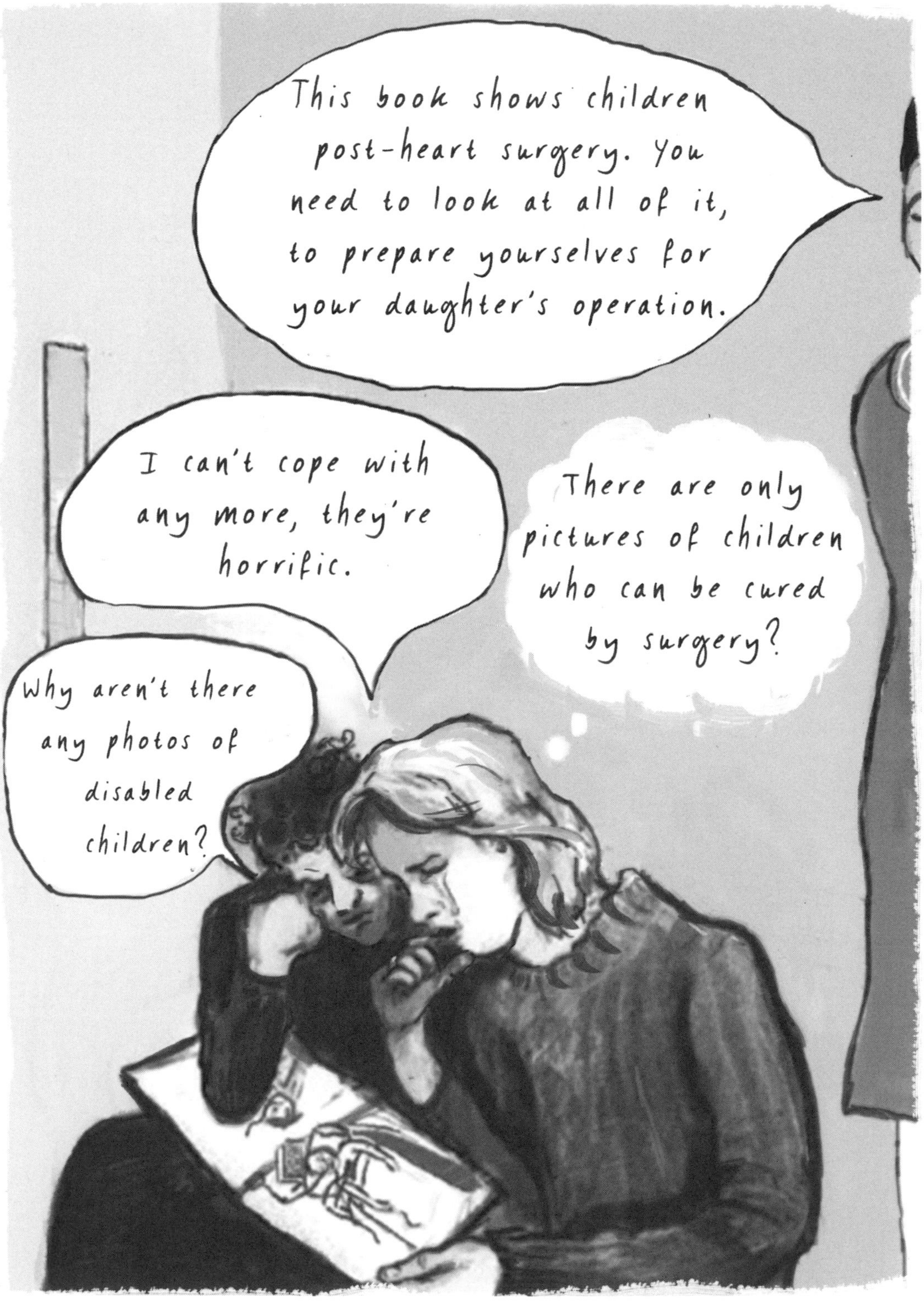
This book shows children post-heart surgery. You need to look at all of it, to prepare yourselves for your daughter's operation.
I can't cope with any more, they're horrific.
There are only pictures of children who can be cured by surgery?
Why aren't there any photos of disabled children?

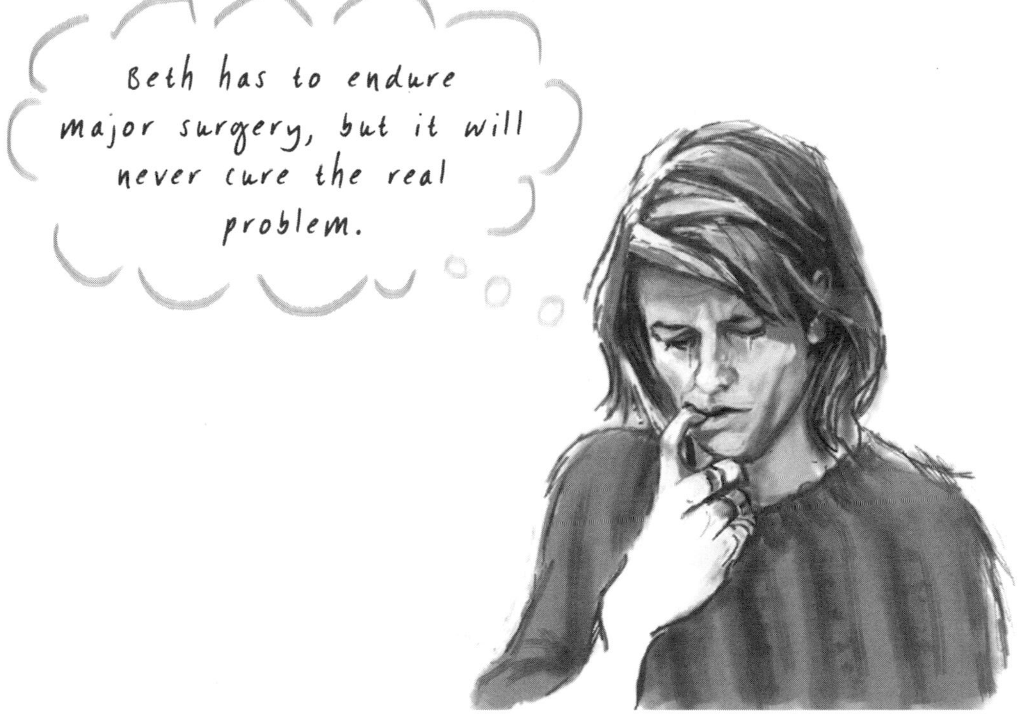
Beth has to endure major surgery, but it will never cure the real problem.

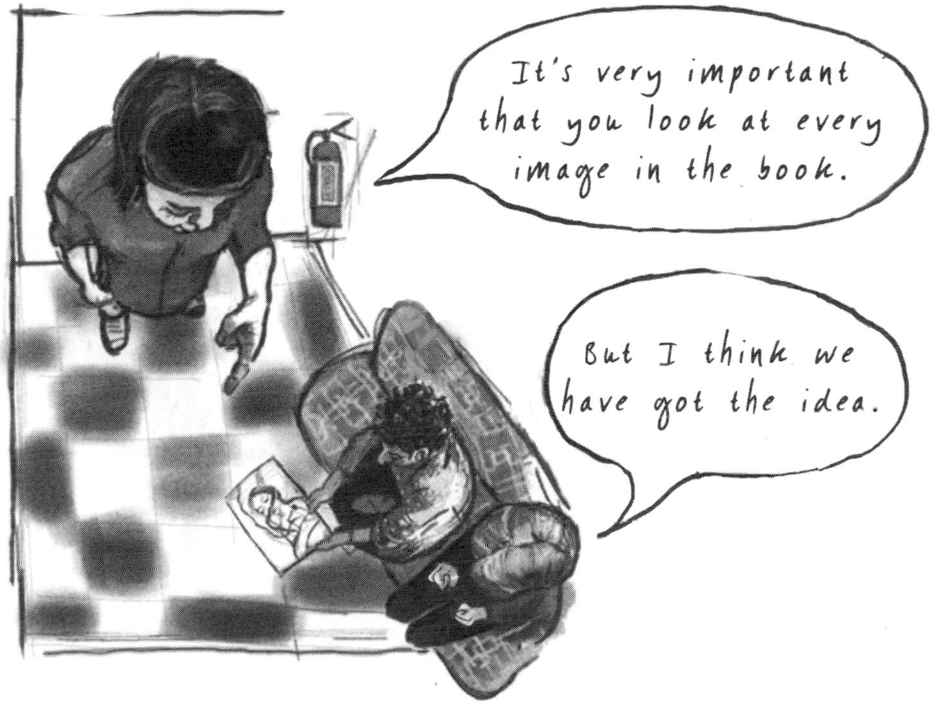
It's very important that you look at every image in the book.
But I think we have got the idea.

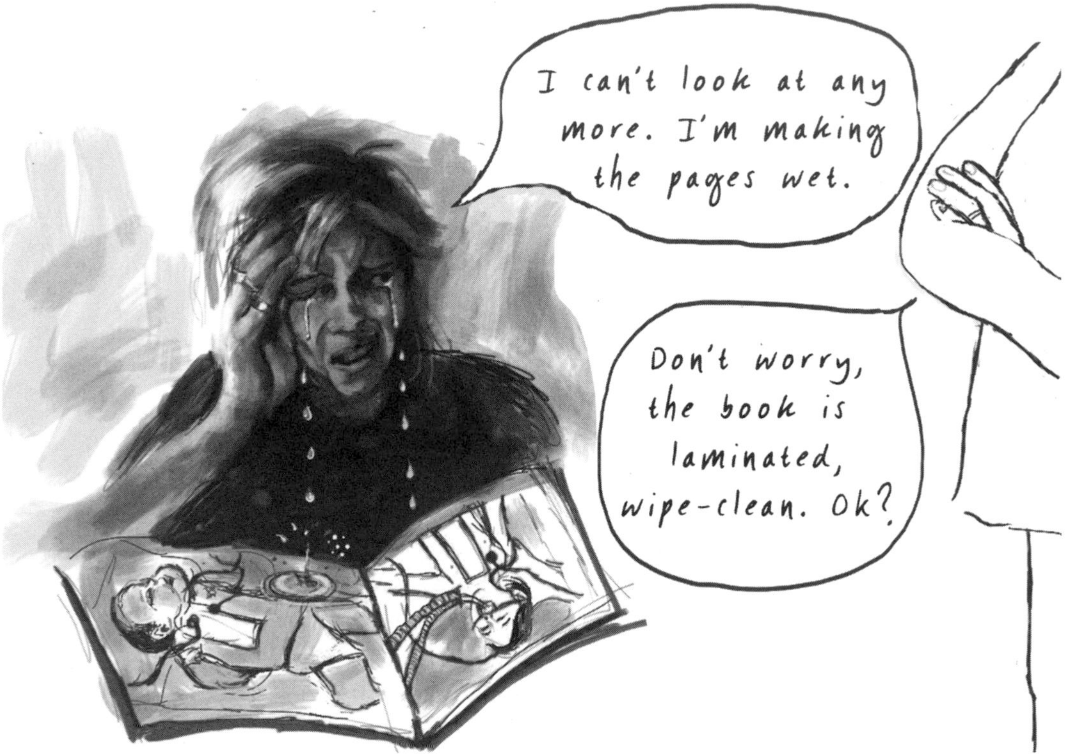
I can't look at any more. I'm making the pages wet.
Don't worry, the book is laminated, wipe-clean. Ok?

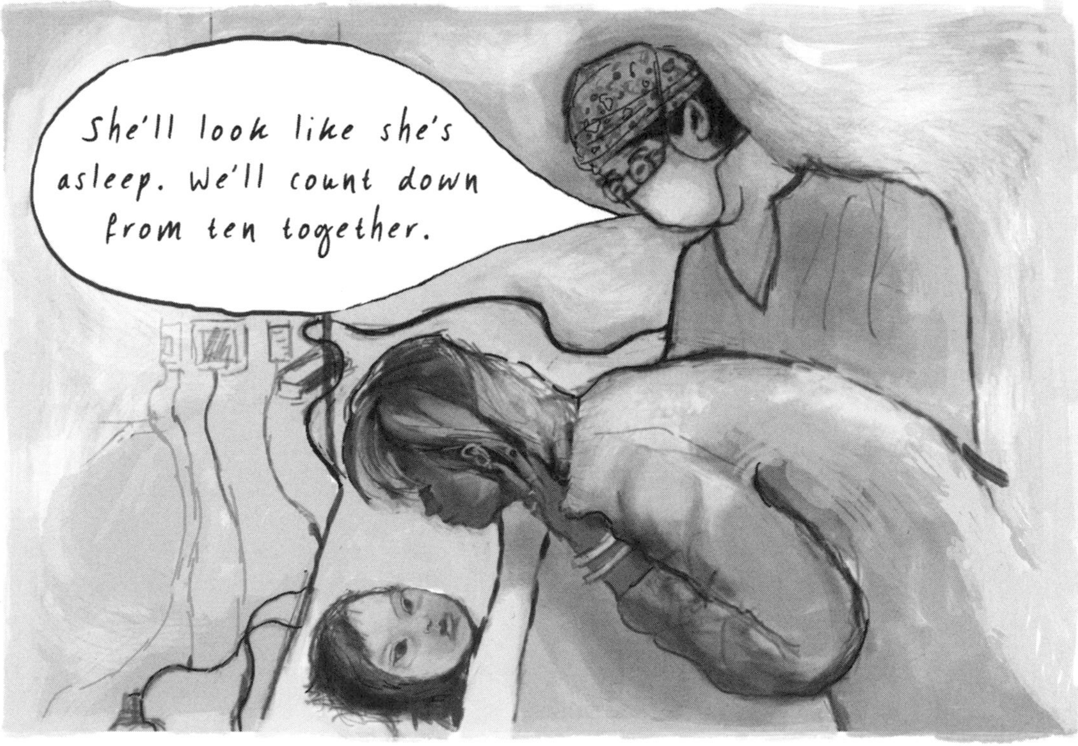
She'll look like she's asleep. We'll count down from ten together.

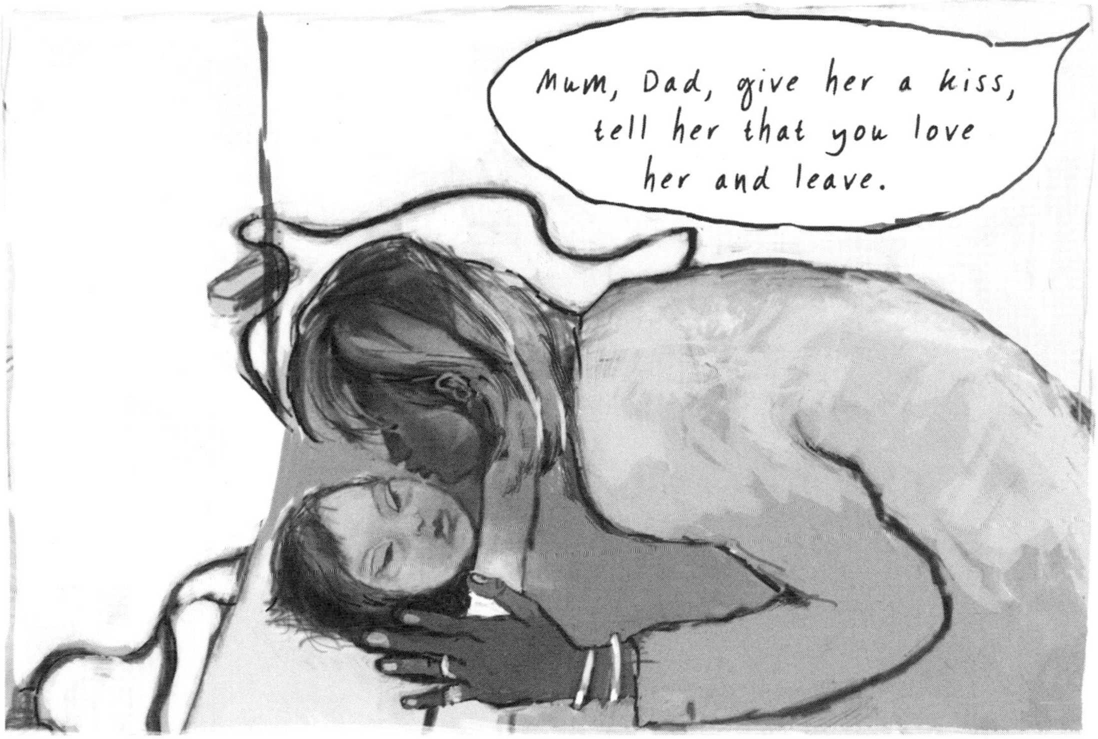
Mum, Dad, give her a kiss, tell her that you love her and leave.

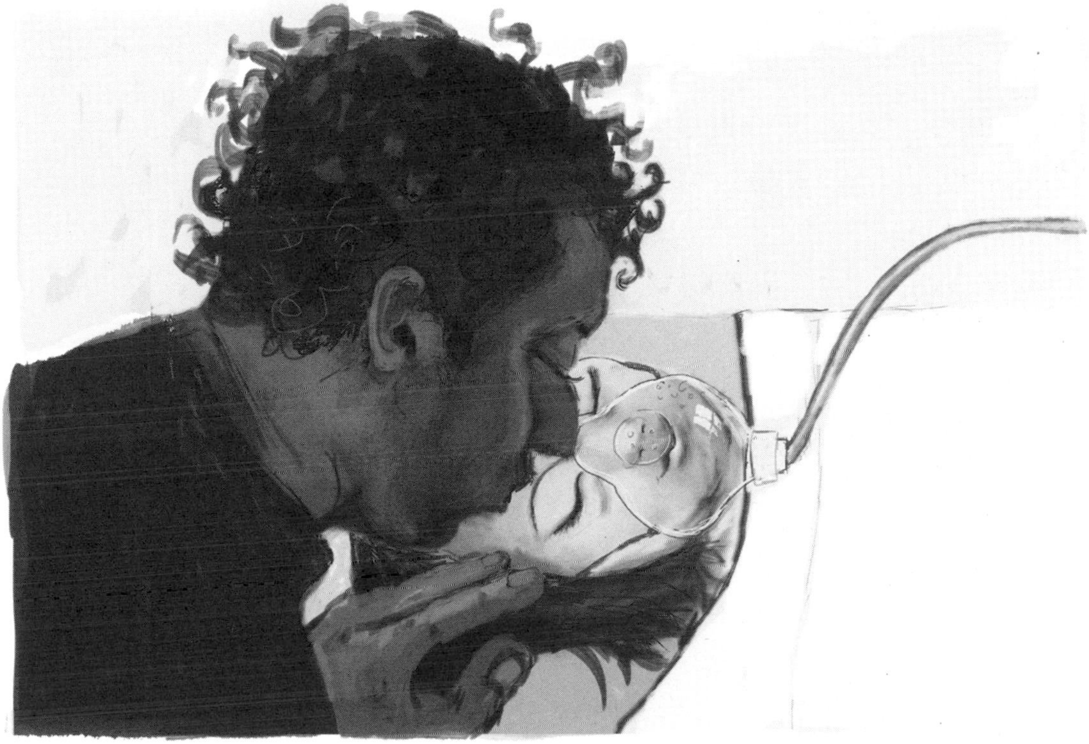

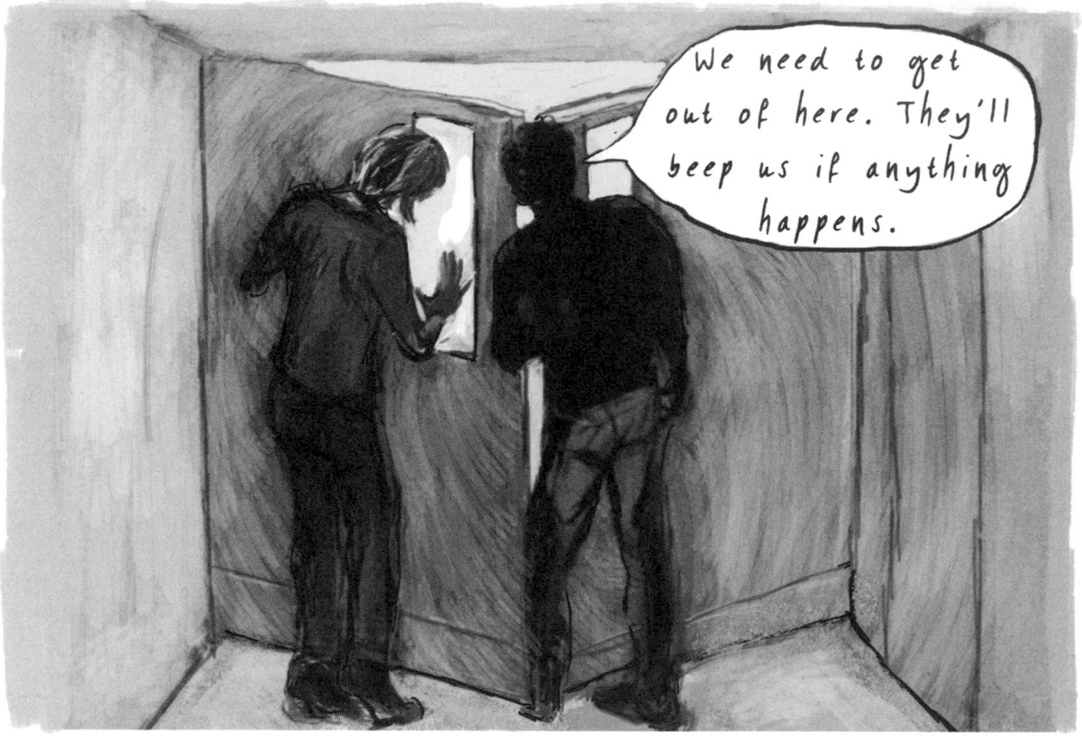
We need to get out of here. They'll beep us if anything happens.

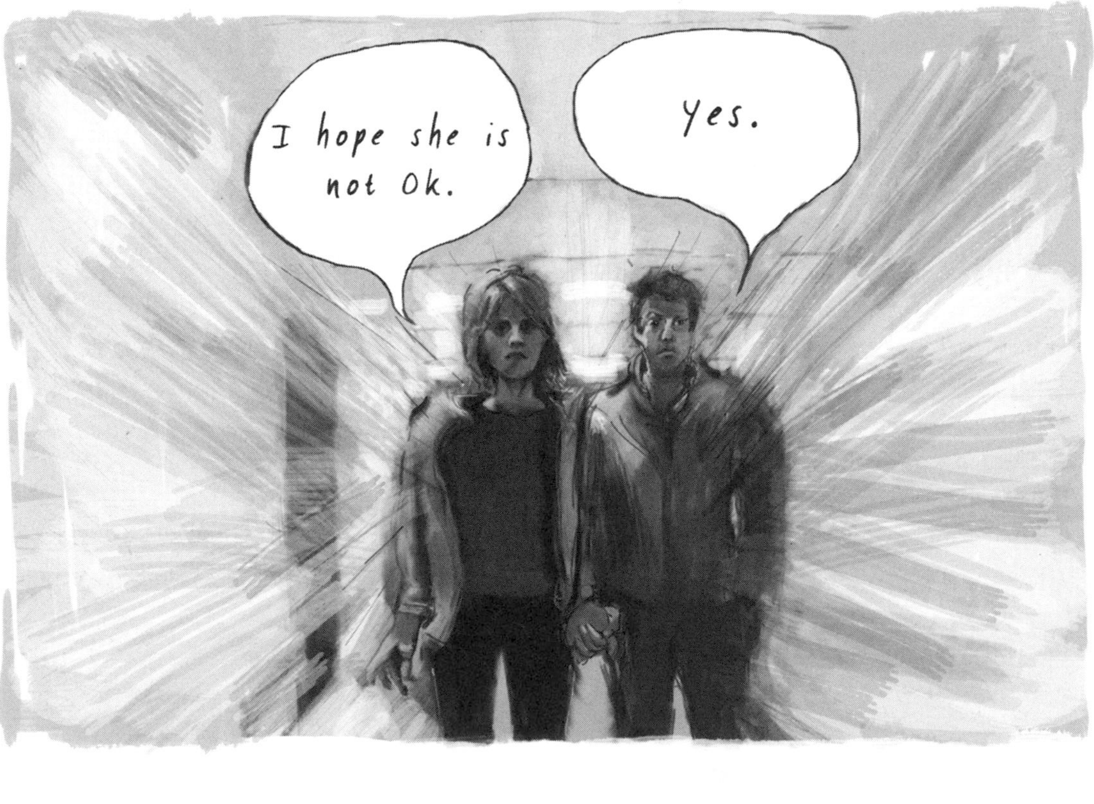
I hope she is not Ok.
Yes.

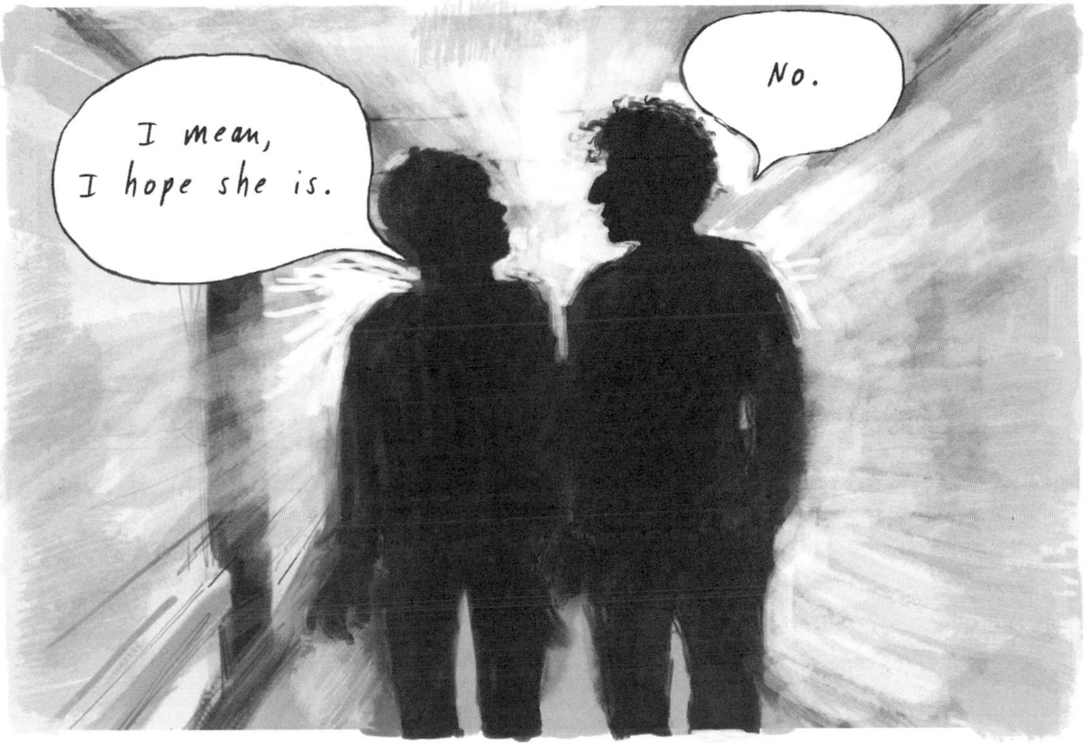
I mean, I hope she is.
No.

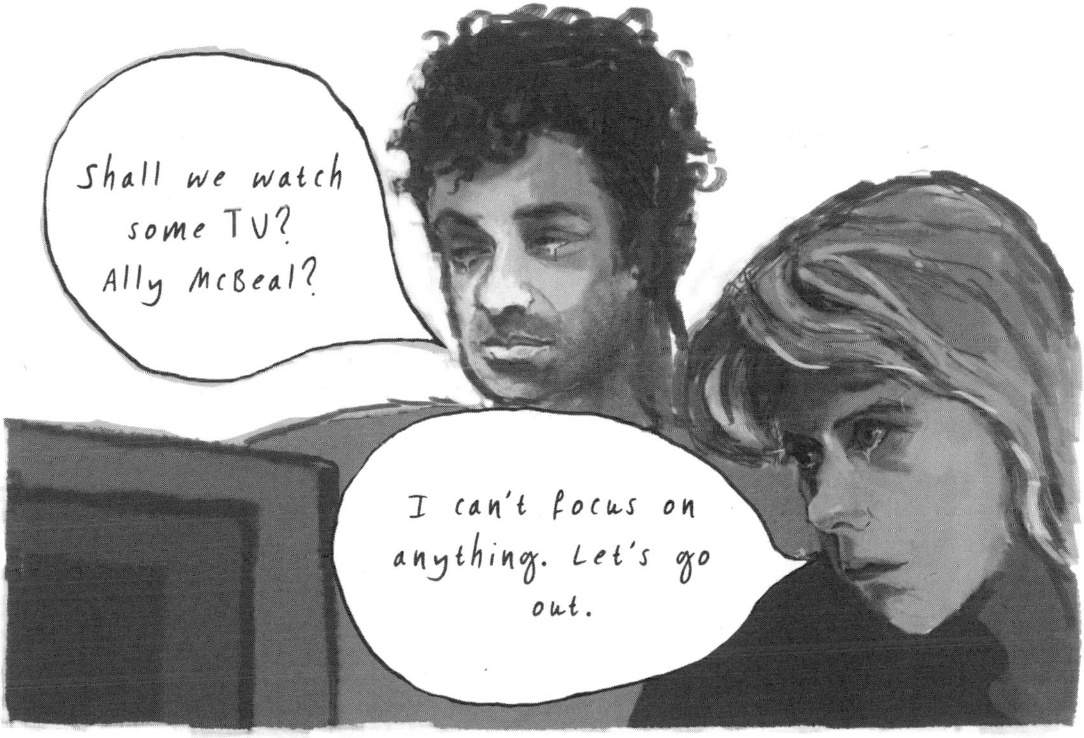
Shall we watch some TV? Ally McBeal?
I can't focus on anything. Let's go out.

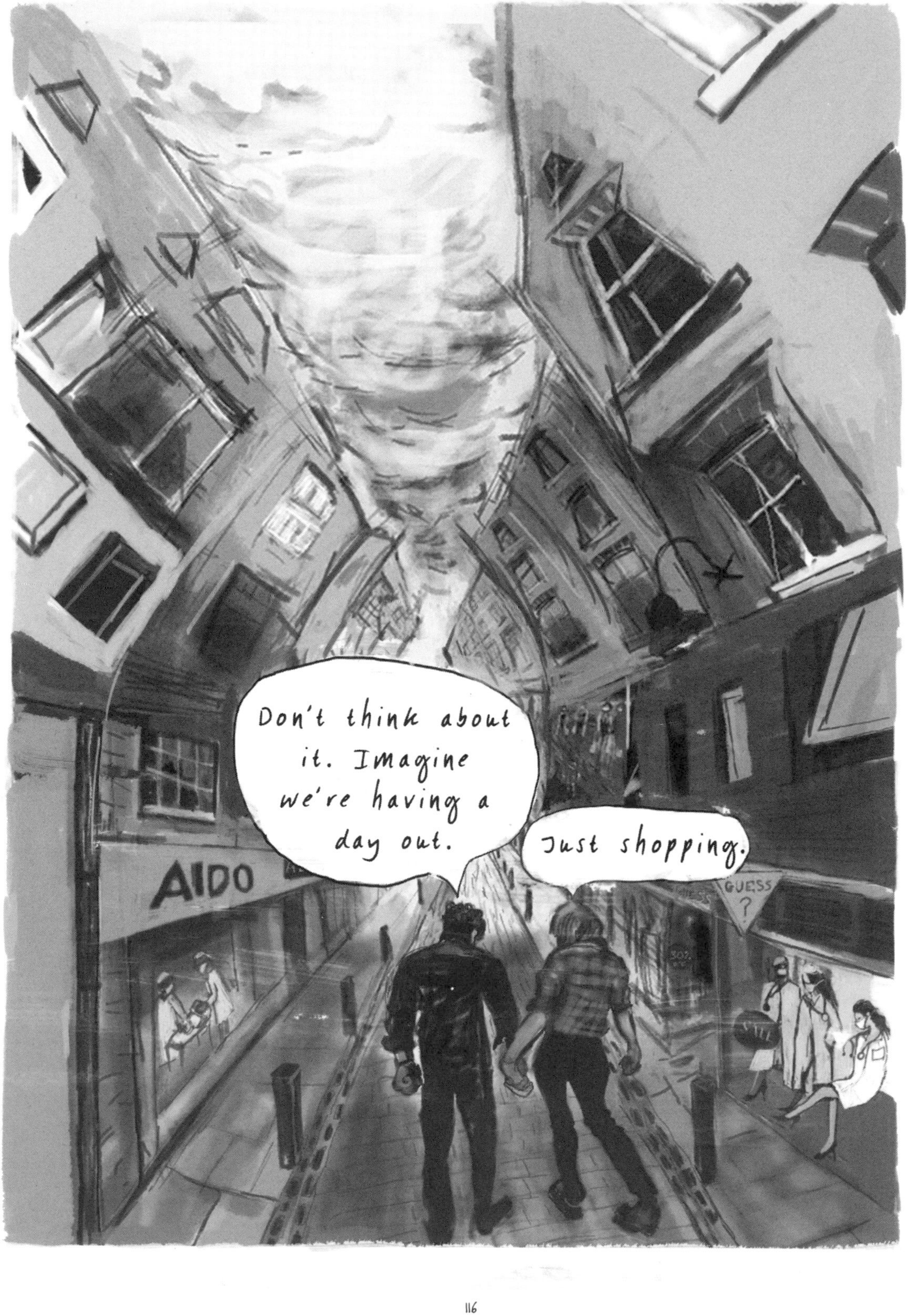
Don't think about it. Imagine we're having a day out.
Just shopping.
AIDO
GUESS ?

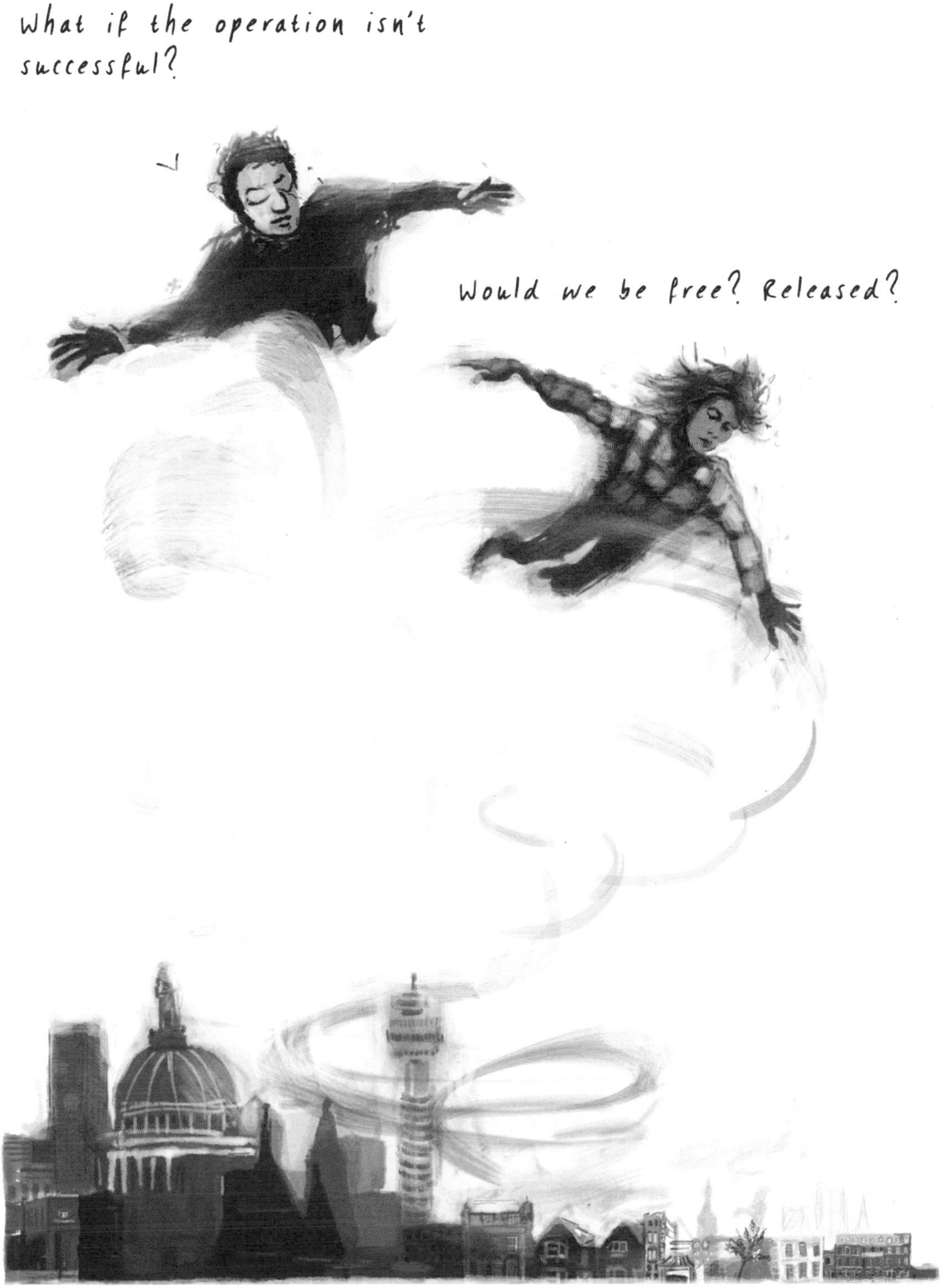
What if the operation isn't successful?
Would we be free? Released?

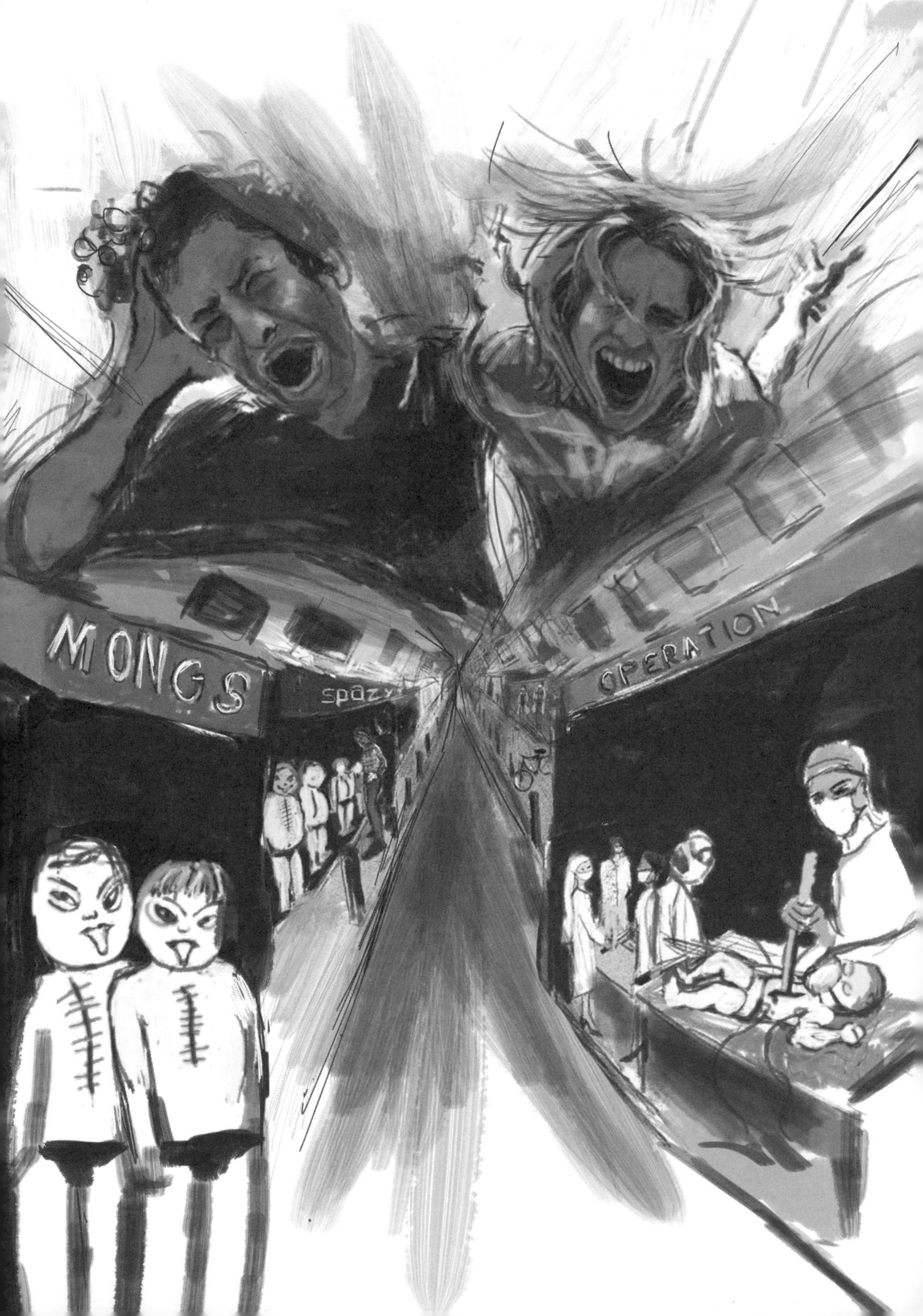
MONGS
spazy
OPERATION

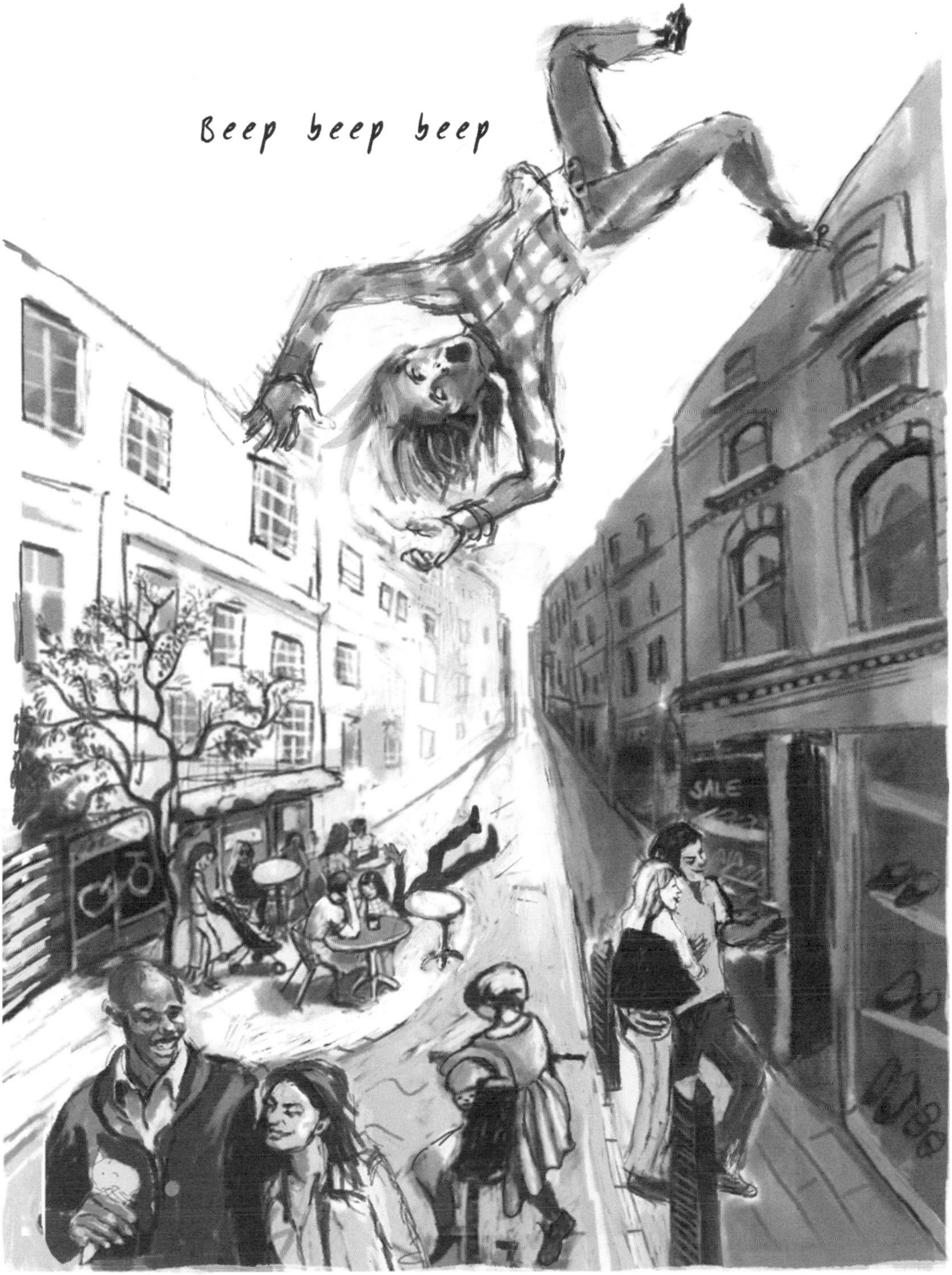
Beep beep beep
SALE

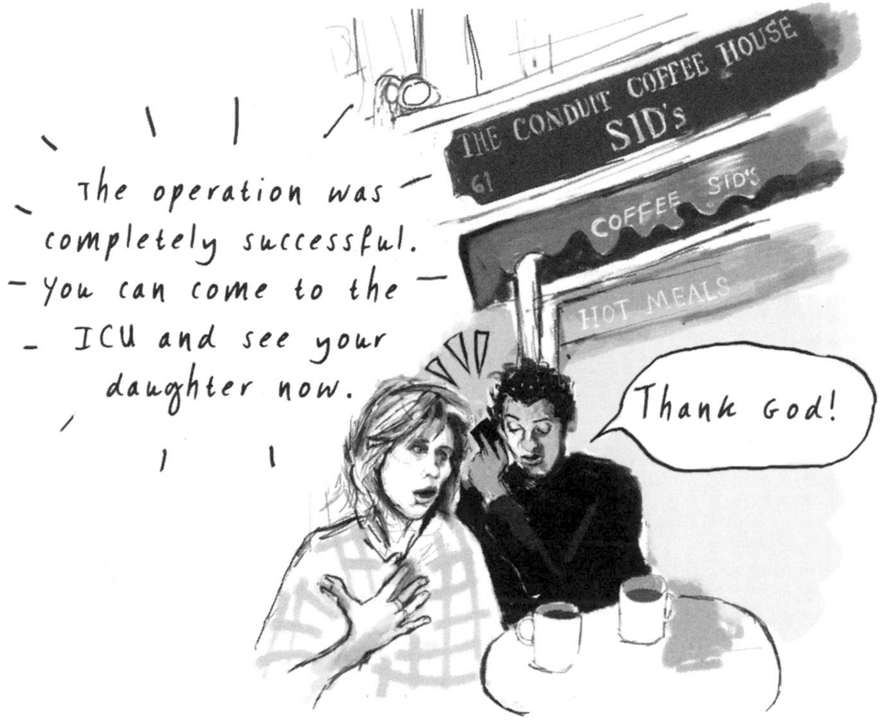
THE CONDUIT COFFEE HOUSE
SID's
61
COFFEE SID'S
HOT MEALS
The operation was completely successful. You can come to the ICU and see your daughter now.
Thank God!

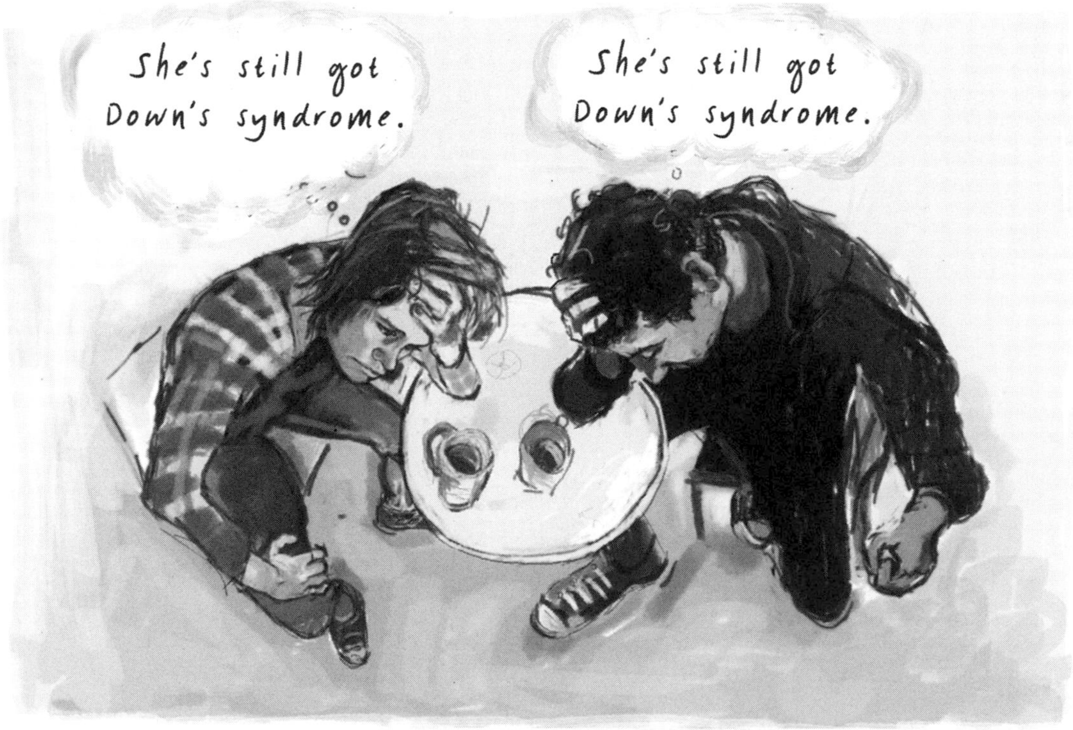
She's still got Down's syndrome.
She's still got Down's syndrome.

Part Three

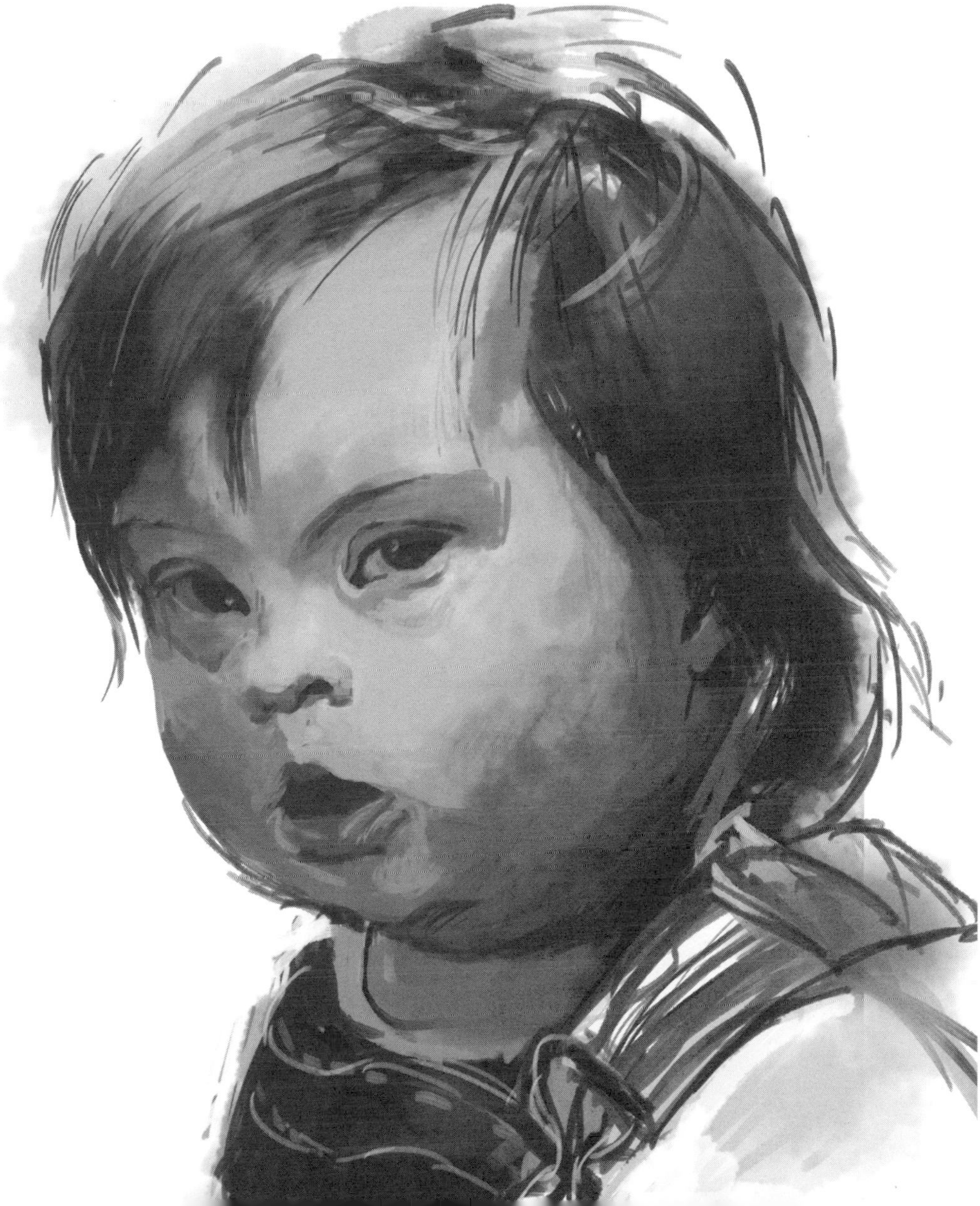

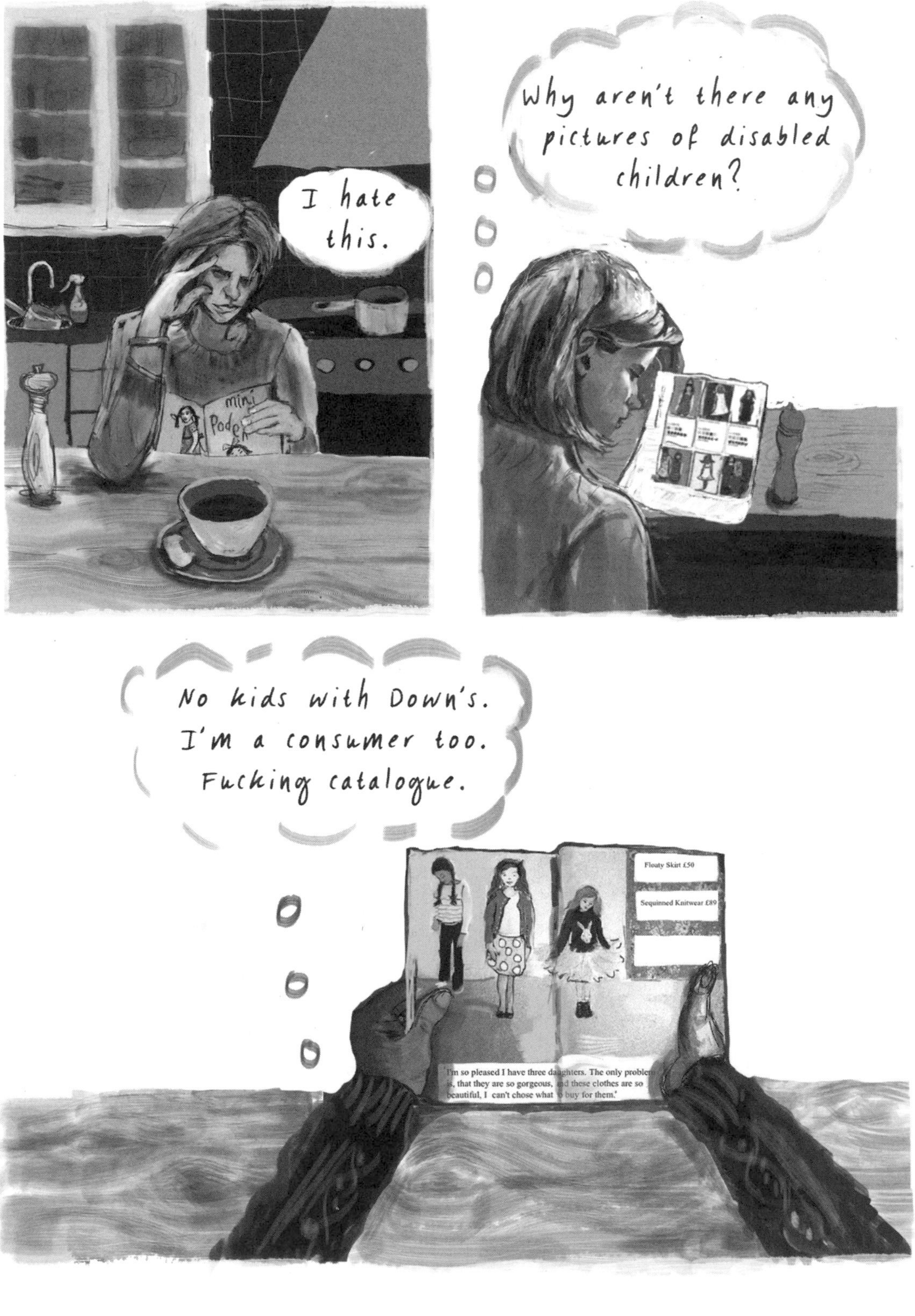
I hate this.
Why aren't there any pictures of disabled children?
No kids with Down's. I'm a consumer too. Fucking catalogue.
Floaty Skirt £50
Sequinned Knitwear £89
'I'm so pleased I have three daughters. The only proble
is, that they are so gorgeous, and these clothes are so
beautiful, I can't chose what to buy for them.'

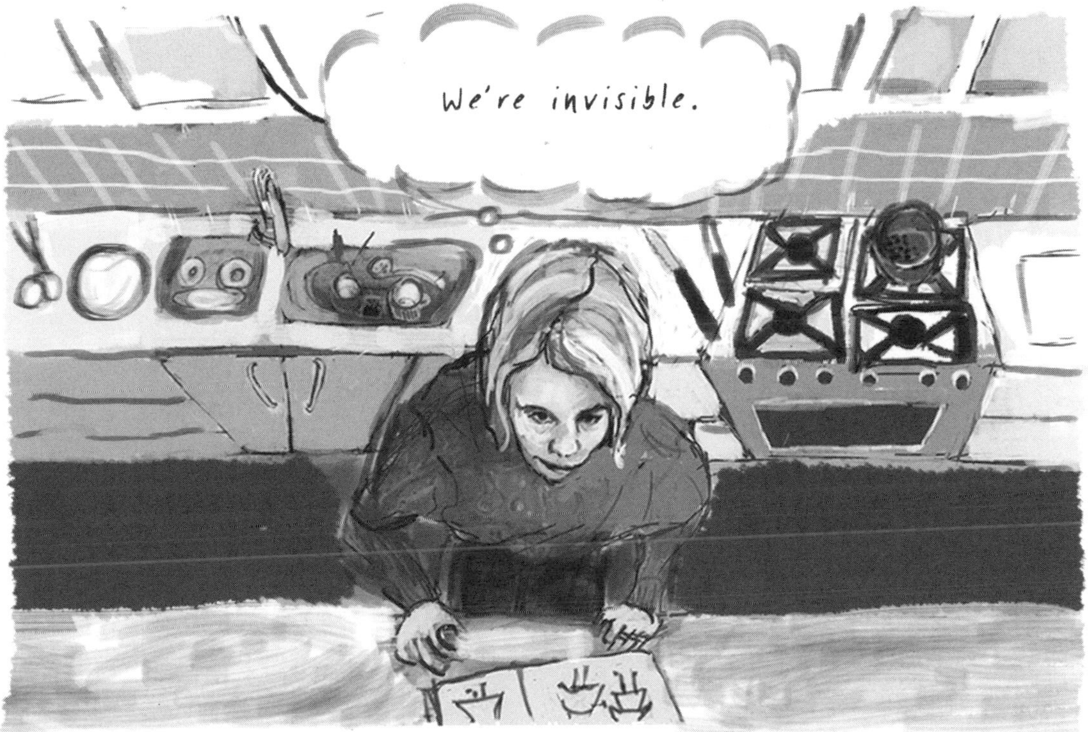
We're invisible.

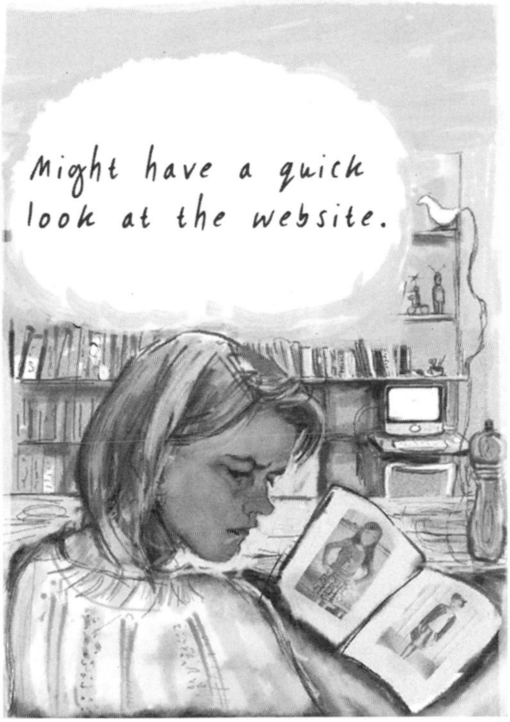
Might have a quick look at the website.

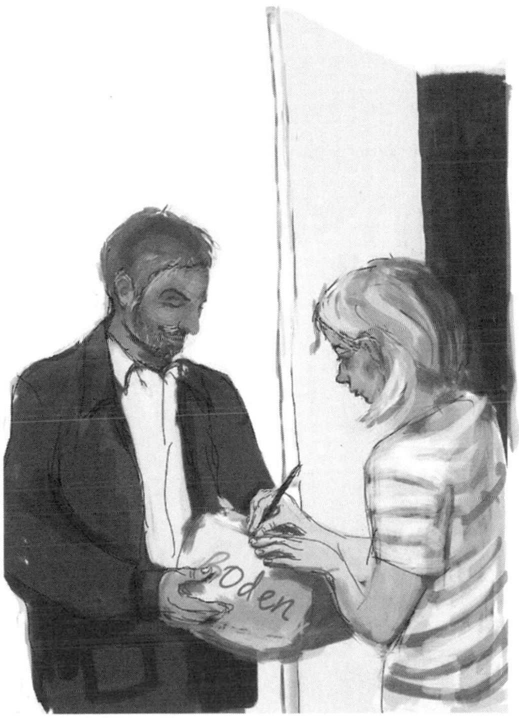
Boden

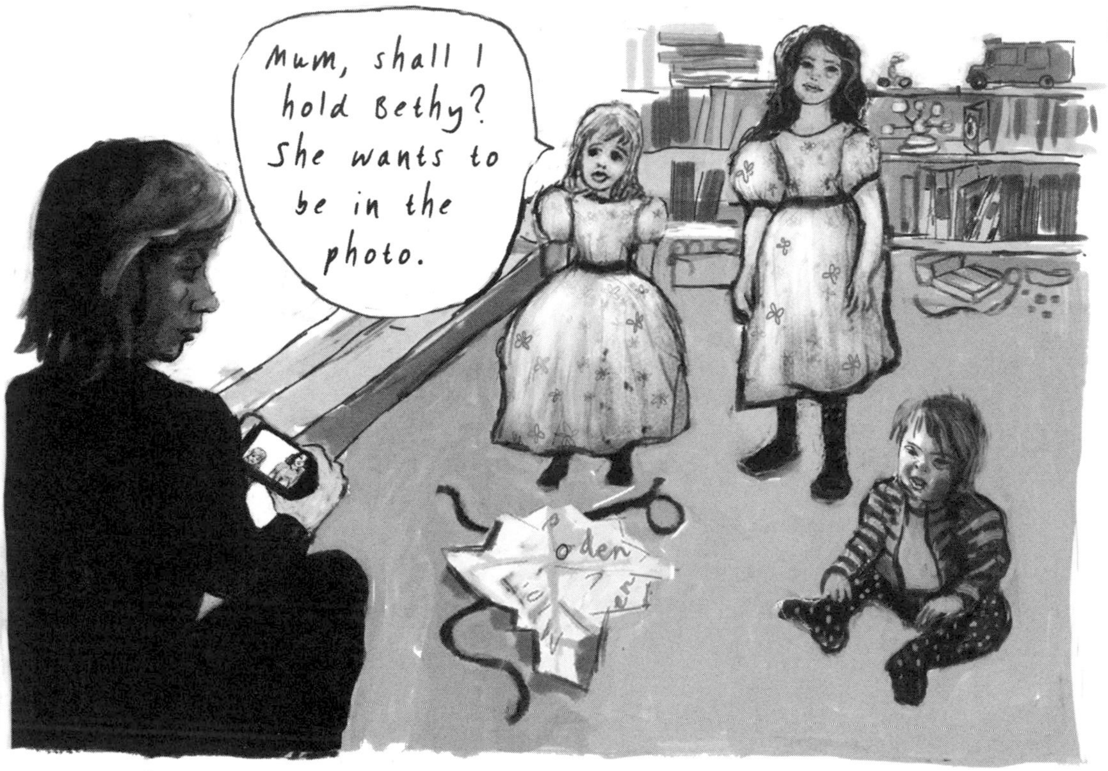
Mum, shall I hold Bethy? She wants to be in the photo.

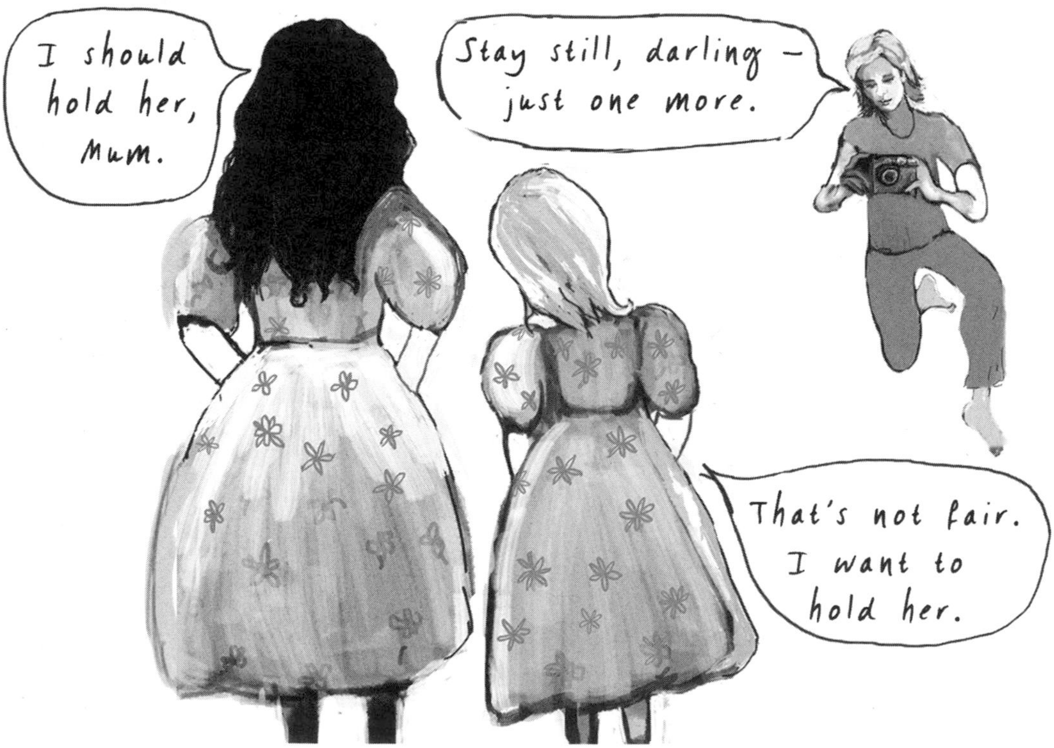
I should hold her, Mum.
Stay still, darling – just one more.
That's not fair. I want to hold her.

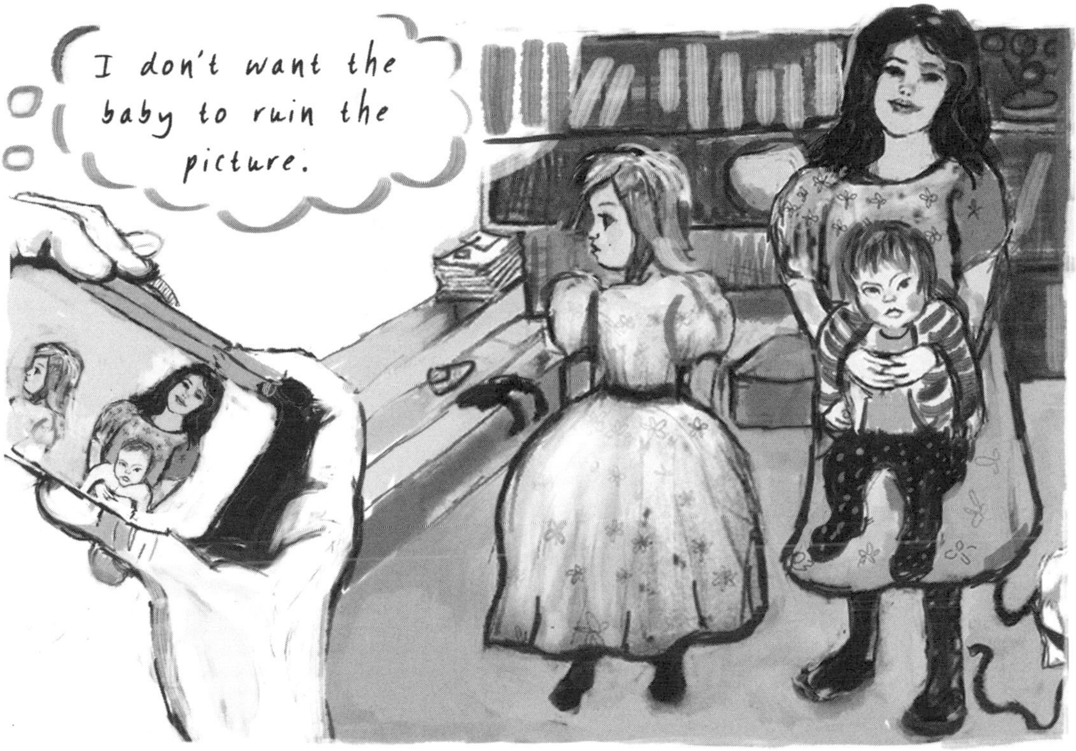
I don't want the baby to ruin the picture.

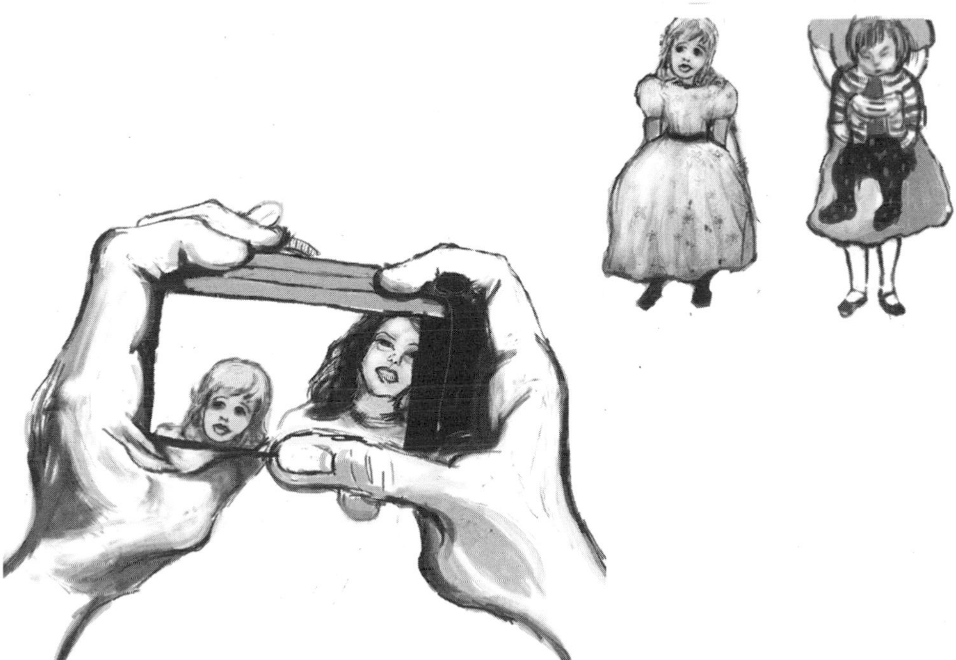

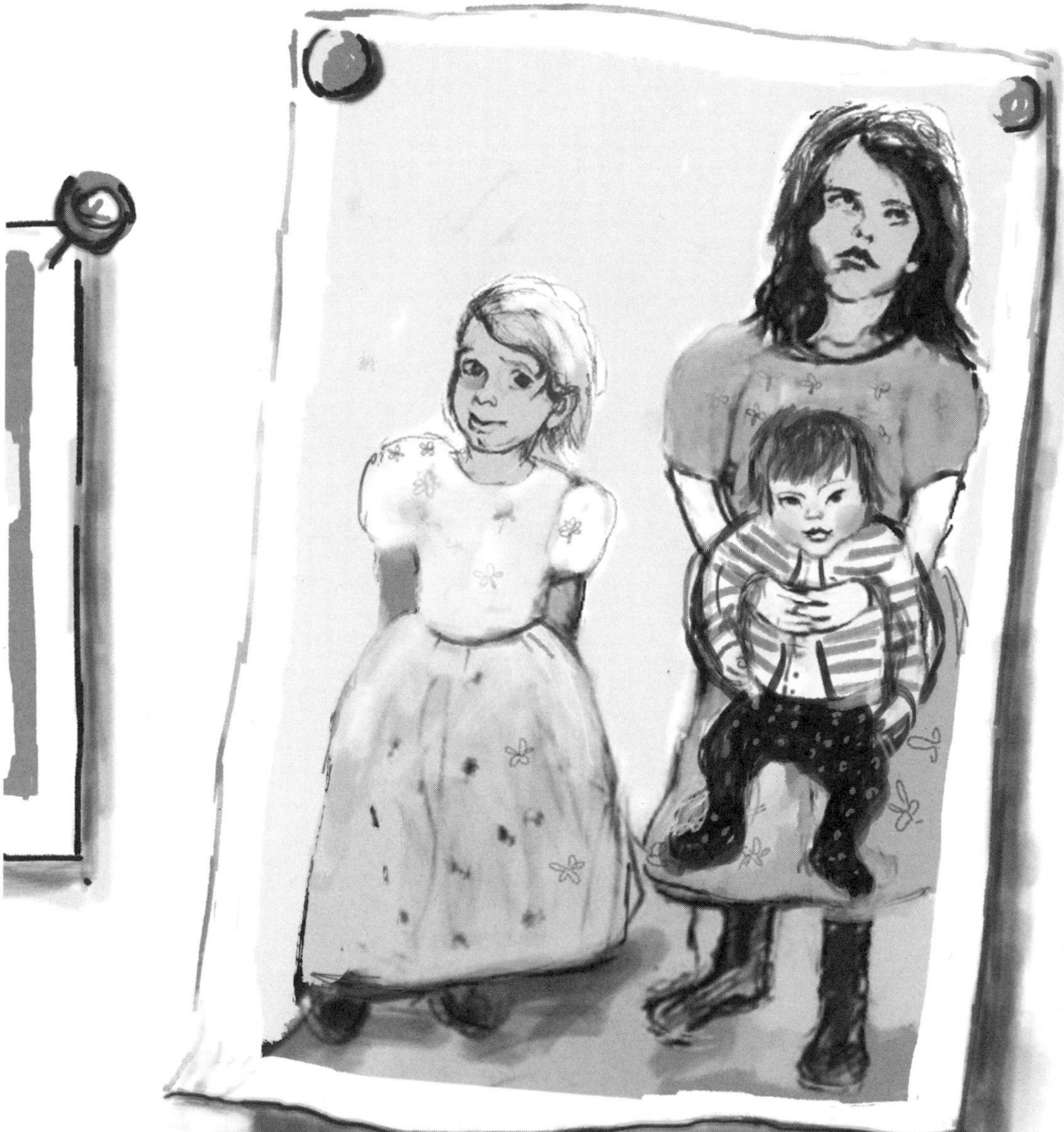

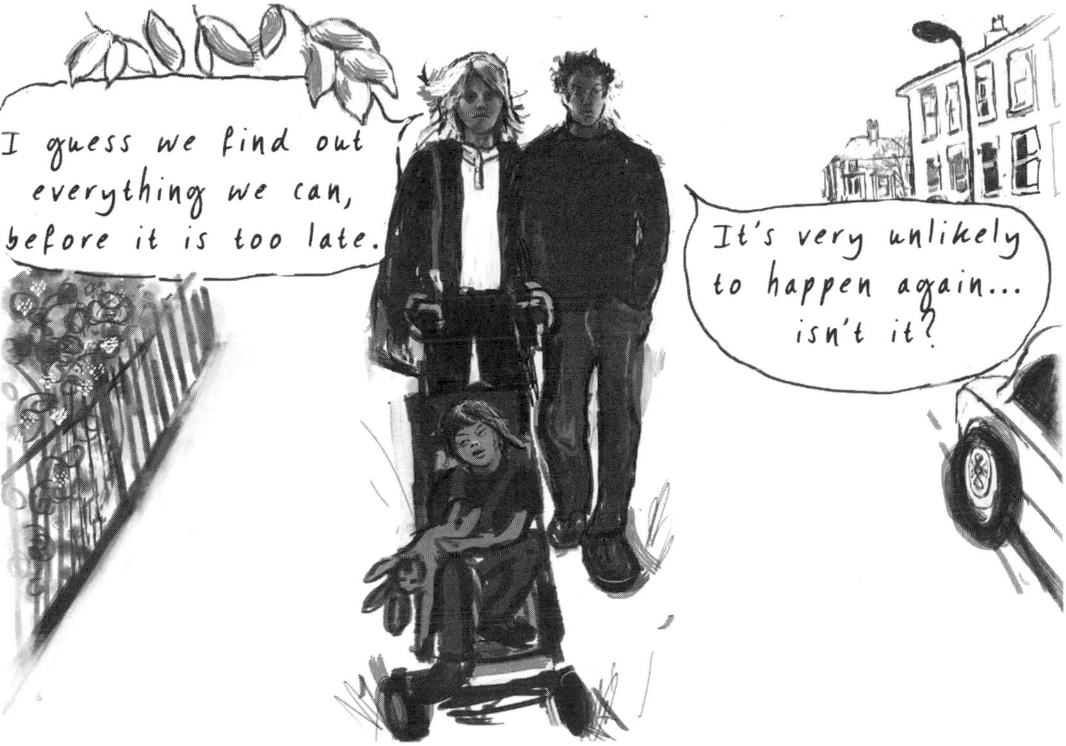
I guess we find out everything we can, before it is too late.
It's very unlikely to happen again... isn't it?

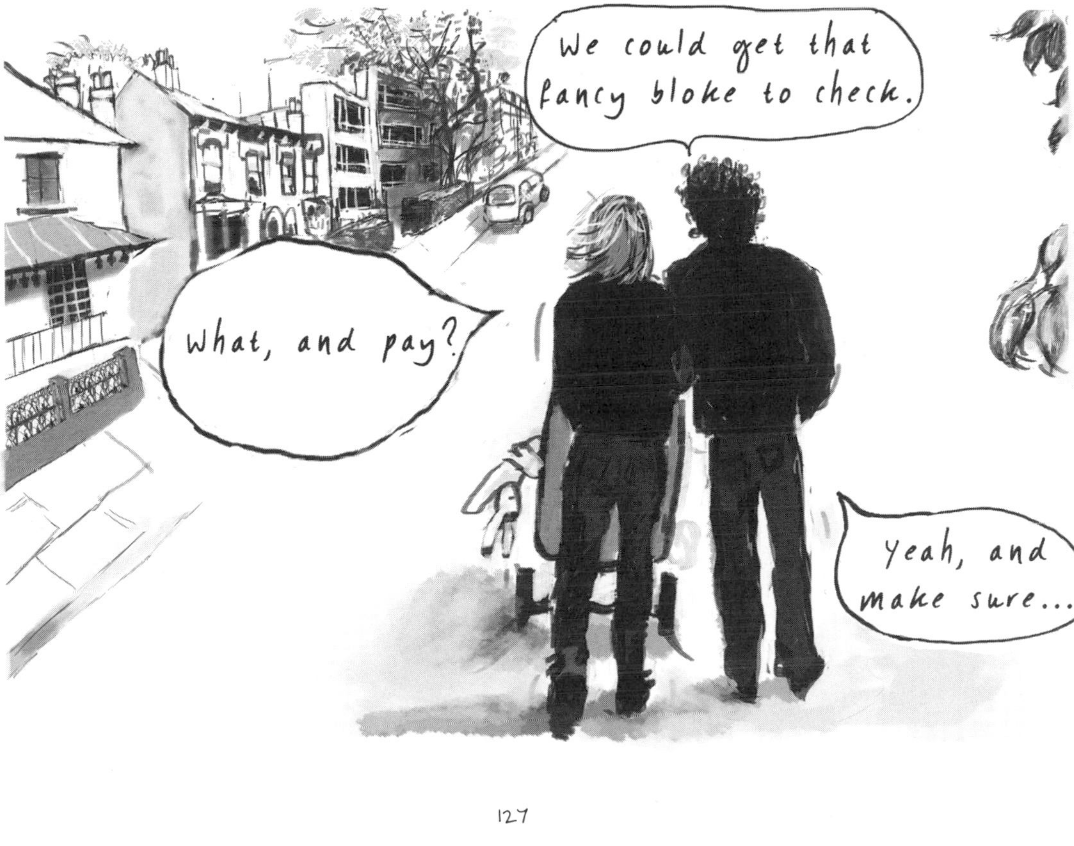
We could get that fancy bloke to check.
What, and pay?
Yeah, and make sure...

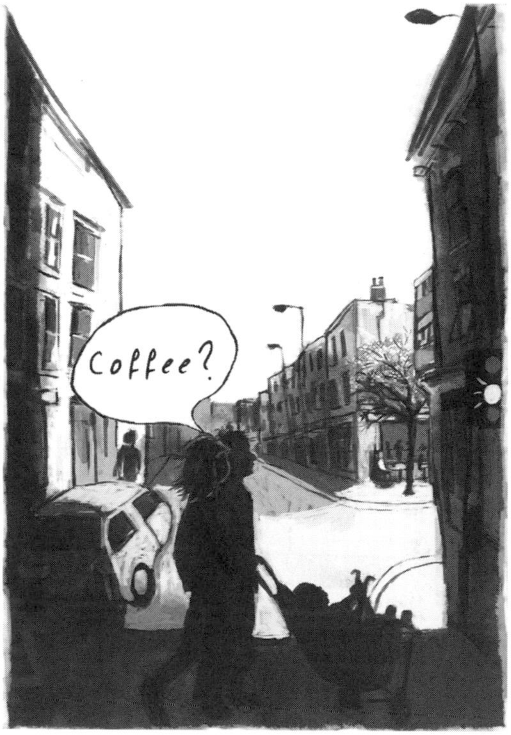
Coffee?

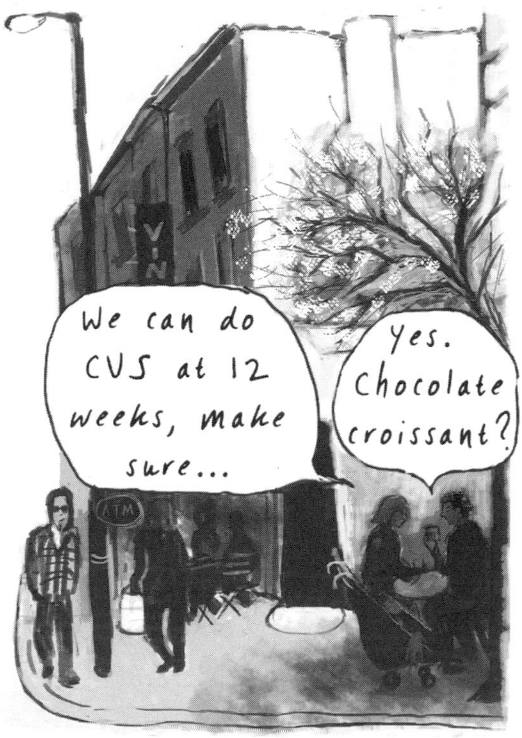
We can do CVS at 12 weeks, make sure...
Yes. Chocolate croissant?
VIN
ATM

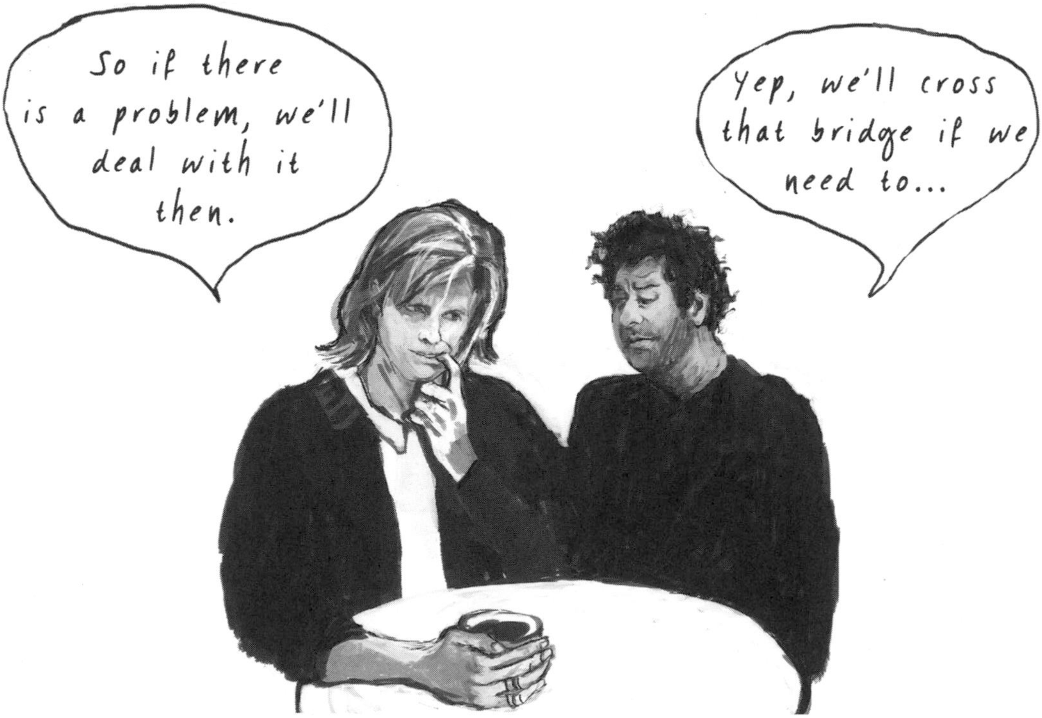
So if there is a problem, we'll deal with it then.
Yep, we'll cross that bridge if we need to...

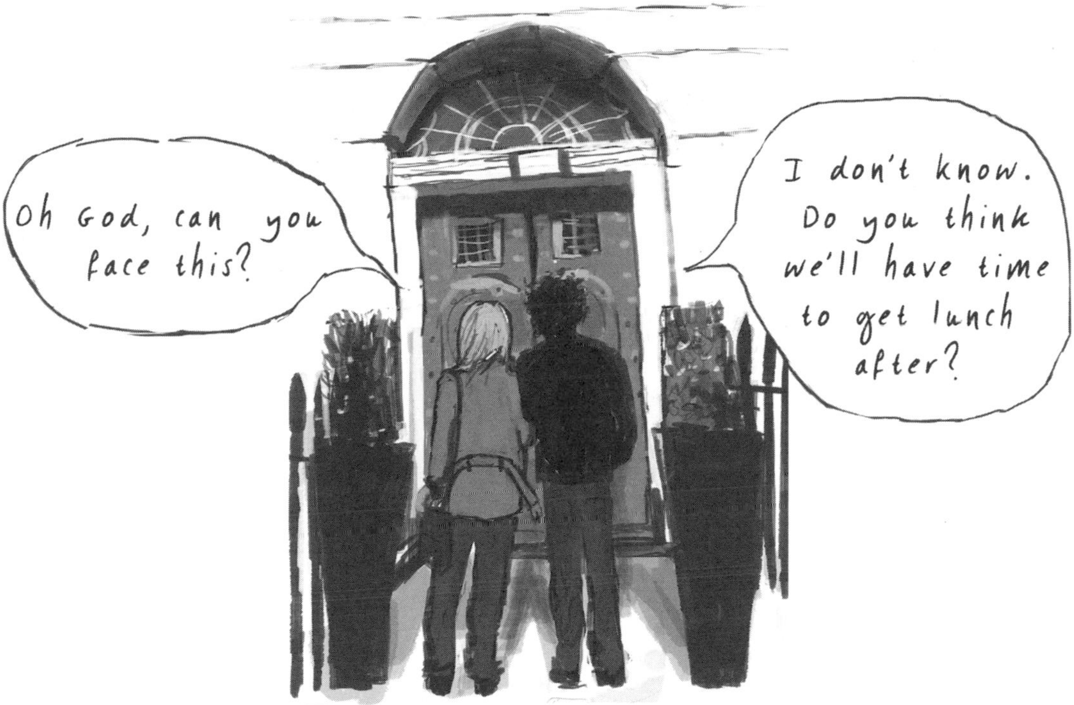

Oh God, can you face this?
I don't know. Do you think we'll have time to get lunch after?

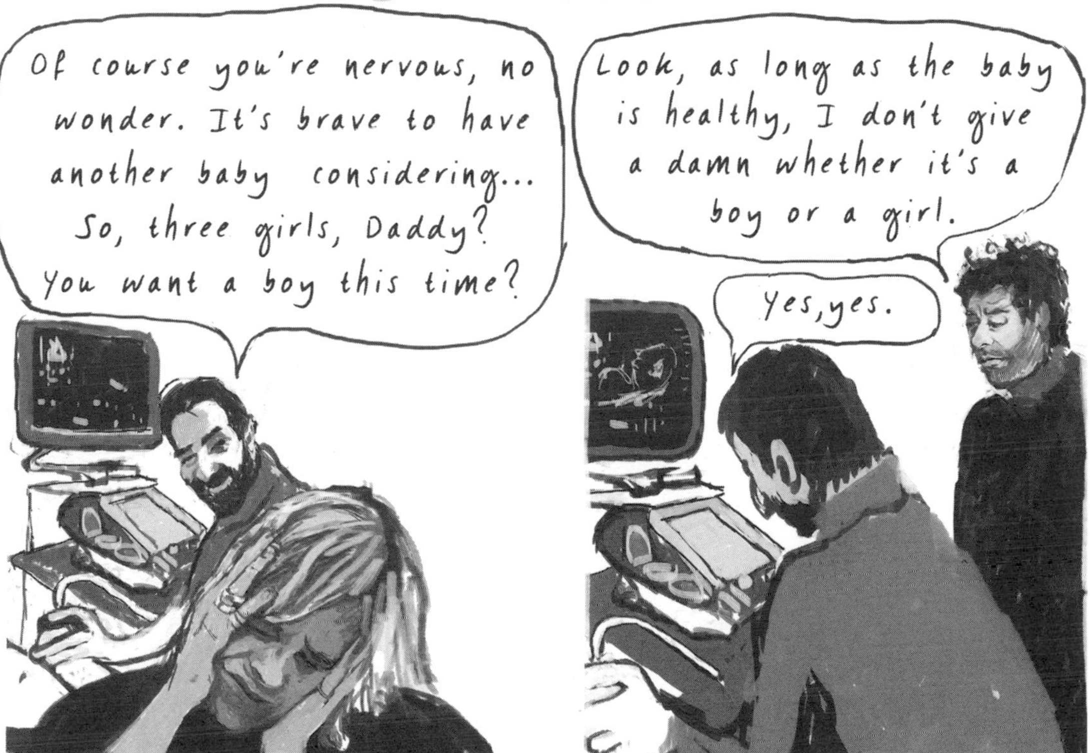

Of course you're nervous, no wonder. It's brave to have another baby considering... So, three girls, Daddy? You want a boy this time?
Look, as long as the baby is healthy, I don't give a damn whether it's a boy or a girl.
Yes, yes.

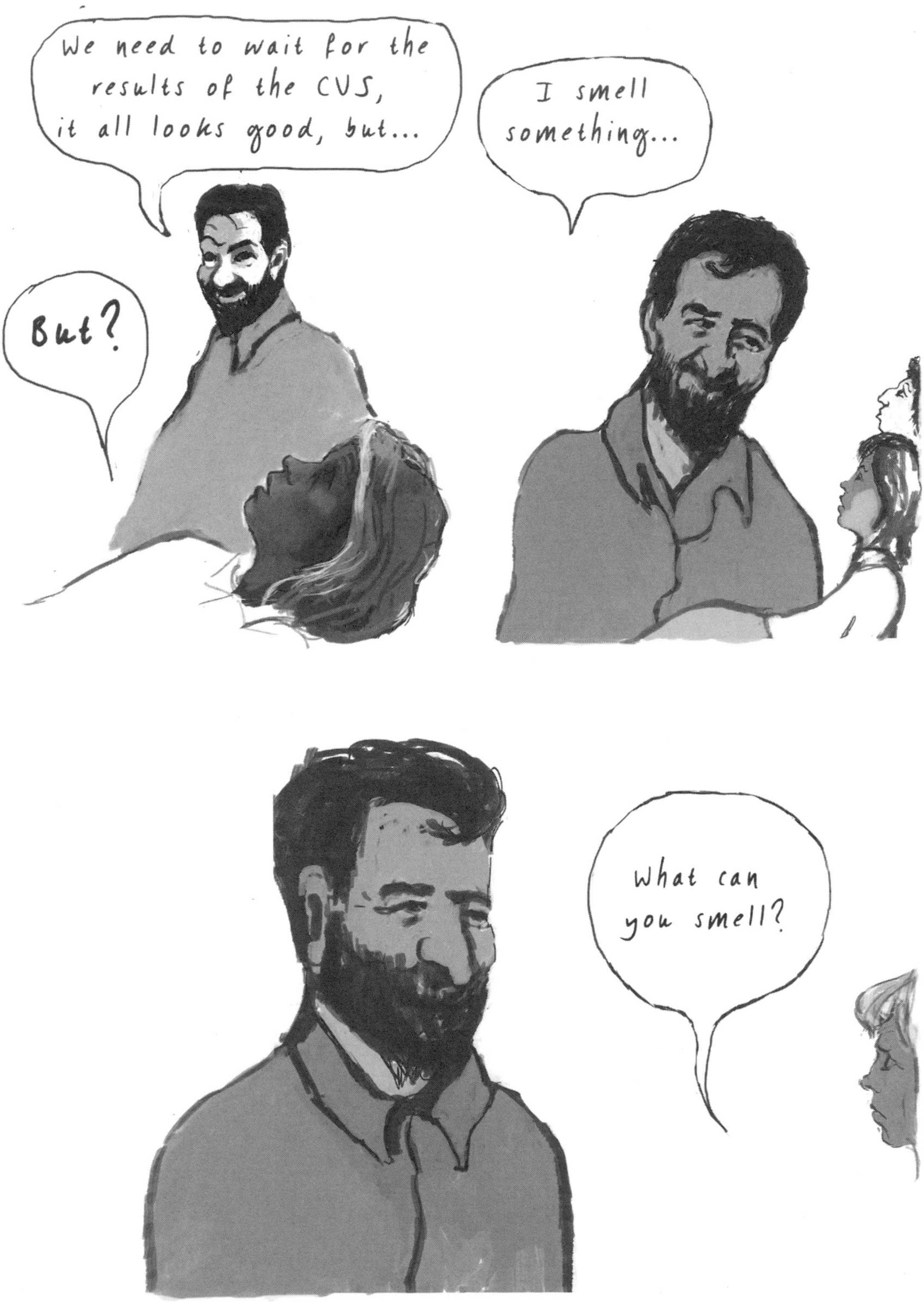
We need to wait for the results of the CVS, it all looks good, but...
But?
I smell something...
What can you smell?

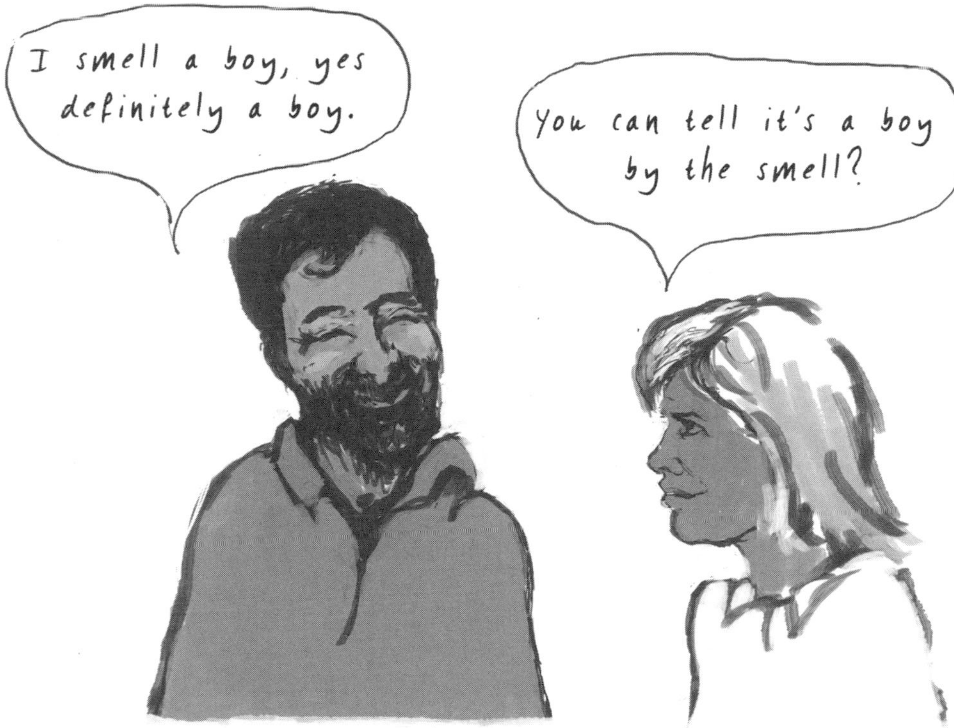
I smell a boy, yes definitely a boy.
You can tell it's a boy by the smell?

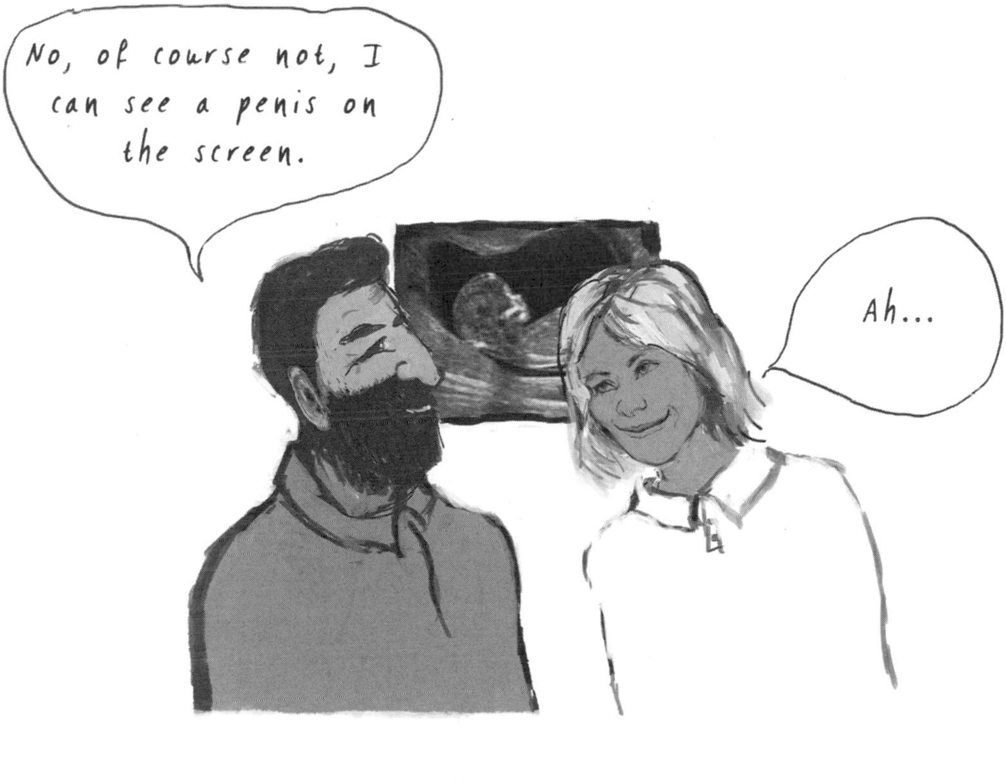
No, of course not, I can see a penis on the screen.
Ah...

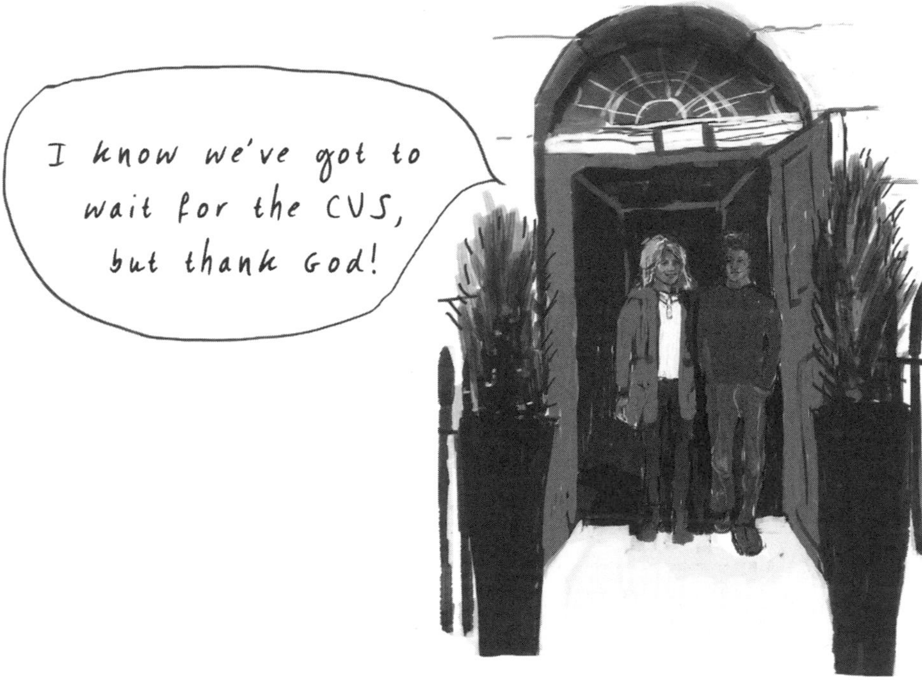
I know we've got to wait for the CVS, but thank God!

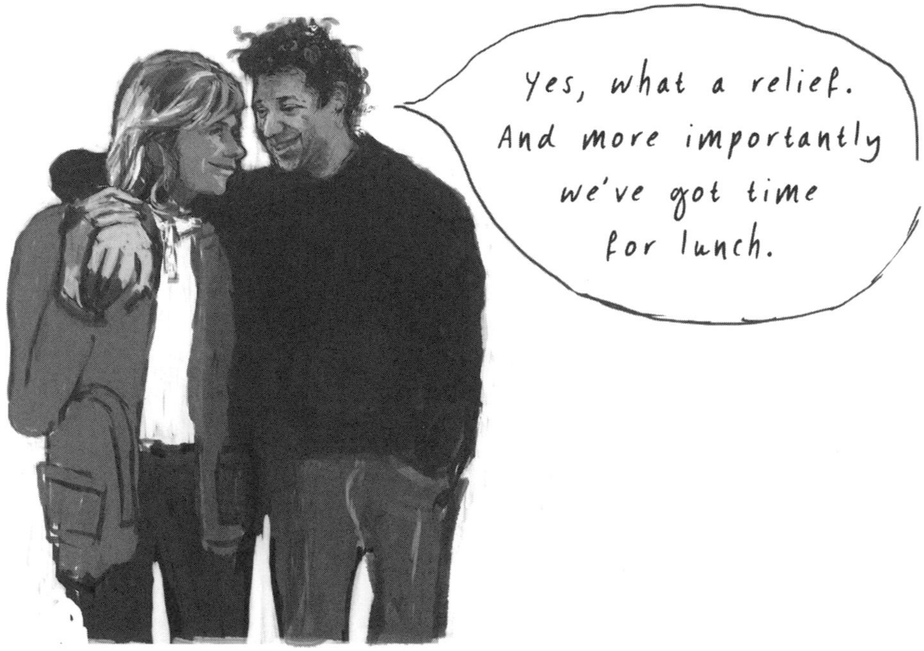
Yes, what a relief. And more importantly we've got time for lunch.

September 2003

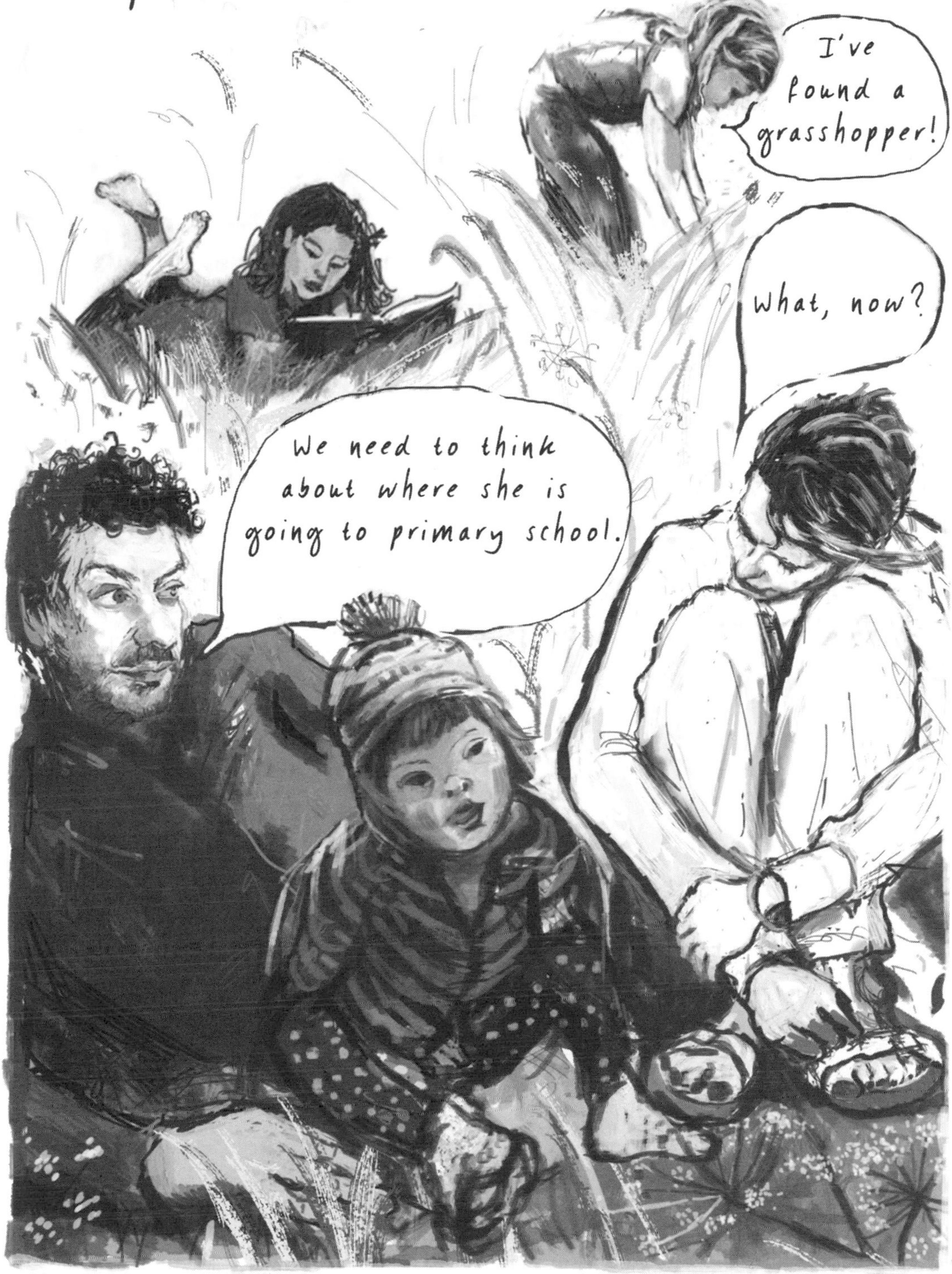
I've found a grasshopper!
What, now?
We need to think about where she is going to primary school.

June 2004

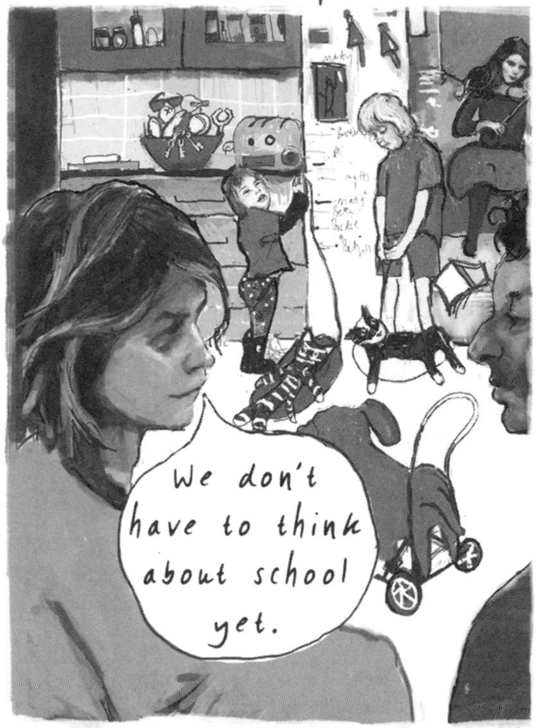
We don't have to think about school yet.

September 2004

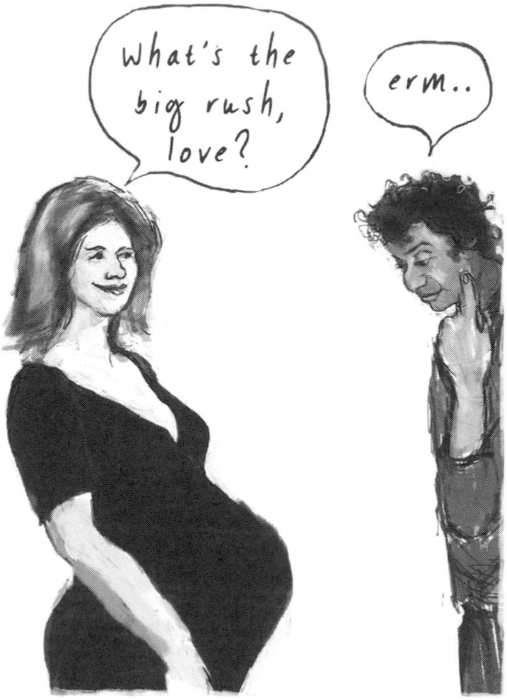
What's the big rush, love?
erm..

October 2004

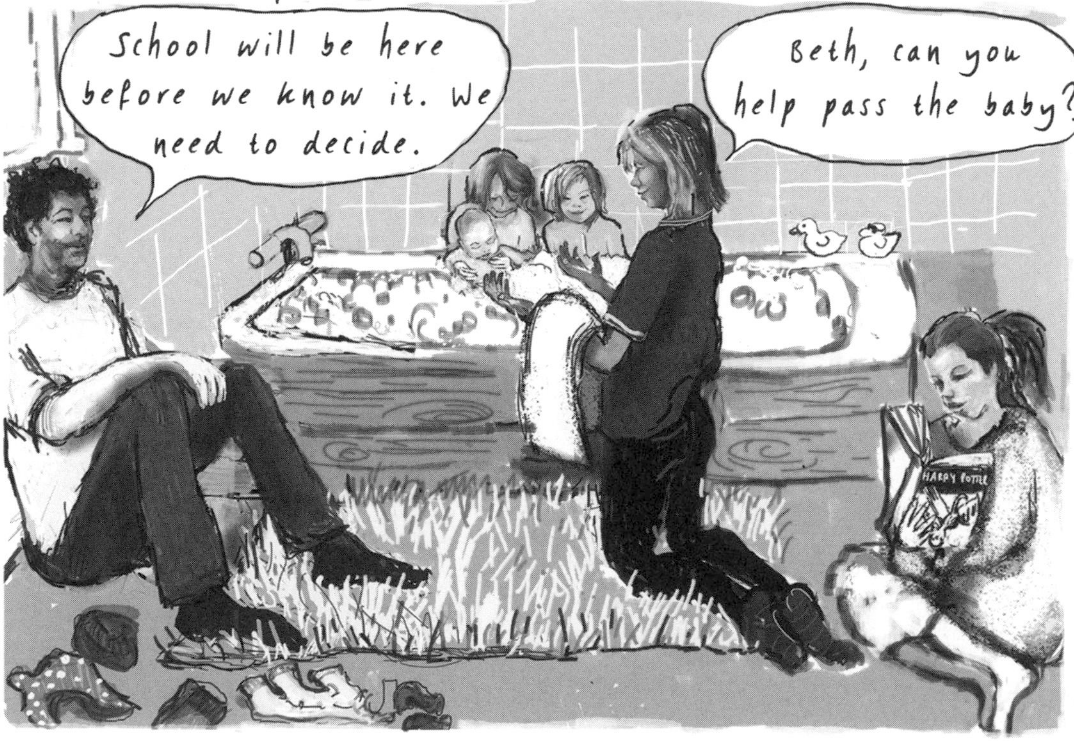
School will be here before we know it. We need to decide.
Beth, can you help pass the baby?
HARRY POTTER

July 2005

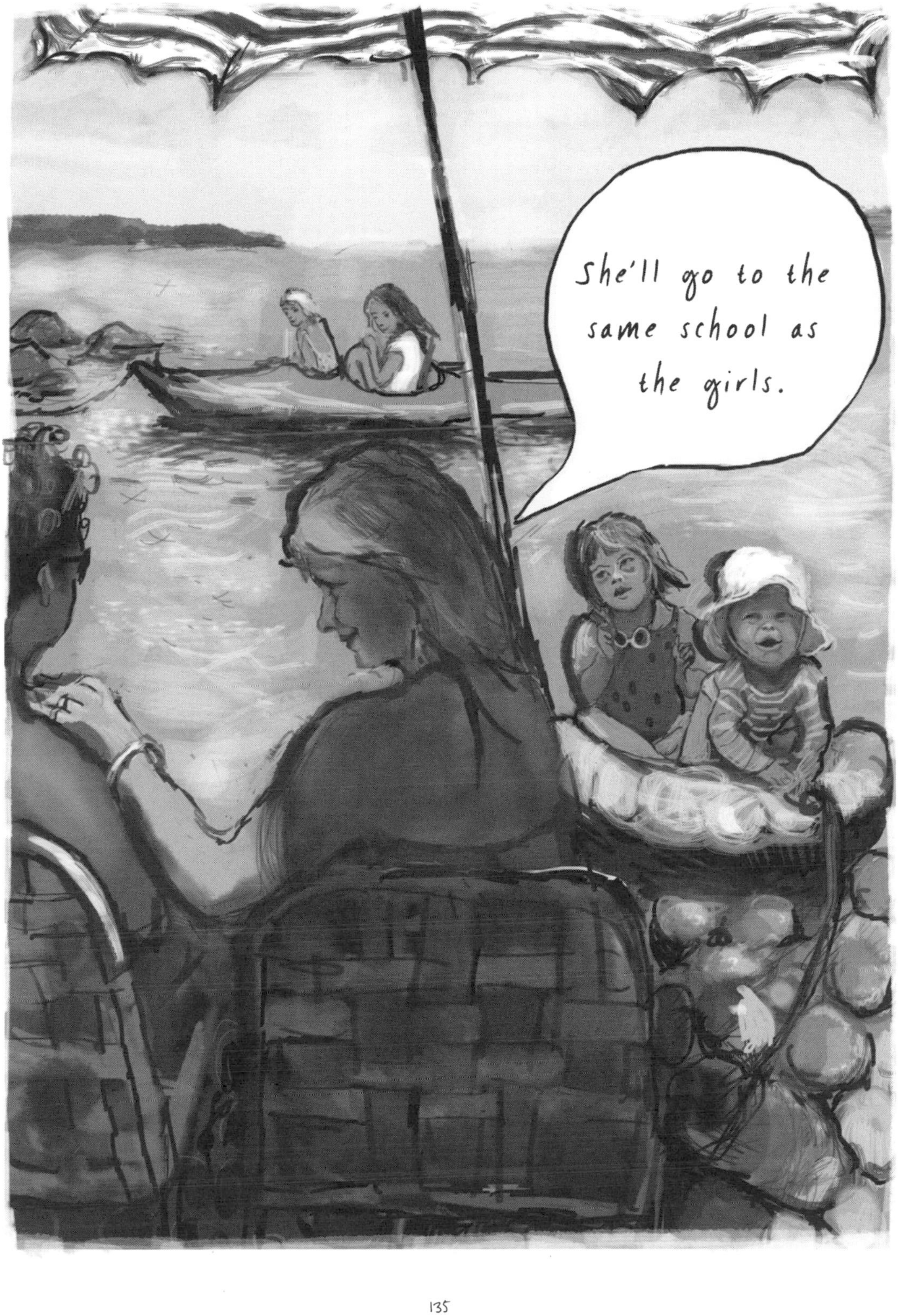
She'll go to the same school as the girls.

October 2006

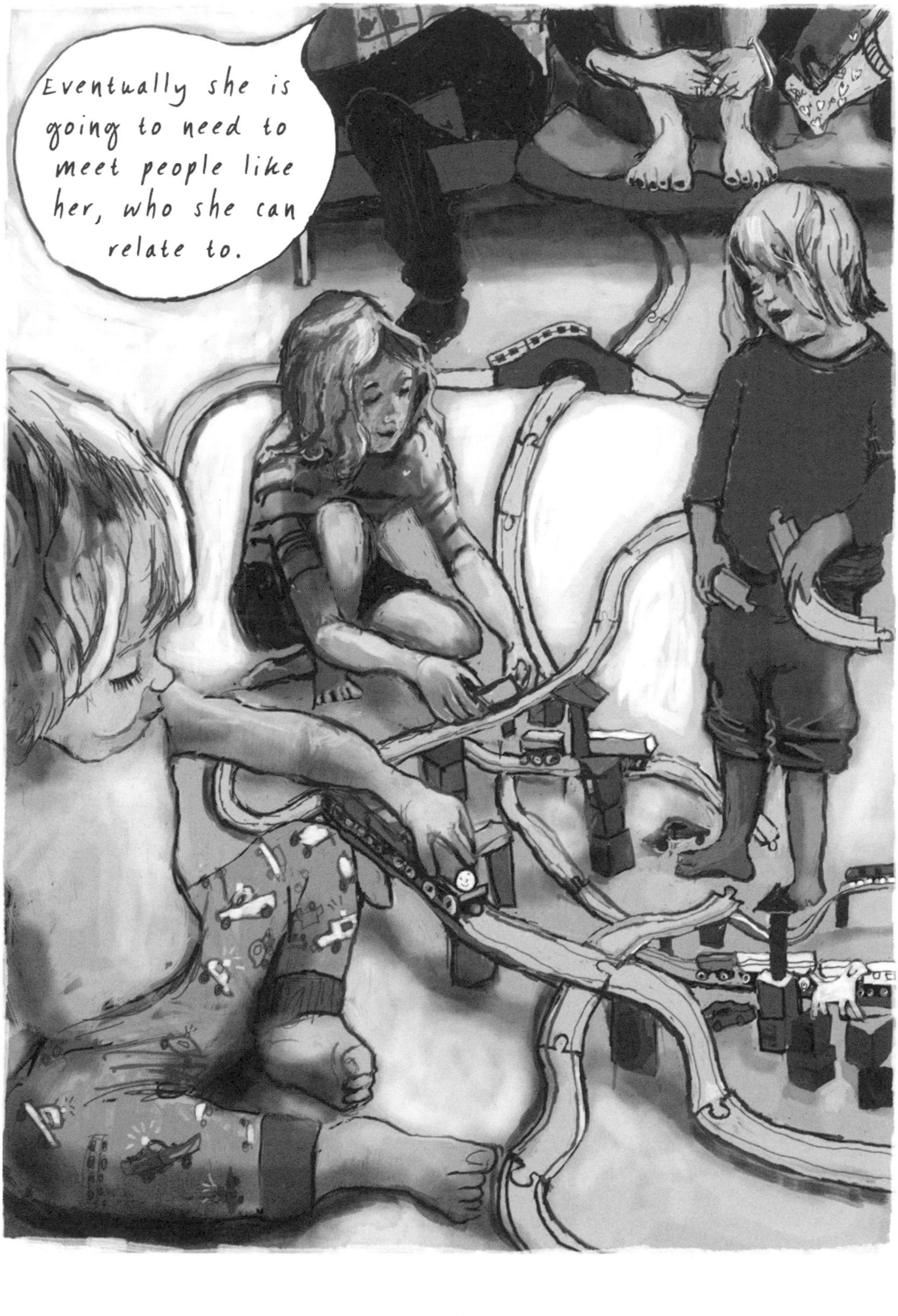
Eventually she is going to need to meet people like her, who she can relate to.

December 2006

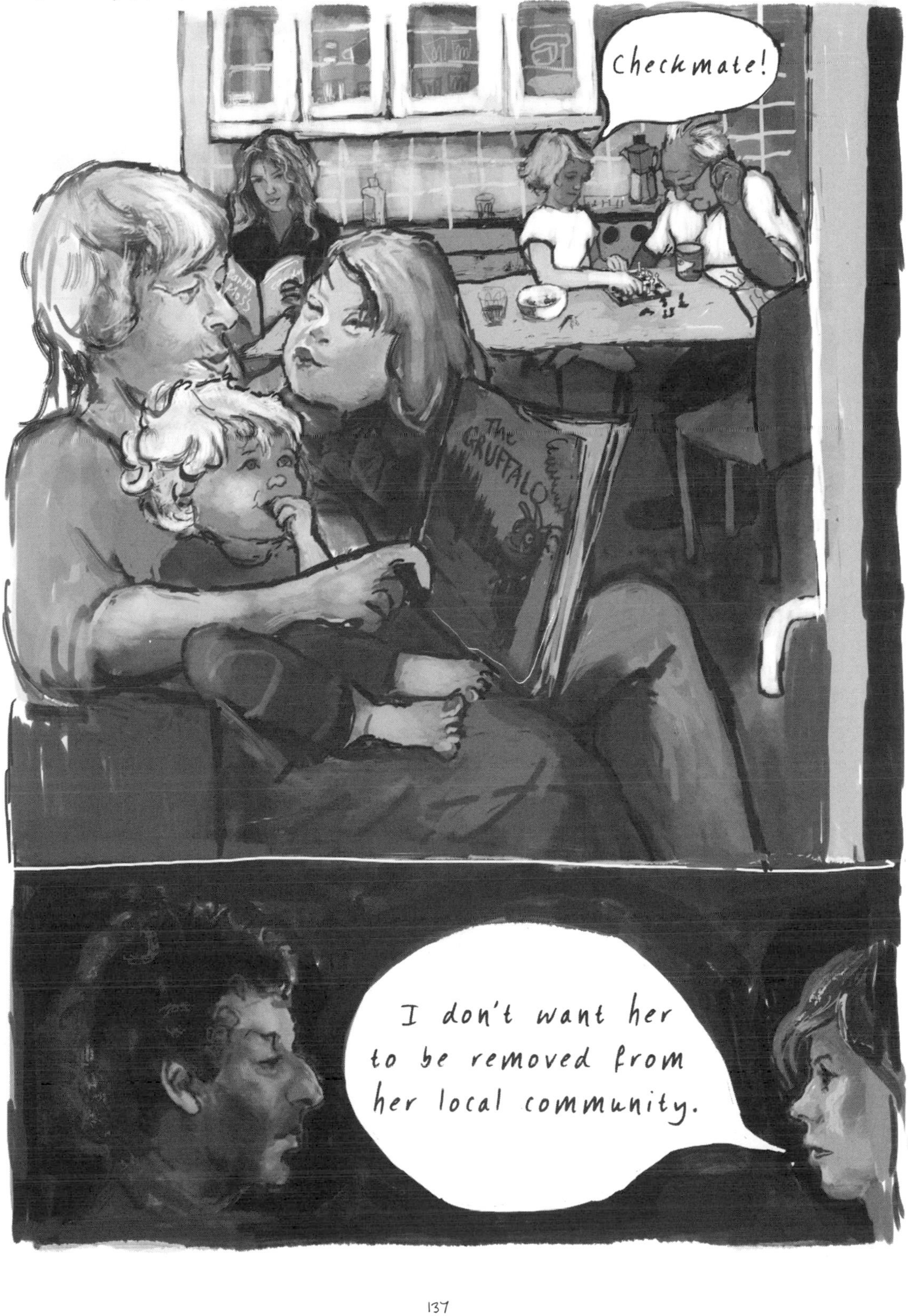
Checkmate!
The GRUFFALO
I don't want her to be removed from her local community.

May 2007

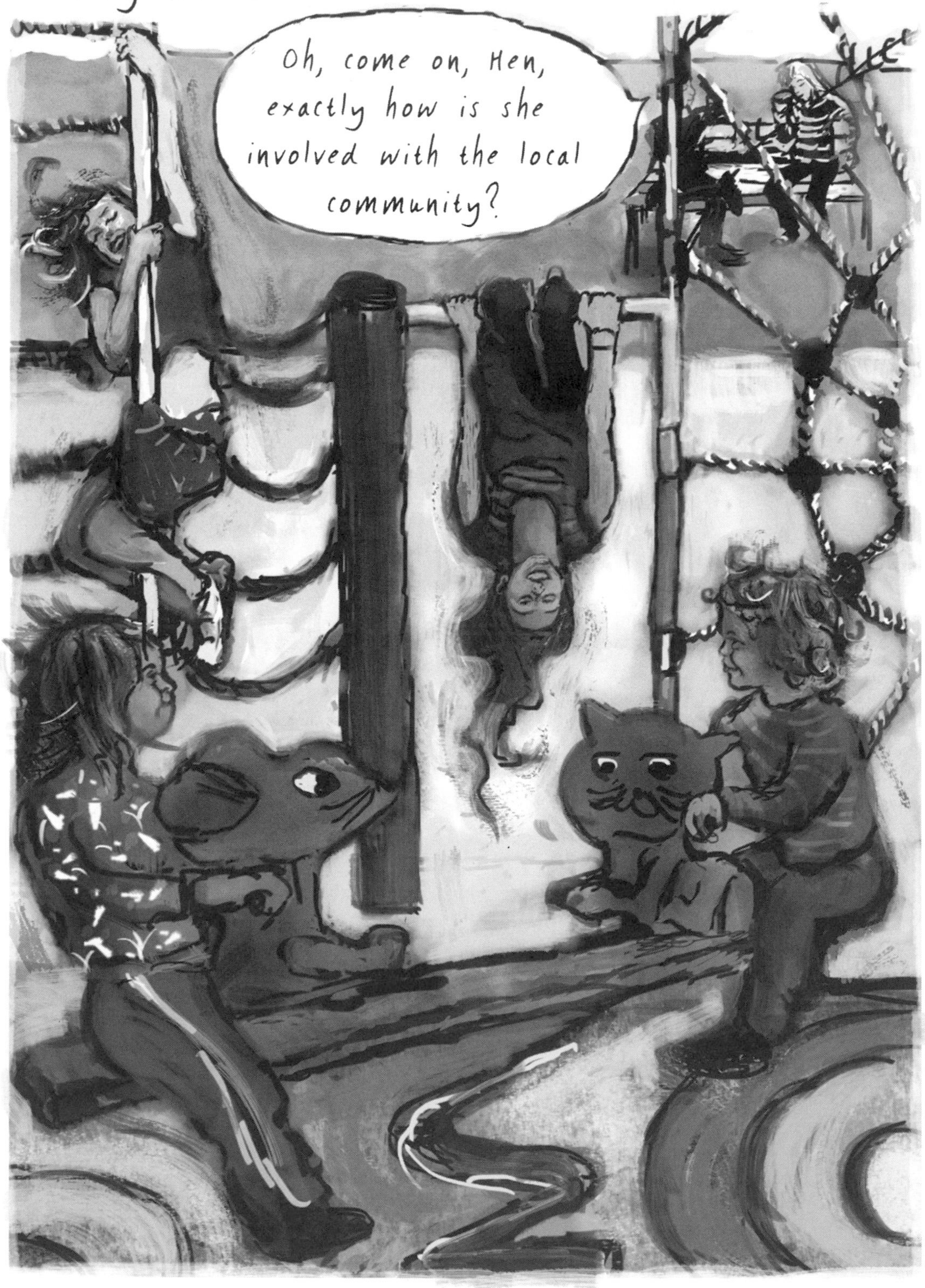
Oh, come on, Hen, exactly how is she involved with the local community?

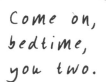

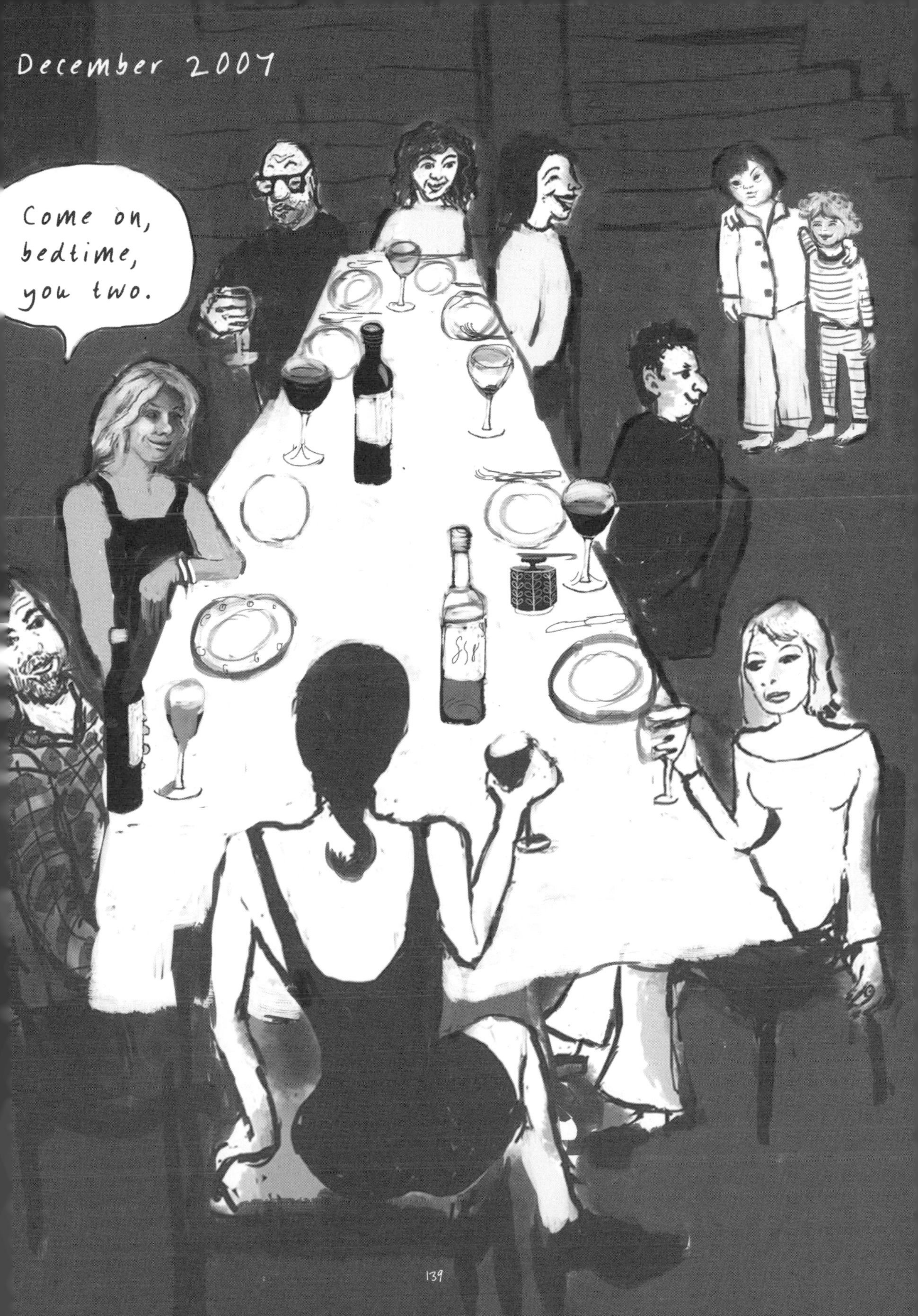

December 2007

Come on,
bedtime,
you two.

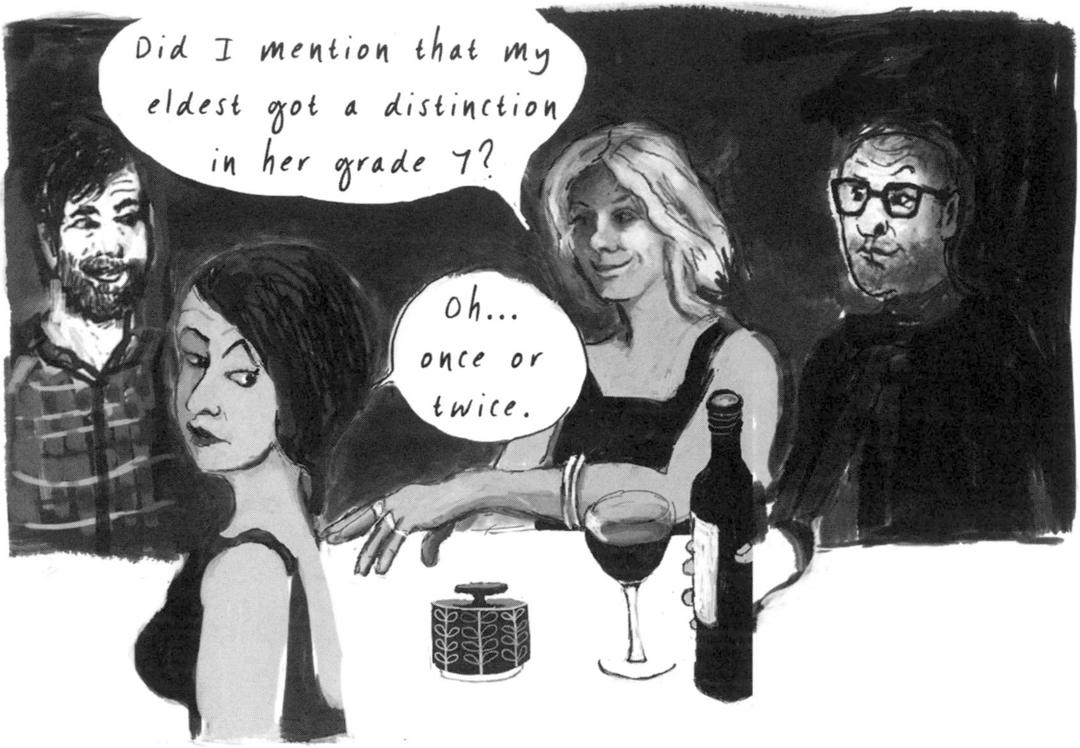
Did I mention that my eldest got a distinction in her grade 7?
Oh... once or twice.

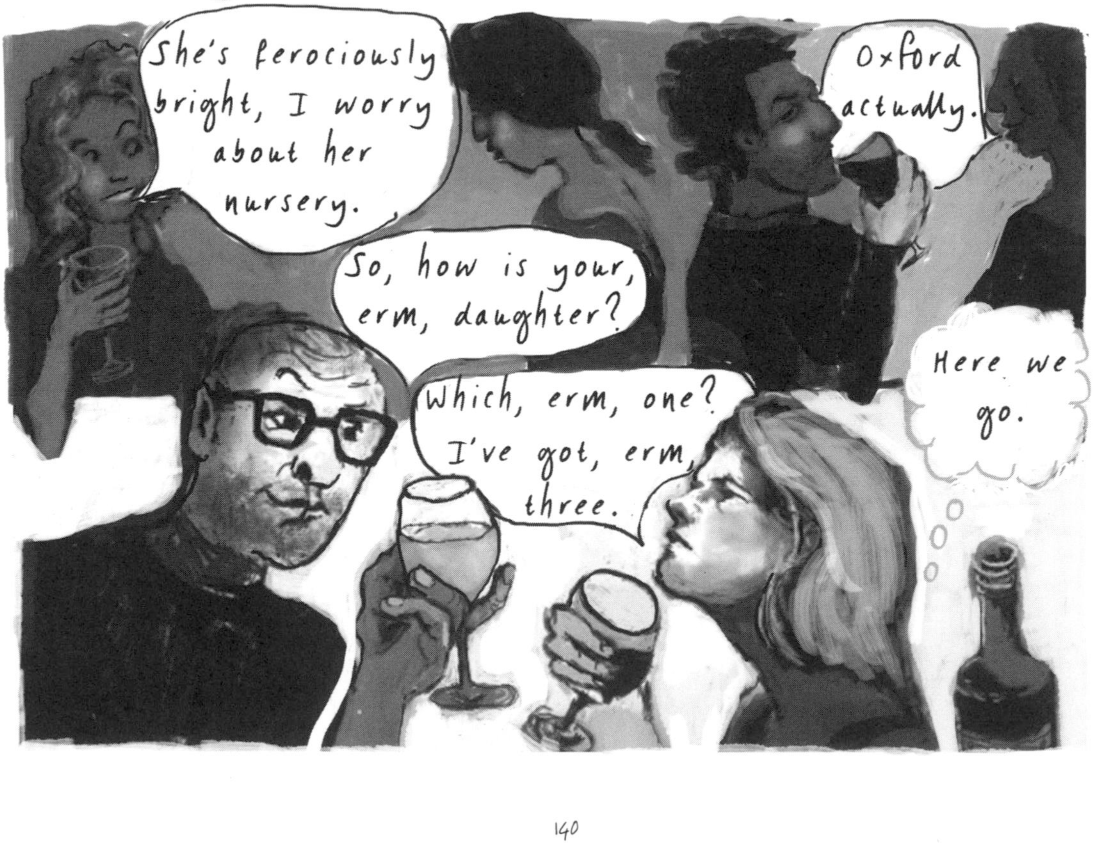
She's ferociously bright, I worry about her nursery.
Oxford actually.
So, how is your, erm, daughter?
Which, erm, one? I've got, erm, three.
Here we go.

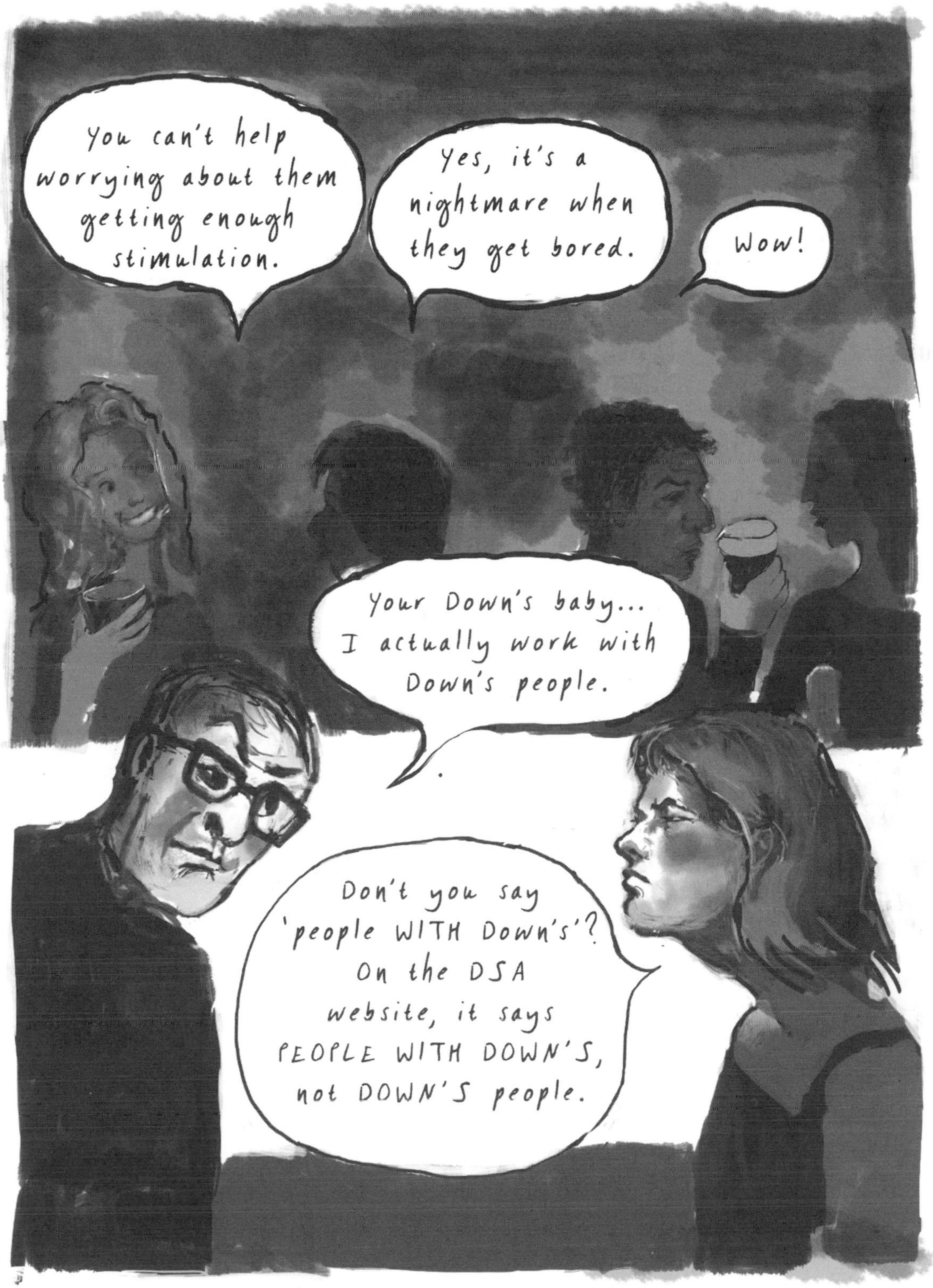
You can't help worrying about them getting enough stimulation.
Yes, it's a nightmare when they get bored.
Wow!
Your Down's baby... I actually work with Down's people.
Don't you say 'people WITH Down's'? On the DSA website, it says PEOPLE WITH DOWN'S, not DOWN'S people.

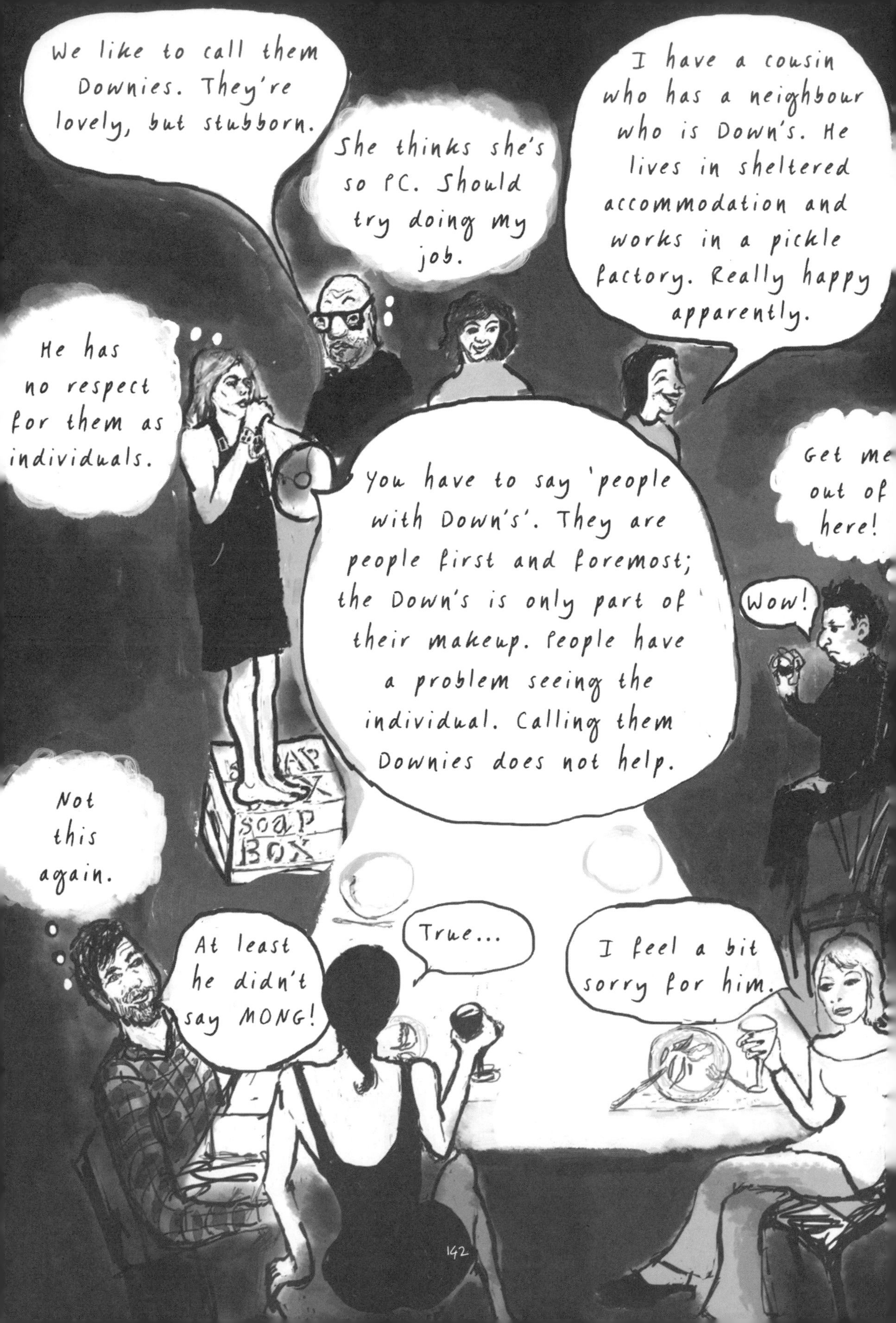
We like to call them Downies. They're lovely, but stubborn.
She thinks she's so PC. Should try doing my job.
I have a cousin who has a neighbour who is Down's. He lives in sheltered accommodation and works in a pickle factory. Really happy apparently.
He has no respect for them as individuals.
You have to say 'people with Down's'. They are people first and foremost; the Down's is only part of their makeup. People have a problem seeing the individual. Calling them Downies does not help.
Get me out of here!
Wow!
SOAP BOX
Not this again.
At least he didn't say MONG!
True...
I feel a bit sorry for him.

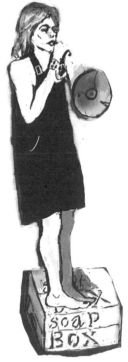

What we call people makes a huge difference to how we see them. It makes a big difference to me, as a mother of a child WITH Down's and my ability to love her.

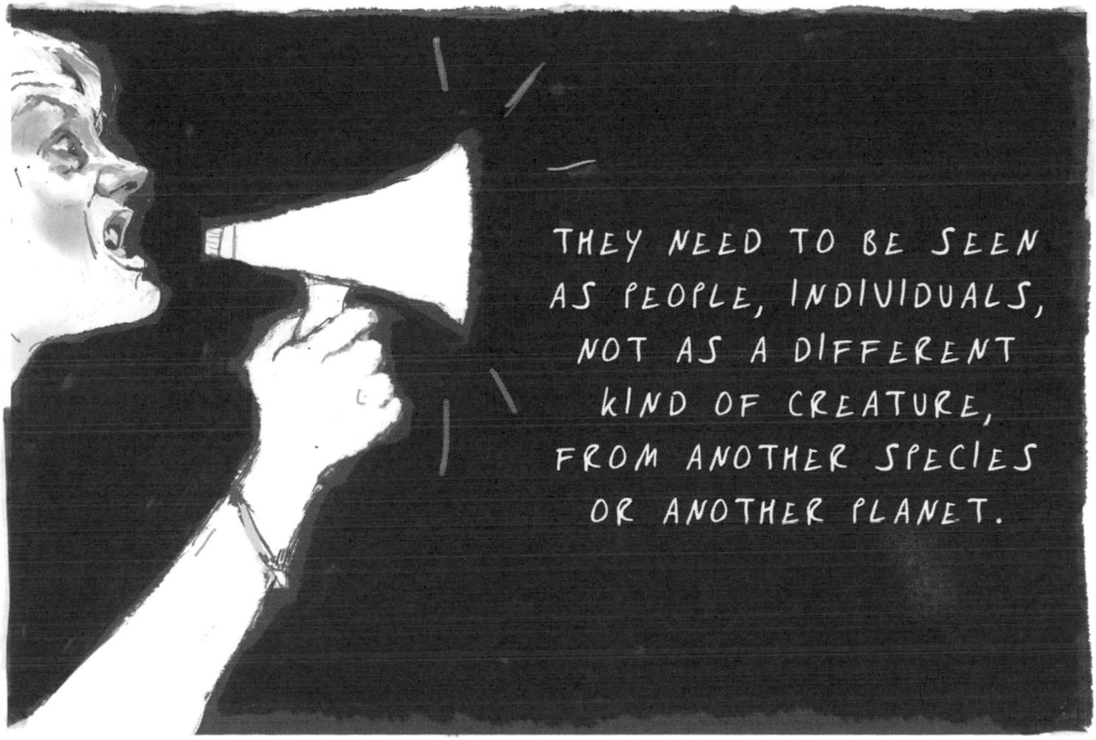

THEY NEED TO BE SEEN AS PEOPLE, INDIVIDUALS, NOT AS A DIFFERENT KIND OF CREATURE, FROM ANOTHER SPECIES OR ANOTHER PLANET.

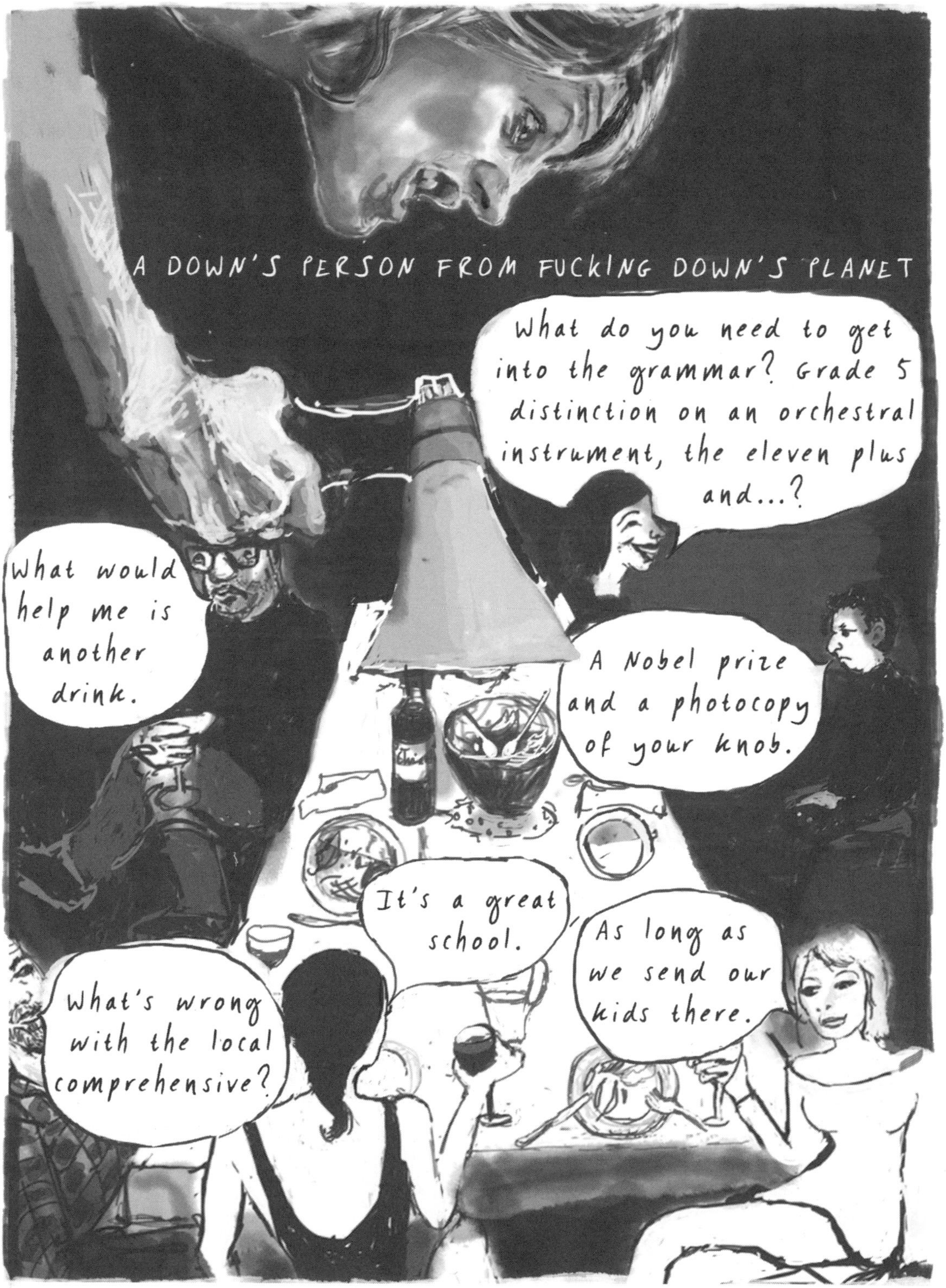
A DOWN'S PERSON FROM FUCKING DOWN'S PLANET
What do you need to get into the grammar? Grade 5 distinction on an orchestral instrument, the eleven plus and...?
What would help me is another drink.
A Nobel prize and a photocopy of your knob.
It's a great school.
As long as we send our kids there.
What's wrong with the local comprehensive?

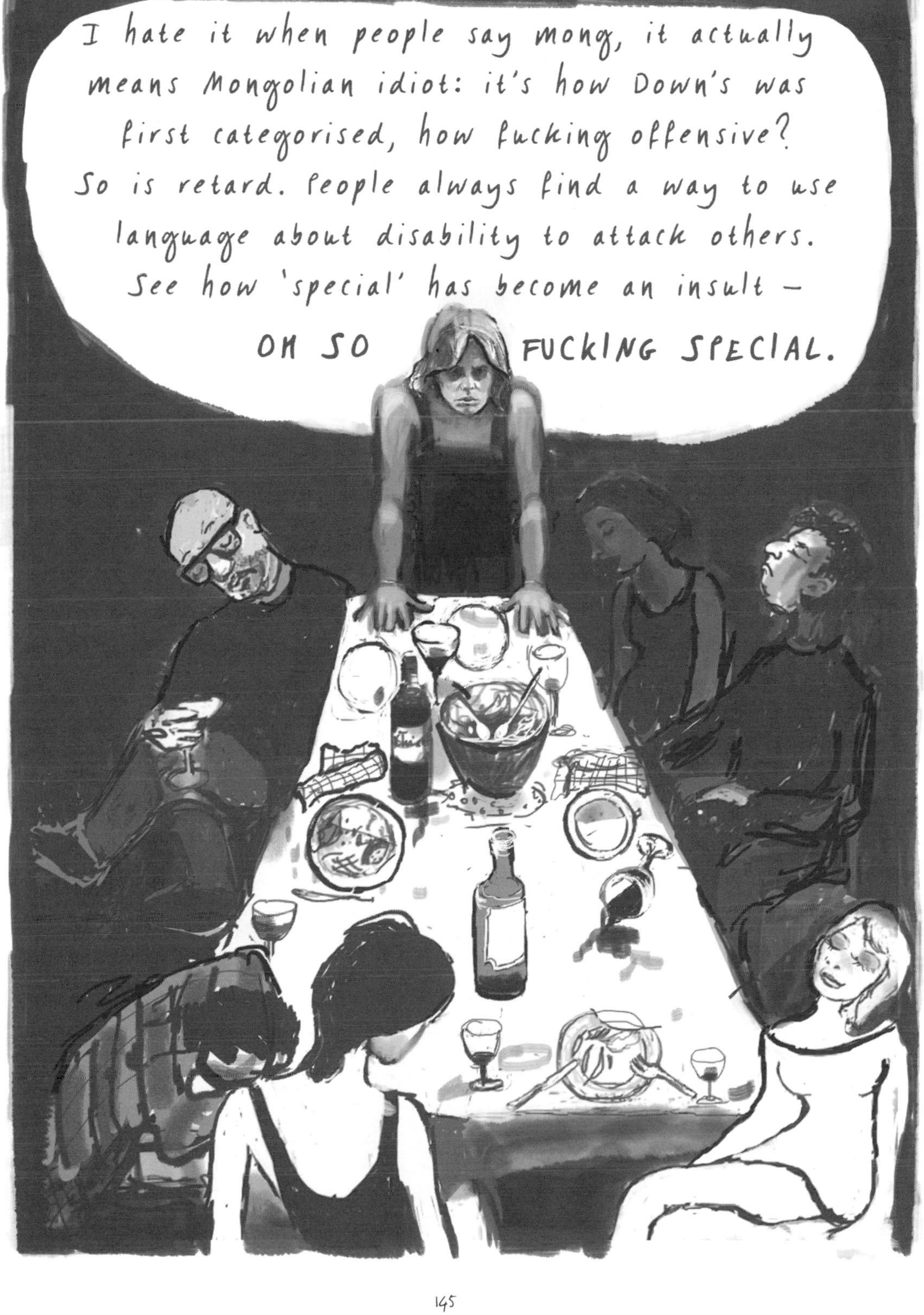
I hate it when people say mong, it actually means Mongolian idiot: it's how Down's was first categorised, how fucking offensive? So is retard. People always find a way to use language about disability to attack others. See how 'special' has become an insult –
OH SO FUCKING SPECIAL.

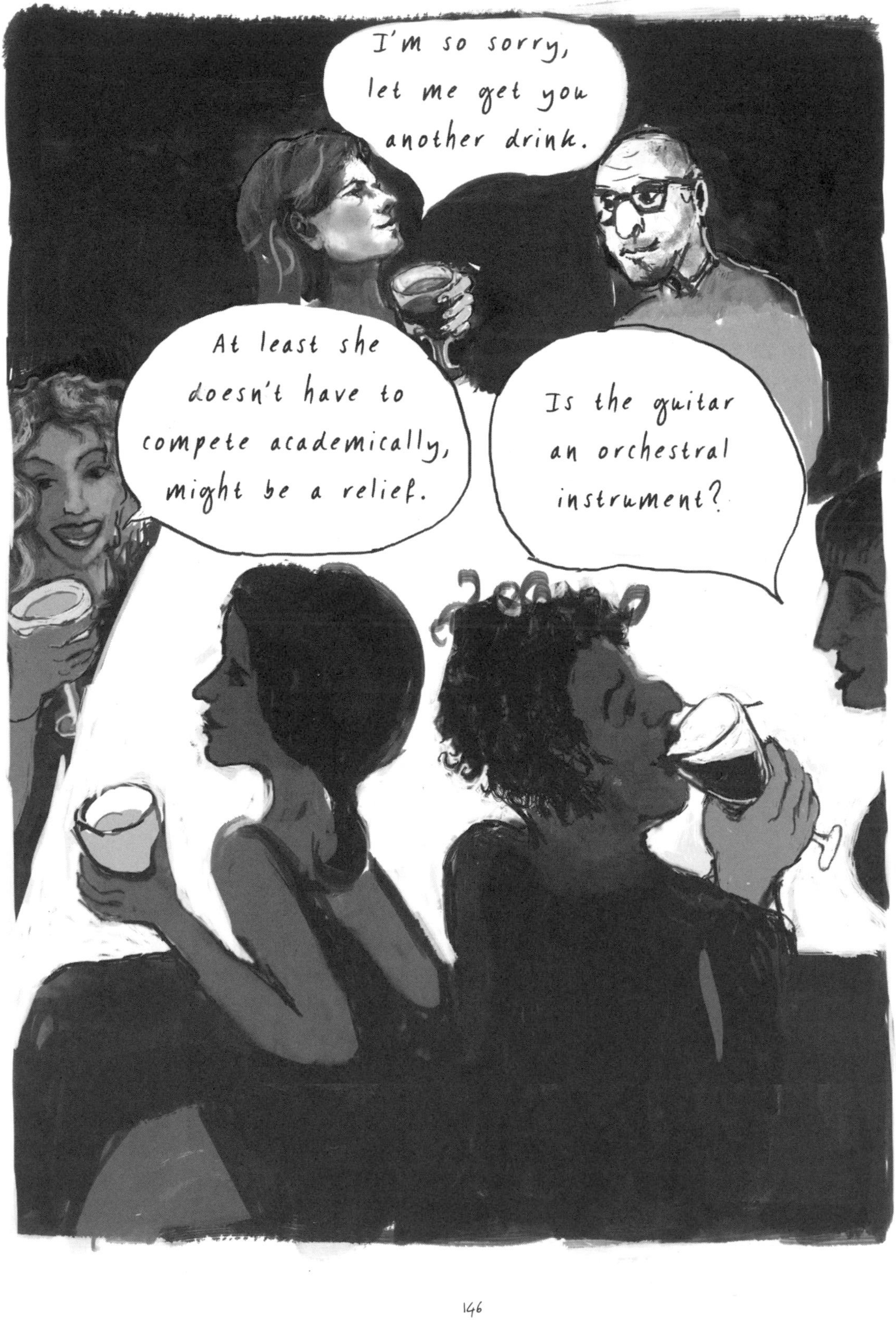
I'm so sorry, let me get you another drink.
At least she doesn't have to compete academically, might be a relief.
Is the guitar an orchestral instrument?

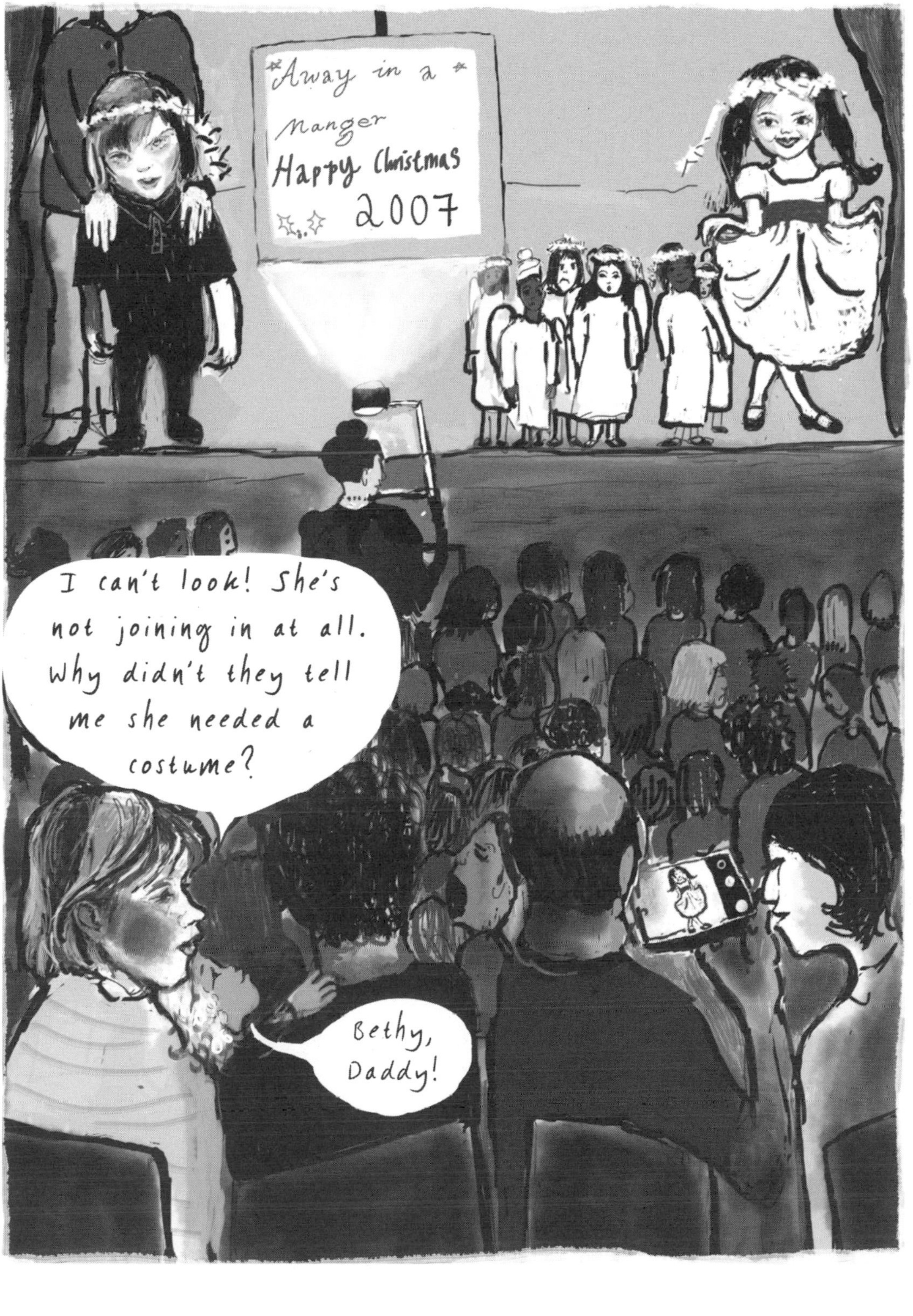
Away in a manger
Happy Christmas 2007
I can't look! She's not joining in at all. Why didn't they tell me she needed a costume?
Bethy, Daddy!

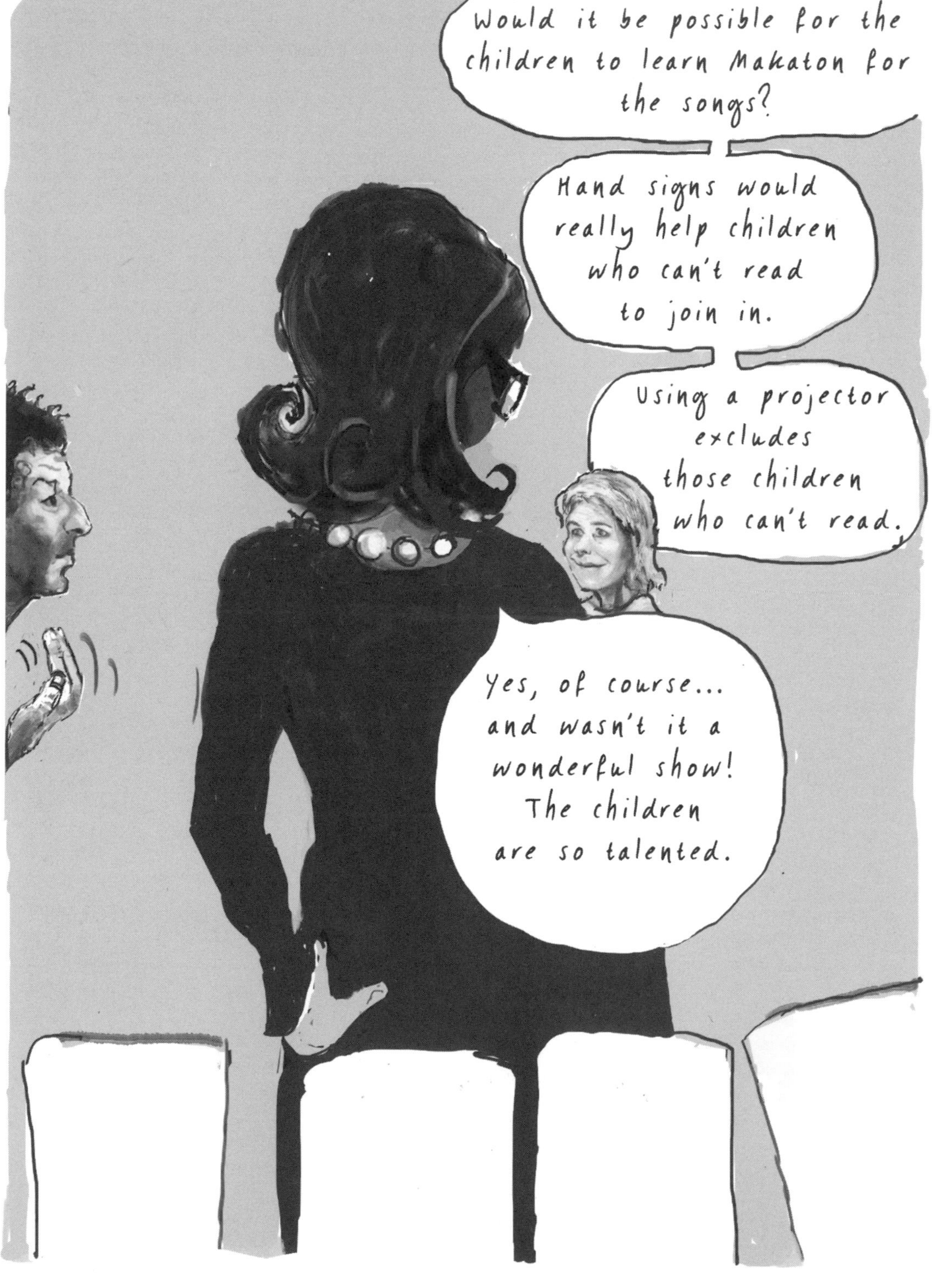
Would it be possible for the children to learn Makaton for the songs?
Hand signs would really help children who can't read to join in.
Using a projector excludes those children who can't read.
Yes, of course... and wasn't it a wonderful show! The children are so talented.

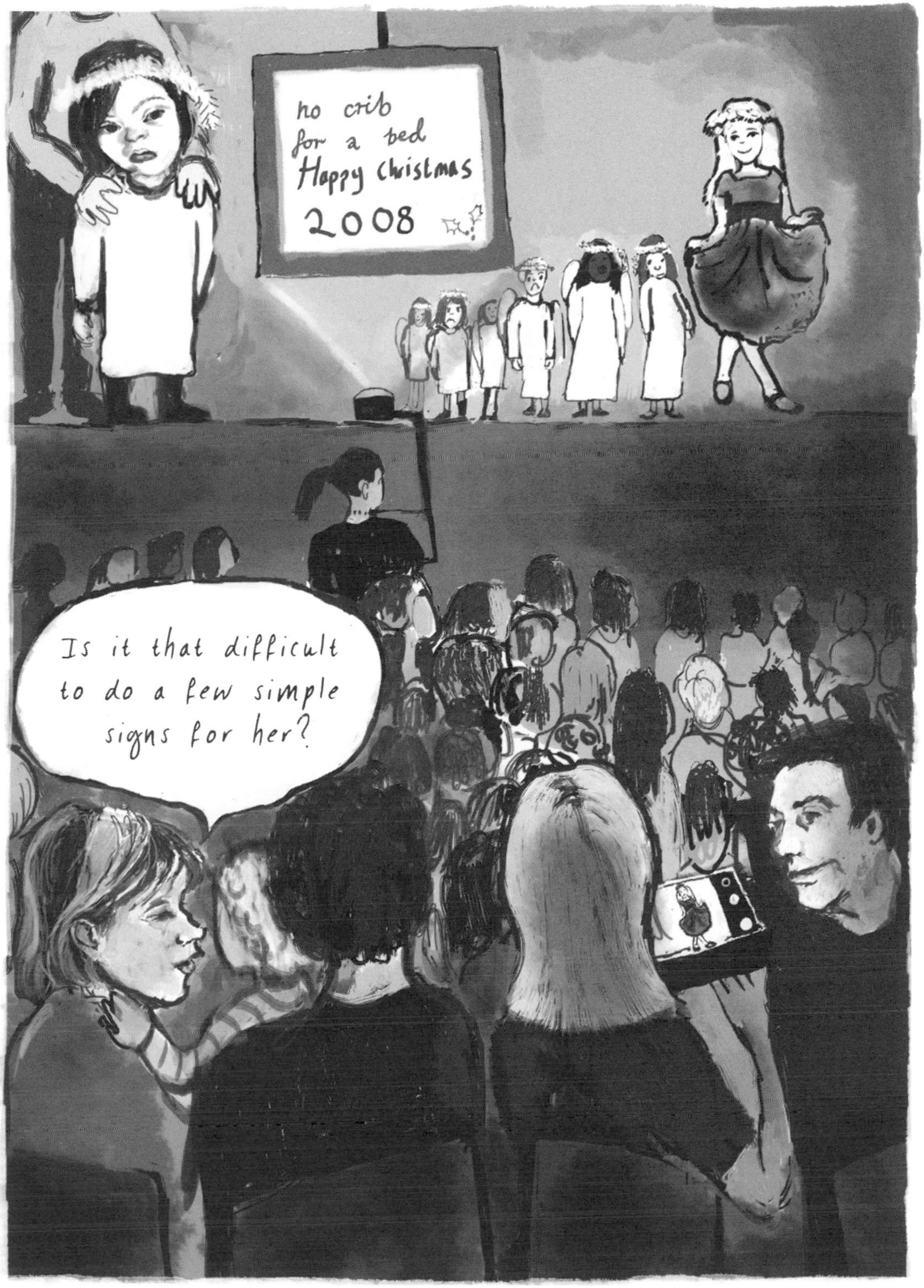
no crib
for a bed
Happy Christmas
2008
Is it that difficult to do a few simple signs for her?

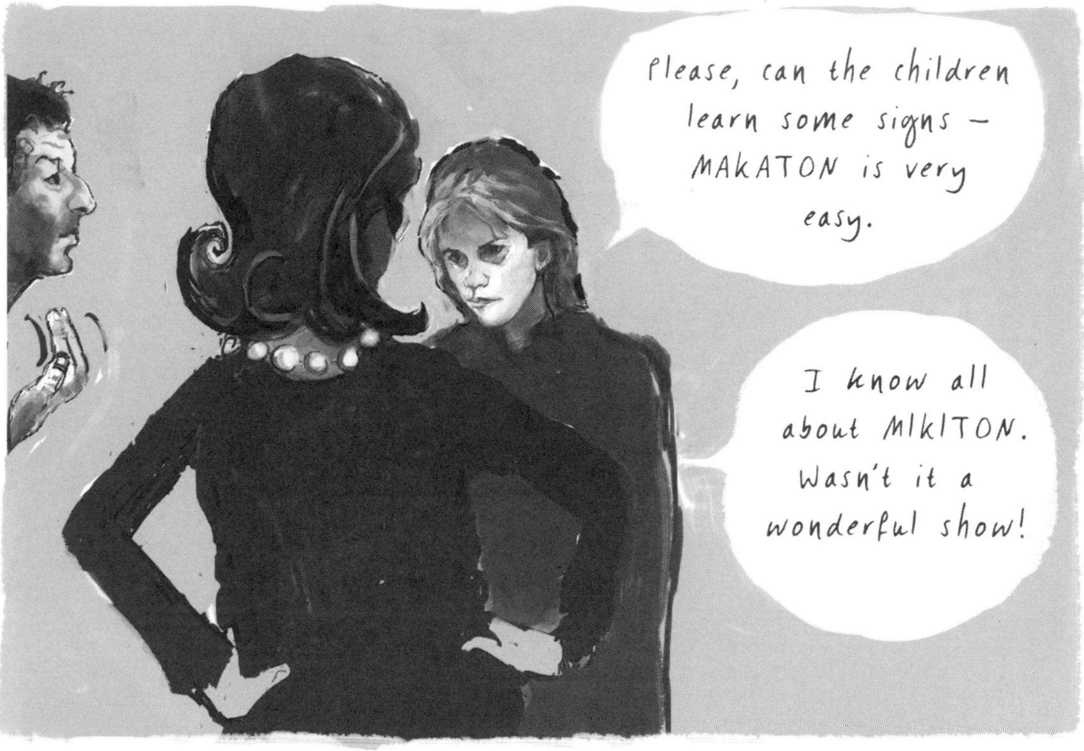
Please, can the children learn some signs – MAKATON is very easy.
I know all about MIKITON. Wasn't it a wonderful show!

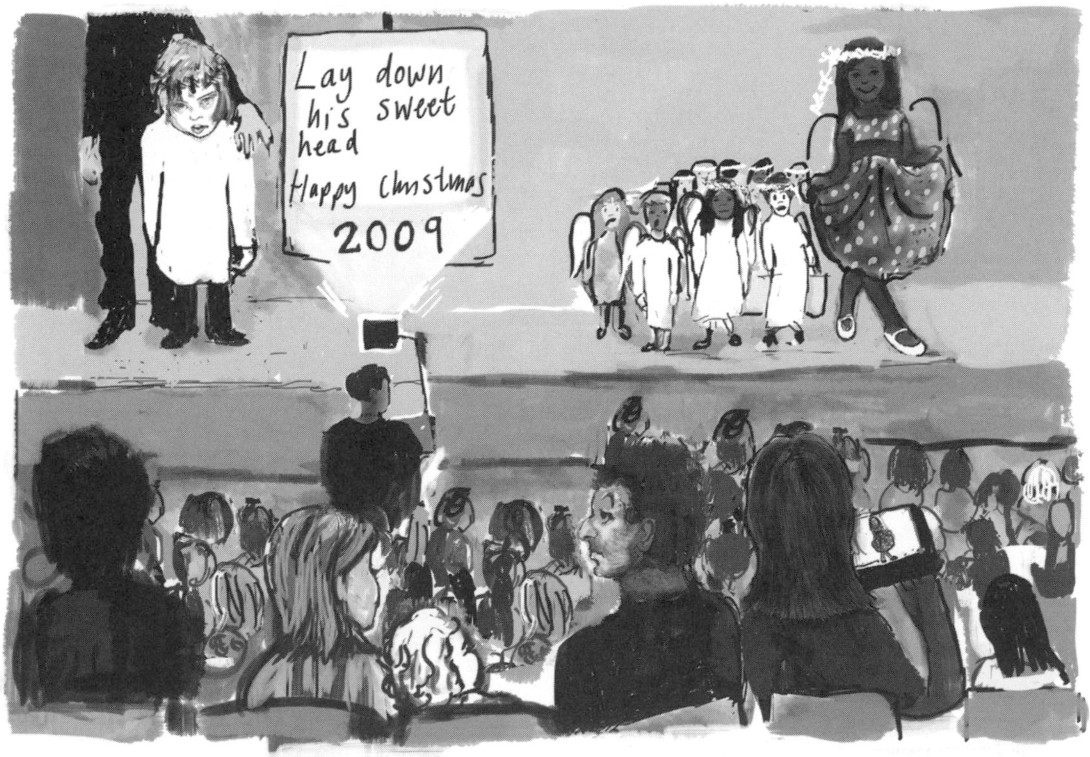
Lay down his sweet head
Happy Christmas
2009

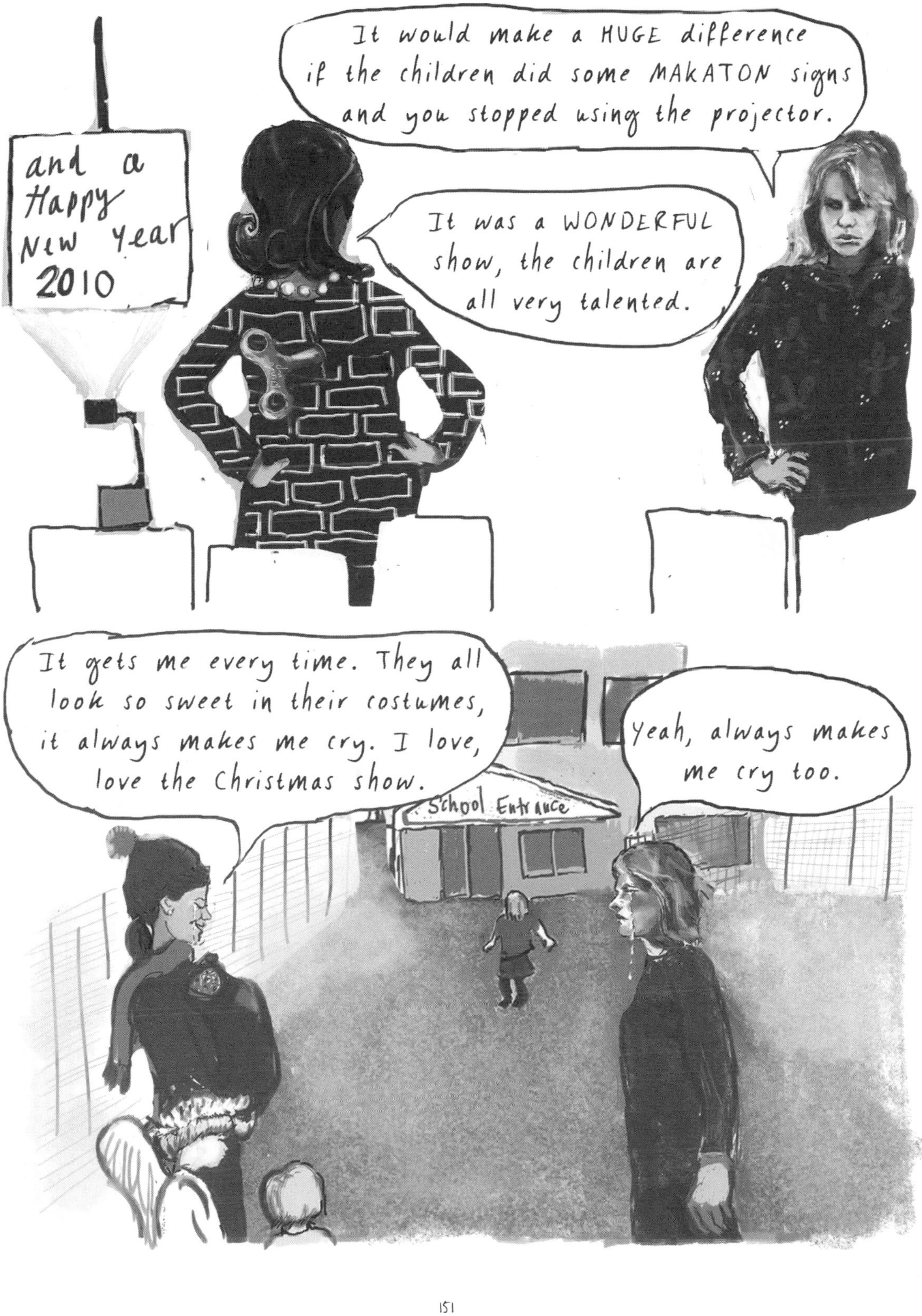
and a Happy New Year 2010
It would make a HUGE difference if the children did some MAKATON signs and you stopped using the projector.
It was a WONDERFUL show, the children are all very talented.
It gets me every time. They all look so sweet in their costumes, it always makes me cry. I love, love the Christmas show.
Yeah, always makes me cry too.
School Entrance

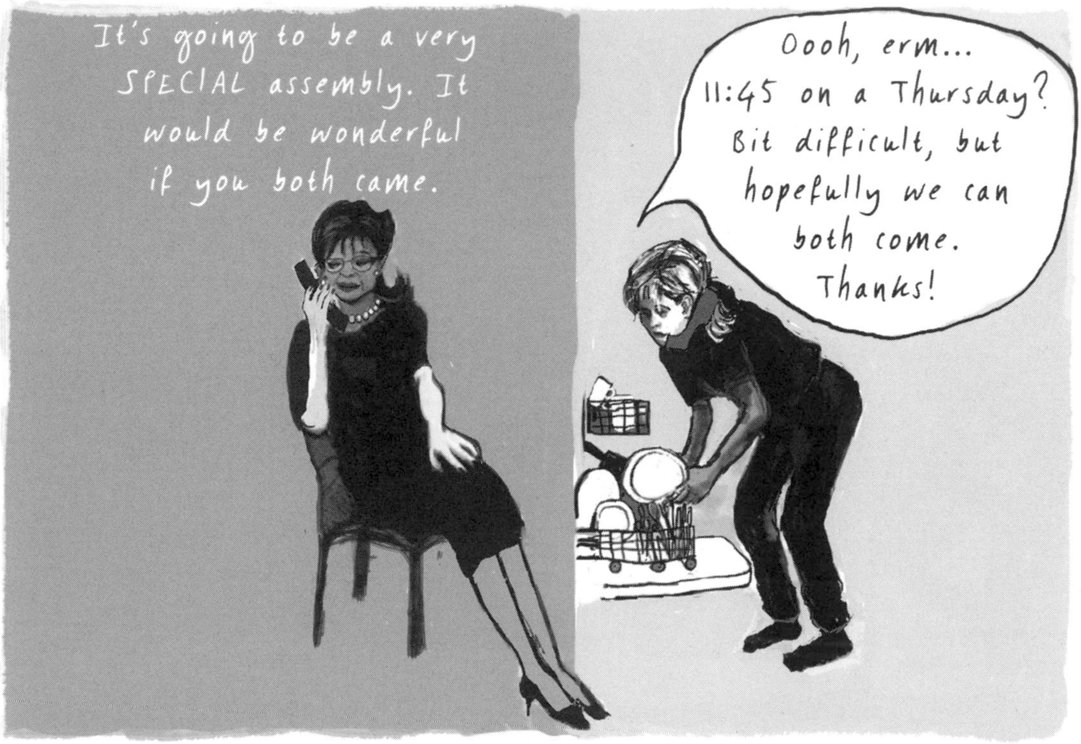
It's going to be a very SPECIAL assembly. It would be wonderful if you both came.
Oooh, erm... 11:45 on a Thursday? Bit difficult, but hopefully we can both come. Thanks!

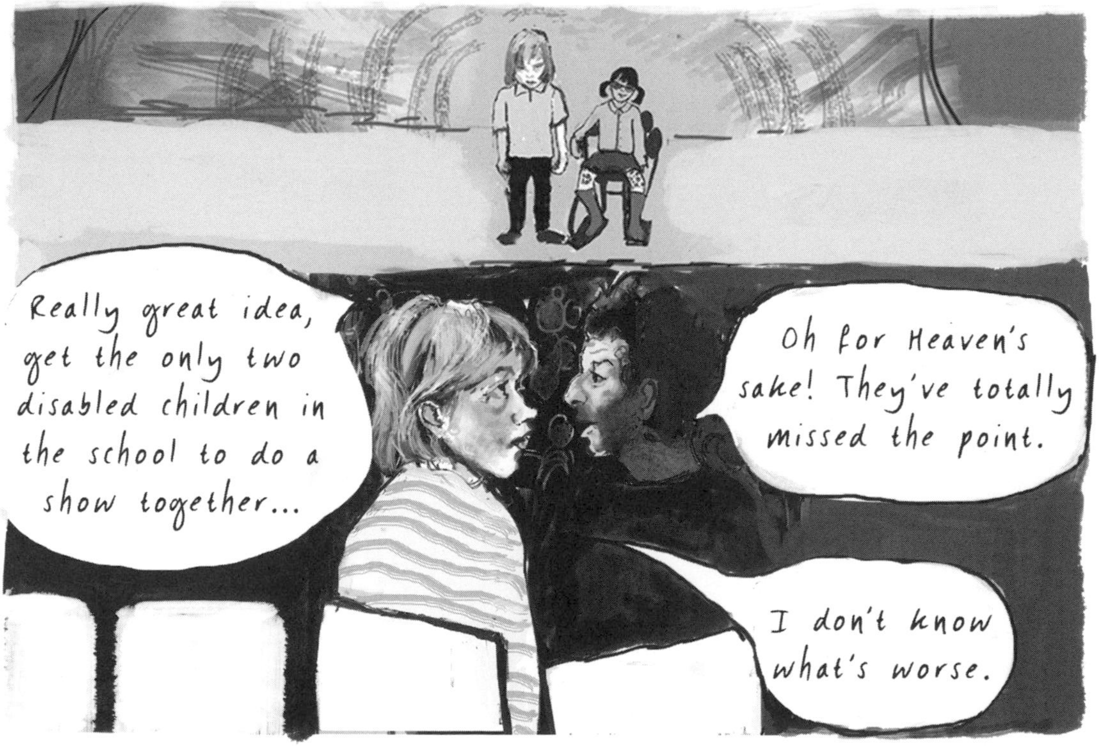
Really great idea, get the only two disabled children in the school to do a show together...
Oh for Heaven's sake! They've totally missed the point.
I don't know what's worse.

June 2011

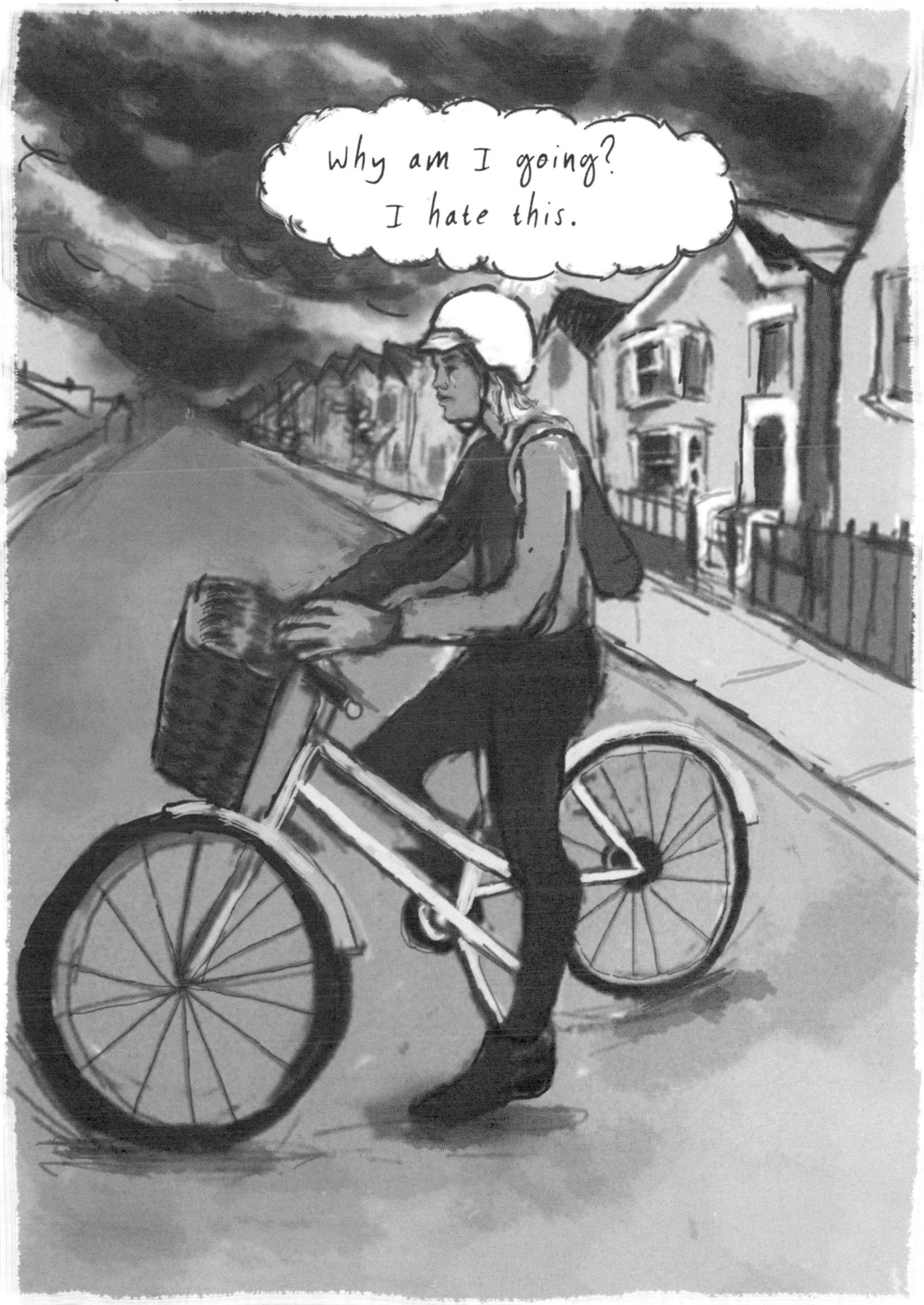
Why am I going?
I hate this.

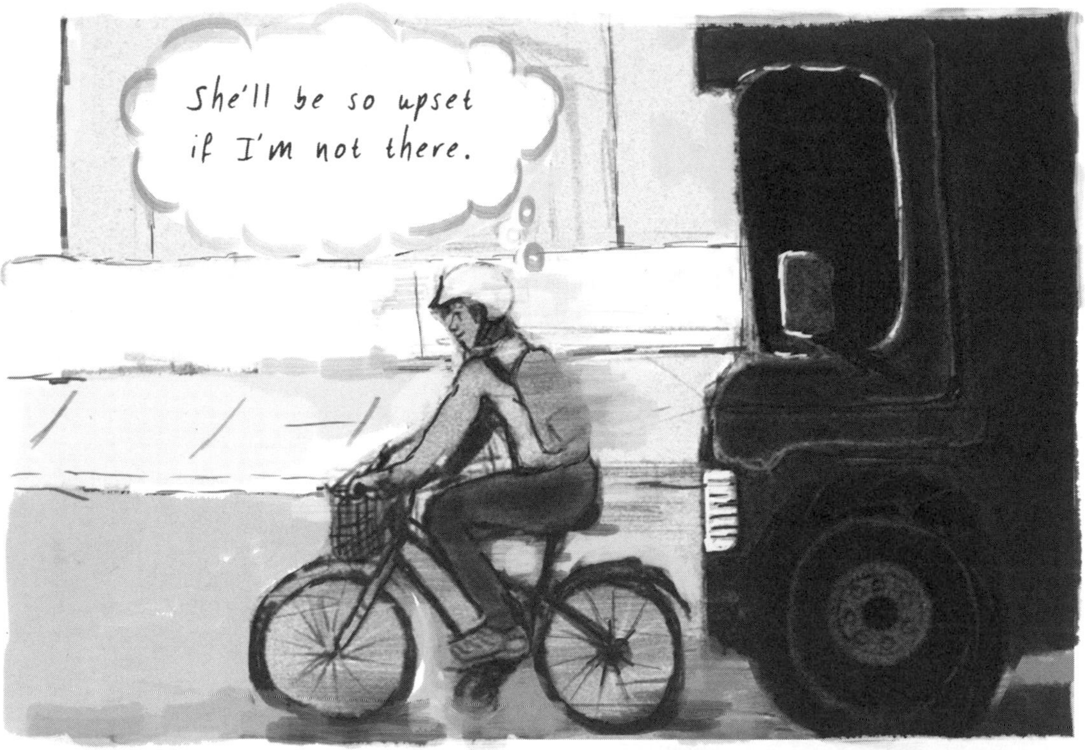
She'll be so upset if I'm not there.

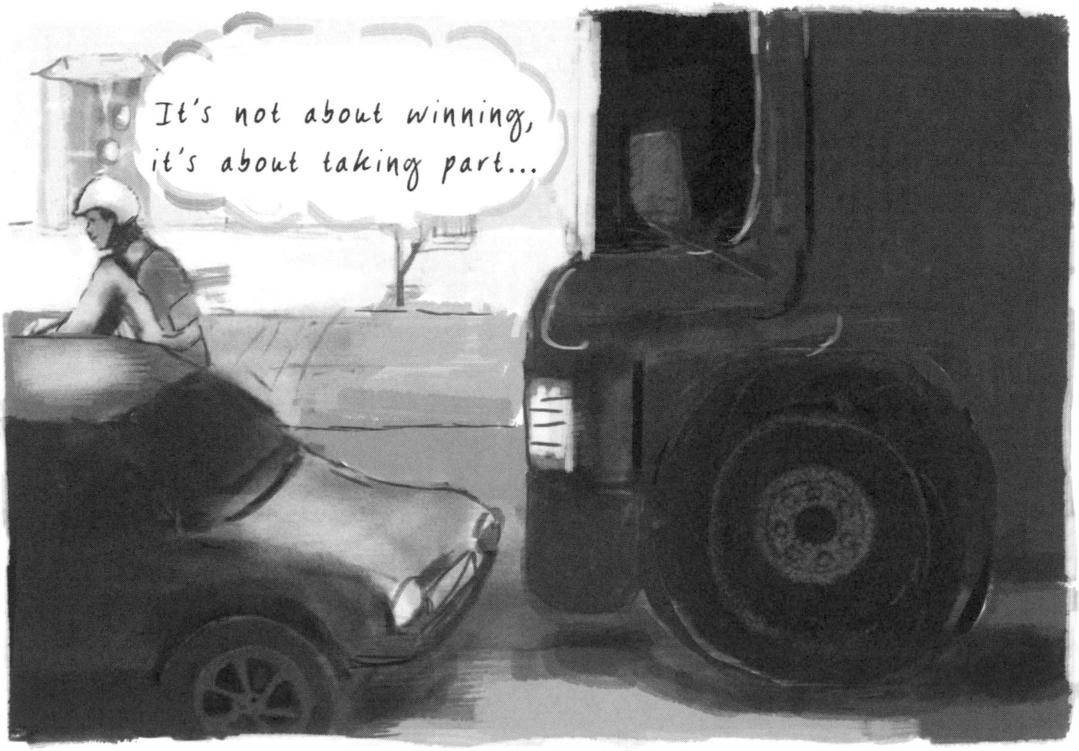
It's not about winning, it's about taking part...

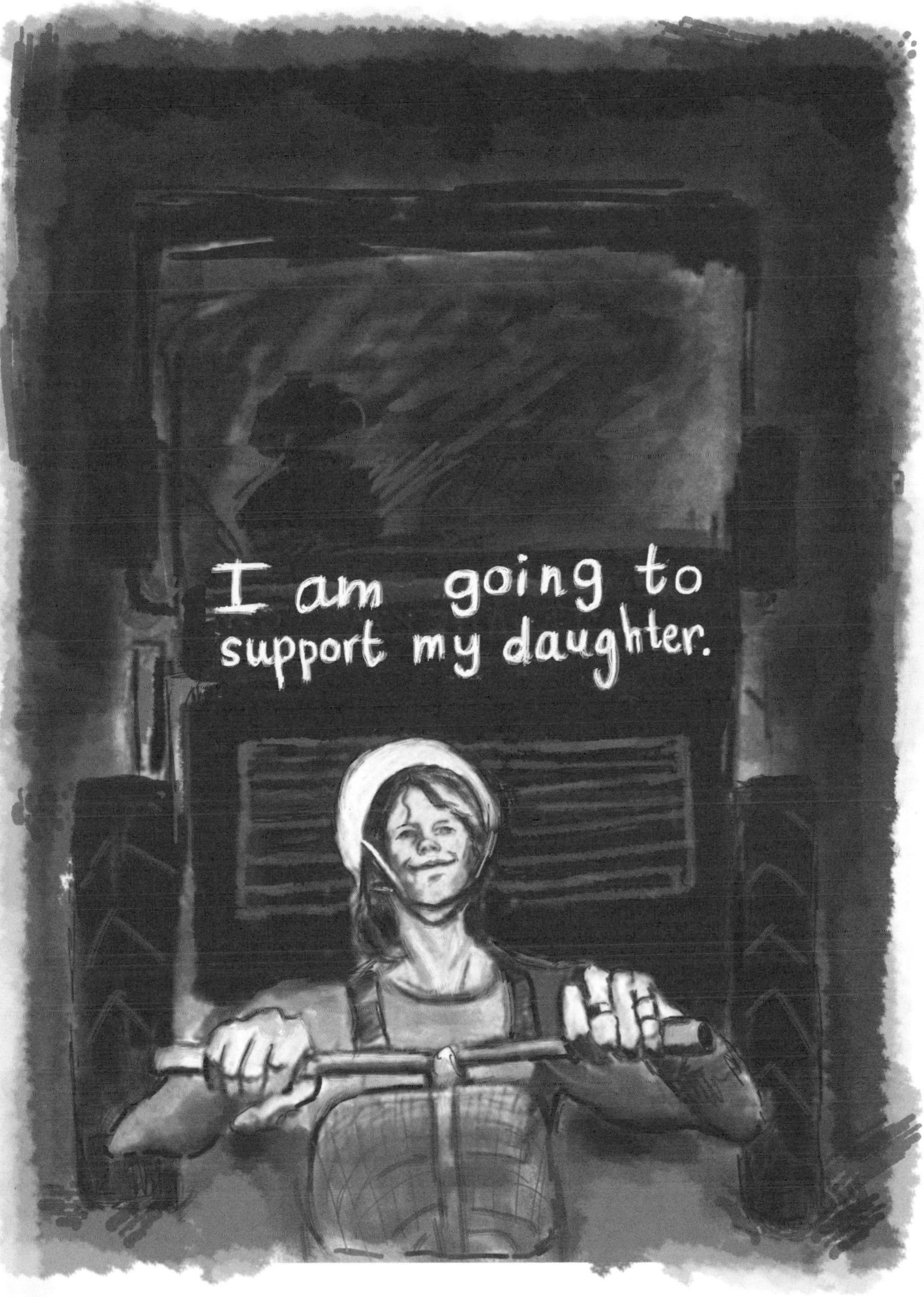
I am going to support my daughter.

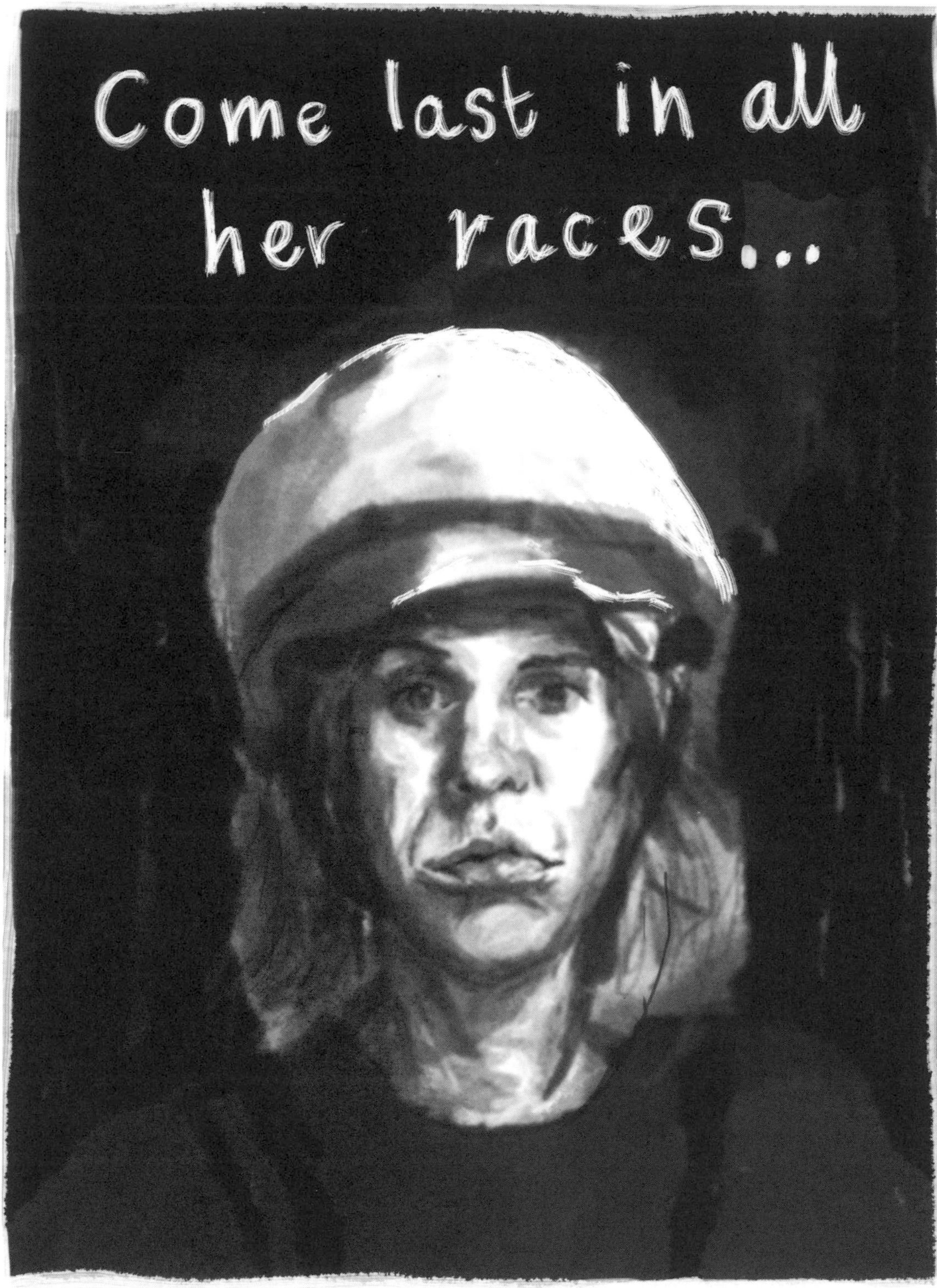
Come last in all her races...

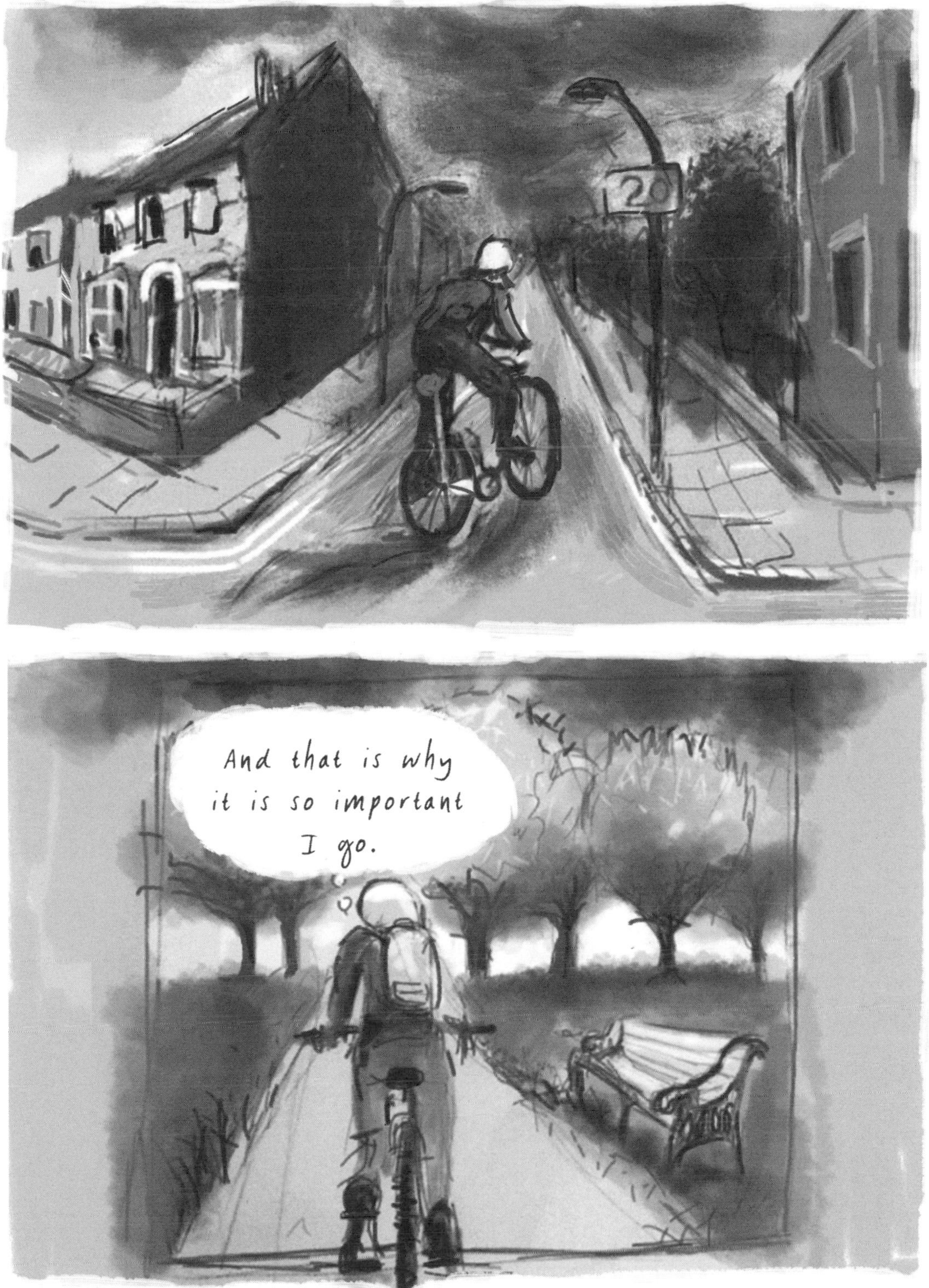
20
And that is why it is so important I go.

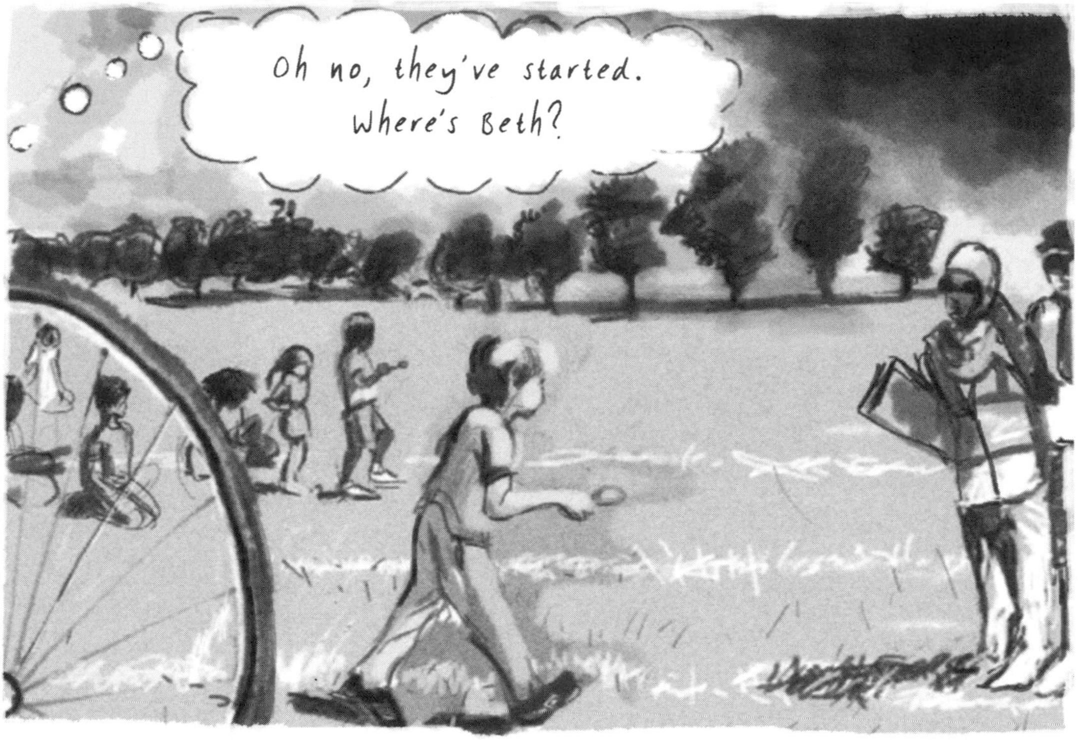
Oh no, they've started.
Where's Beth?

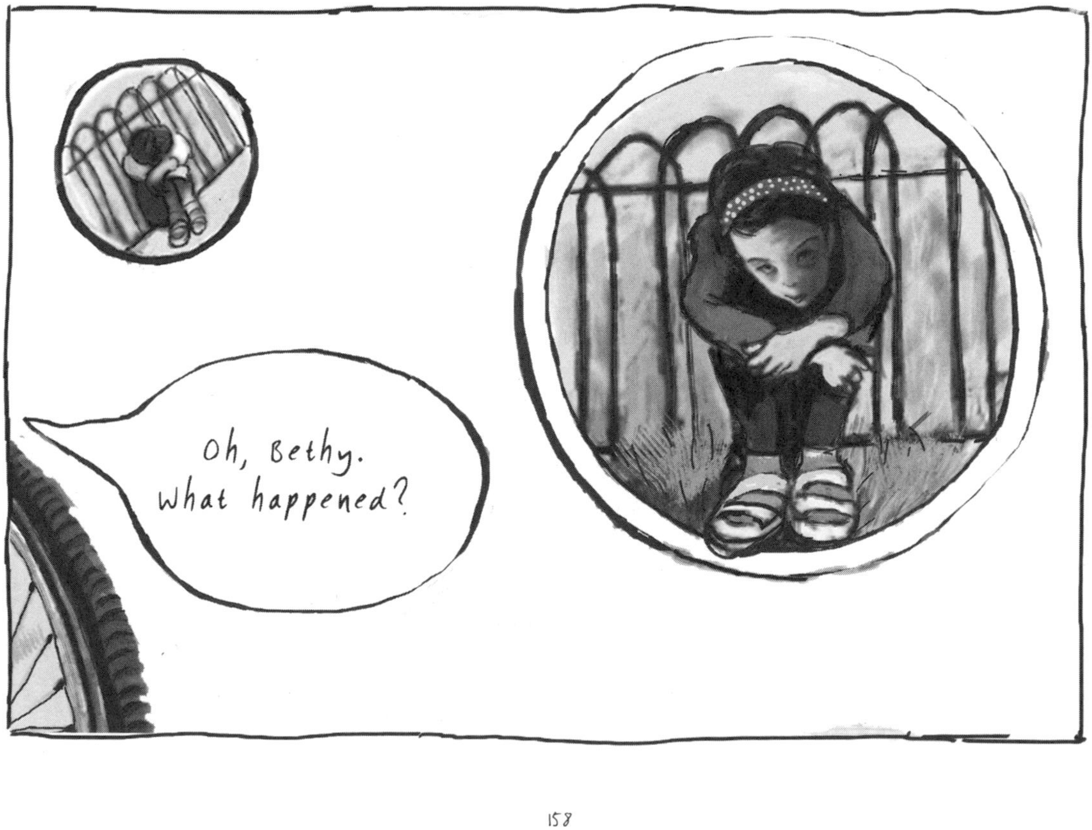
Oh, Bethy.
What happened?

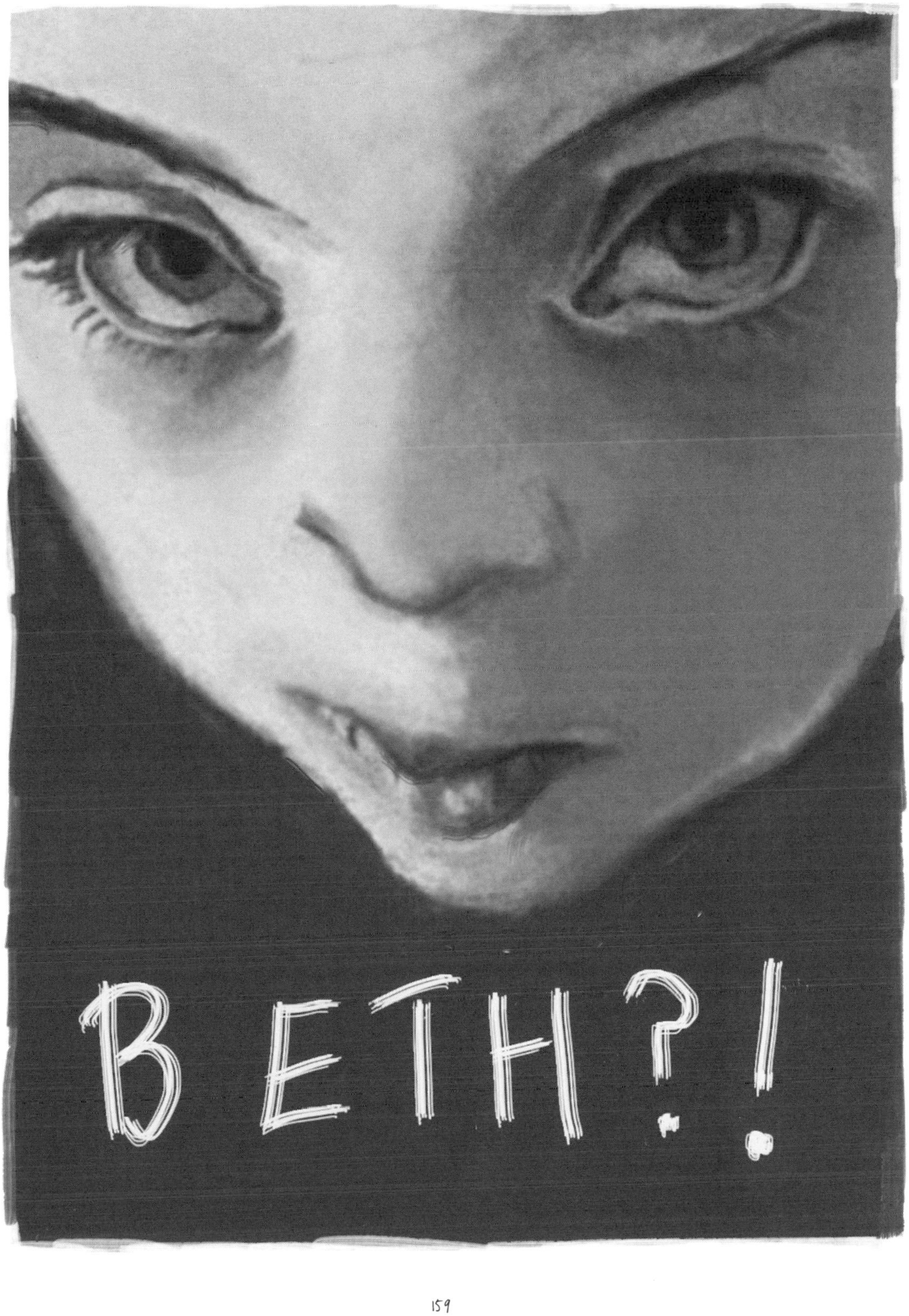
BETH?!

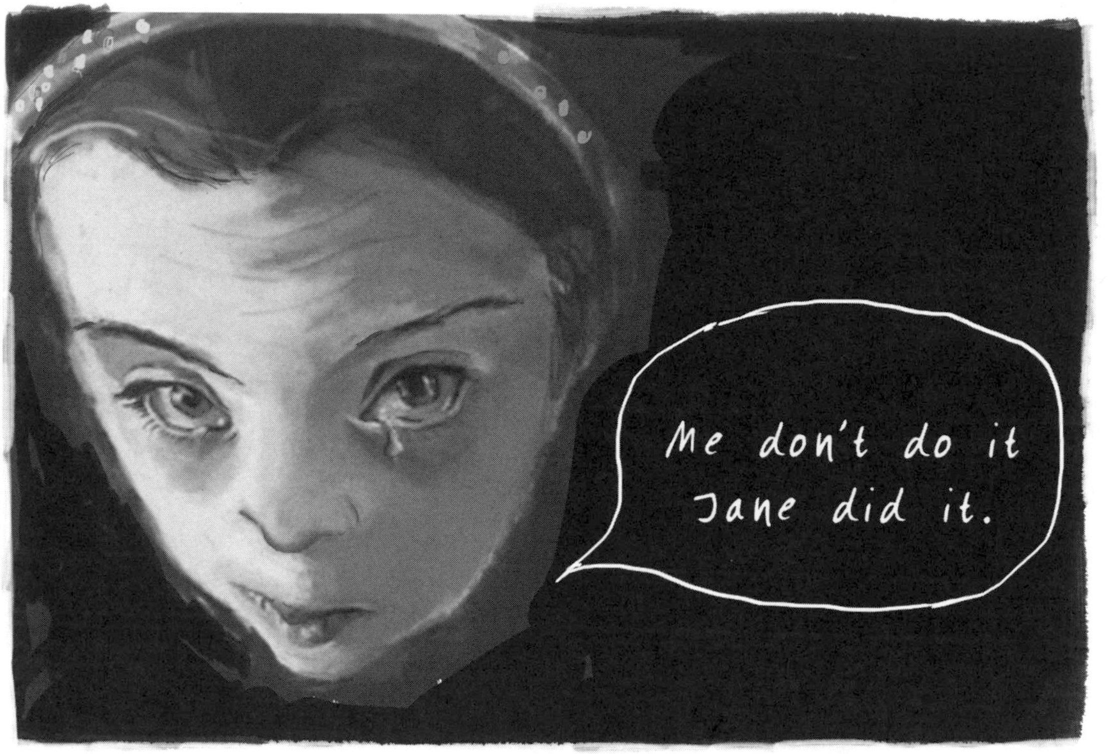
Me don't do it Jane did it.

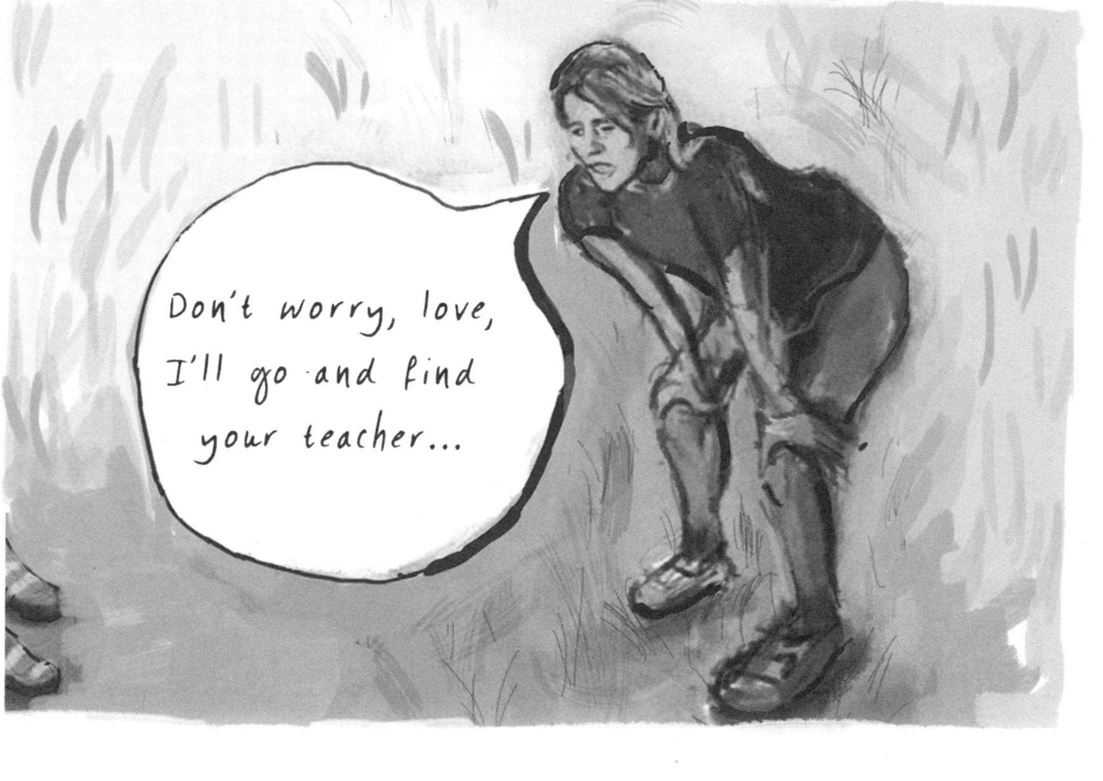
Don't worry, love, I'll go and find your teacher...

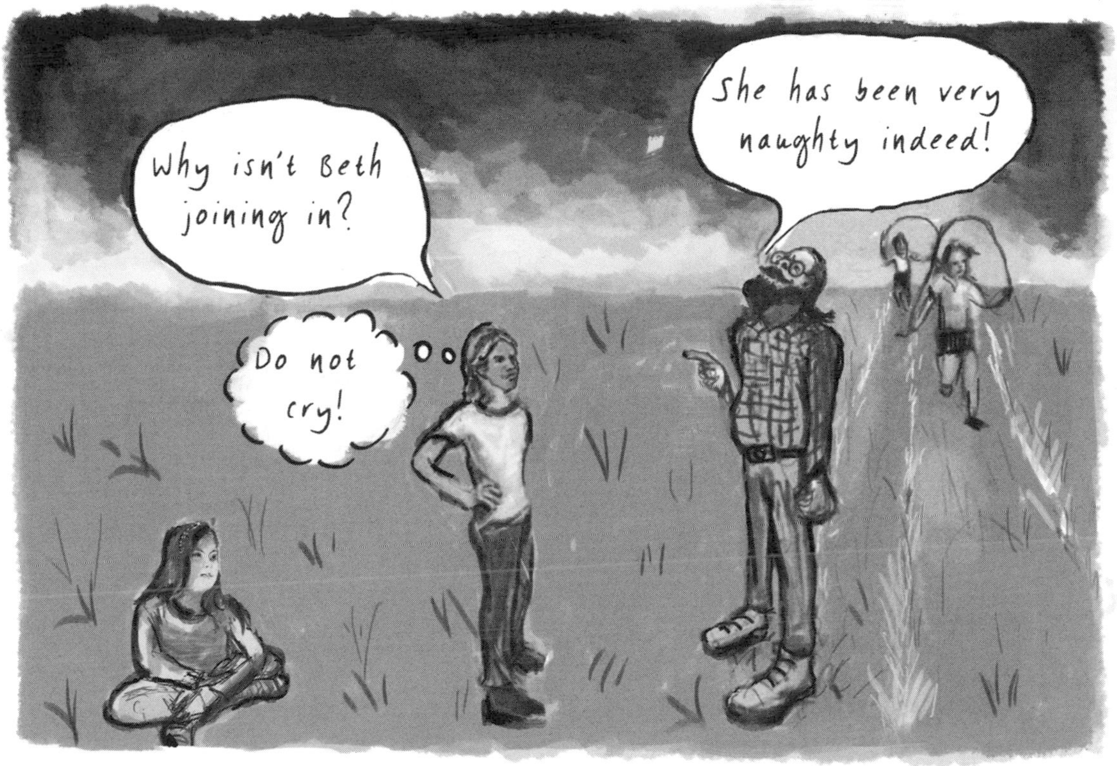
Why isn't Beth joining in?
She has been very naughty indeed!
Do not cry!

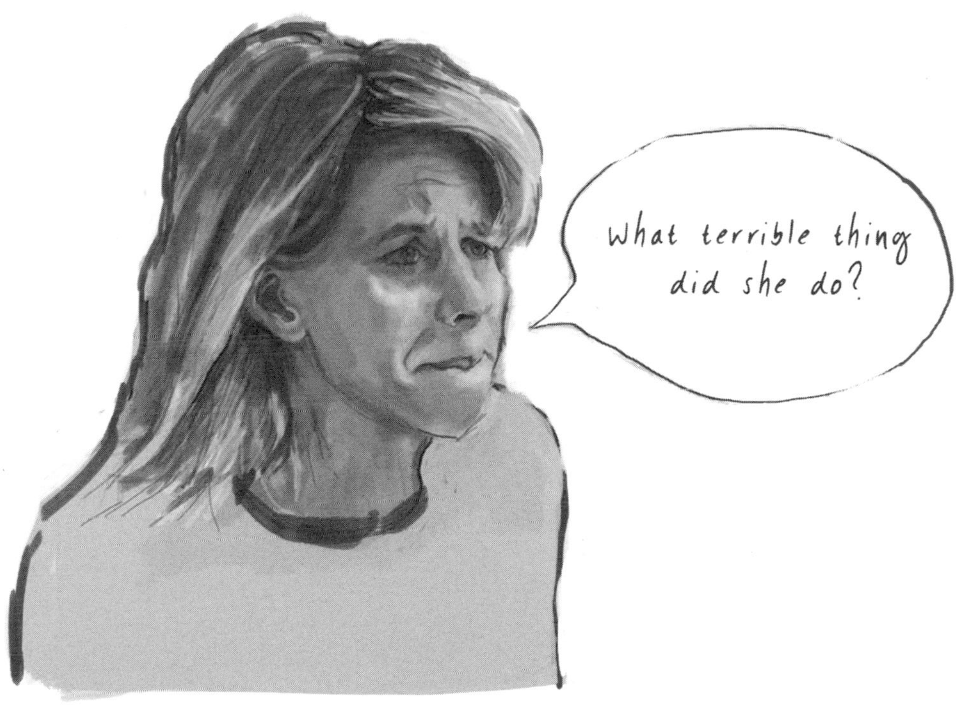
What terrible thing did she do?

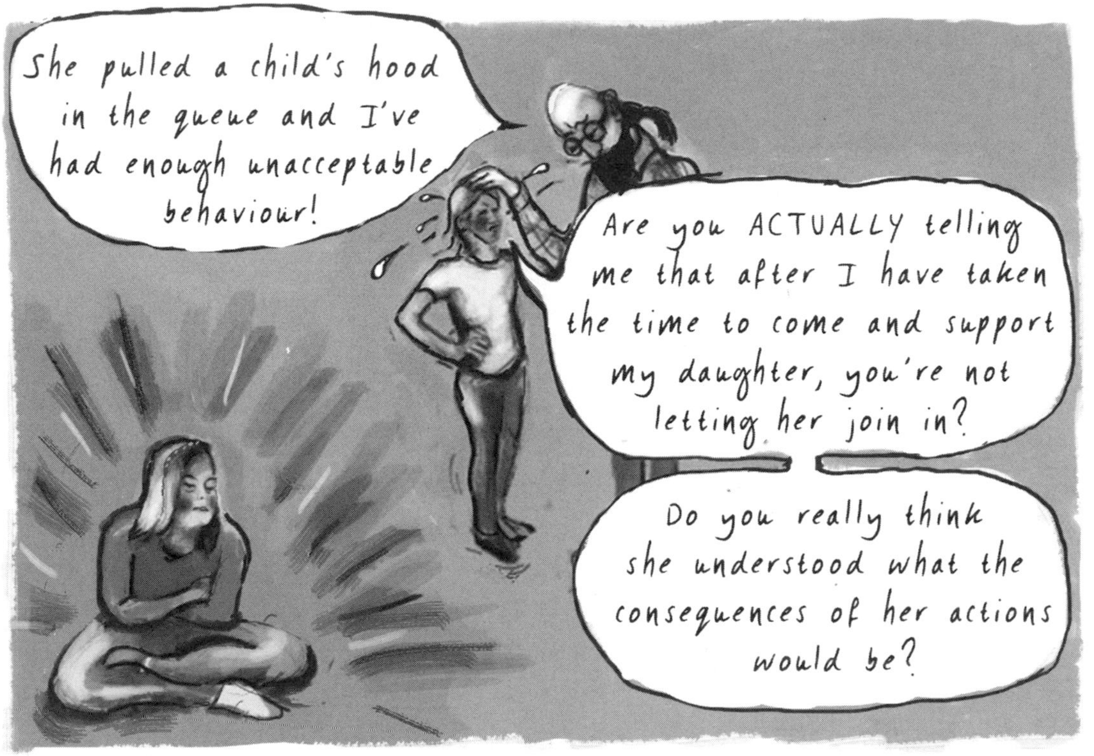
She pulled a child's hood in the queue and I've had enough unacceptable behaviour!
Are you ACTUALLY telling me that after I have taken the time to come and support my daughter, you're not letting her join in?
Do you really think she understood what the consequences of her actions would be?

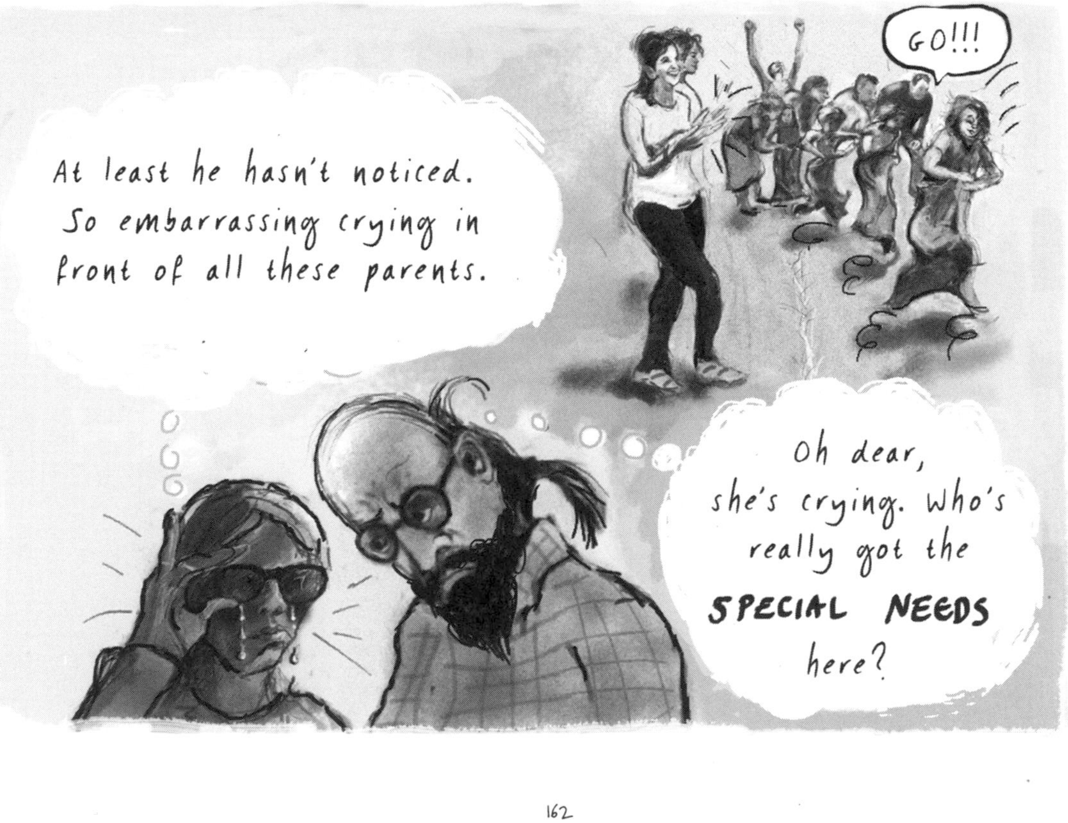
GO!!!
At least he hasn't noticed. So embarrassing crying in front of all these parents.
Oh dear, she's crying. Who's really got the SPECIAL NEEDS here?

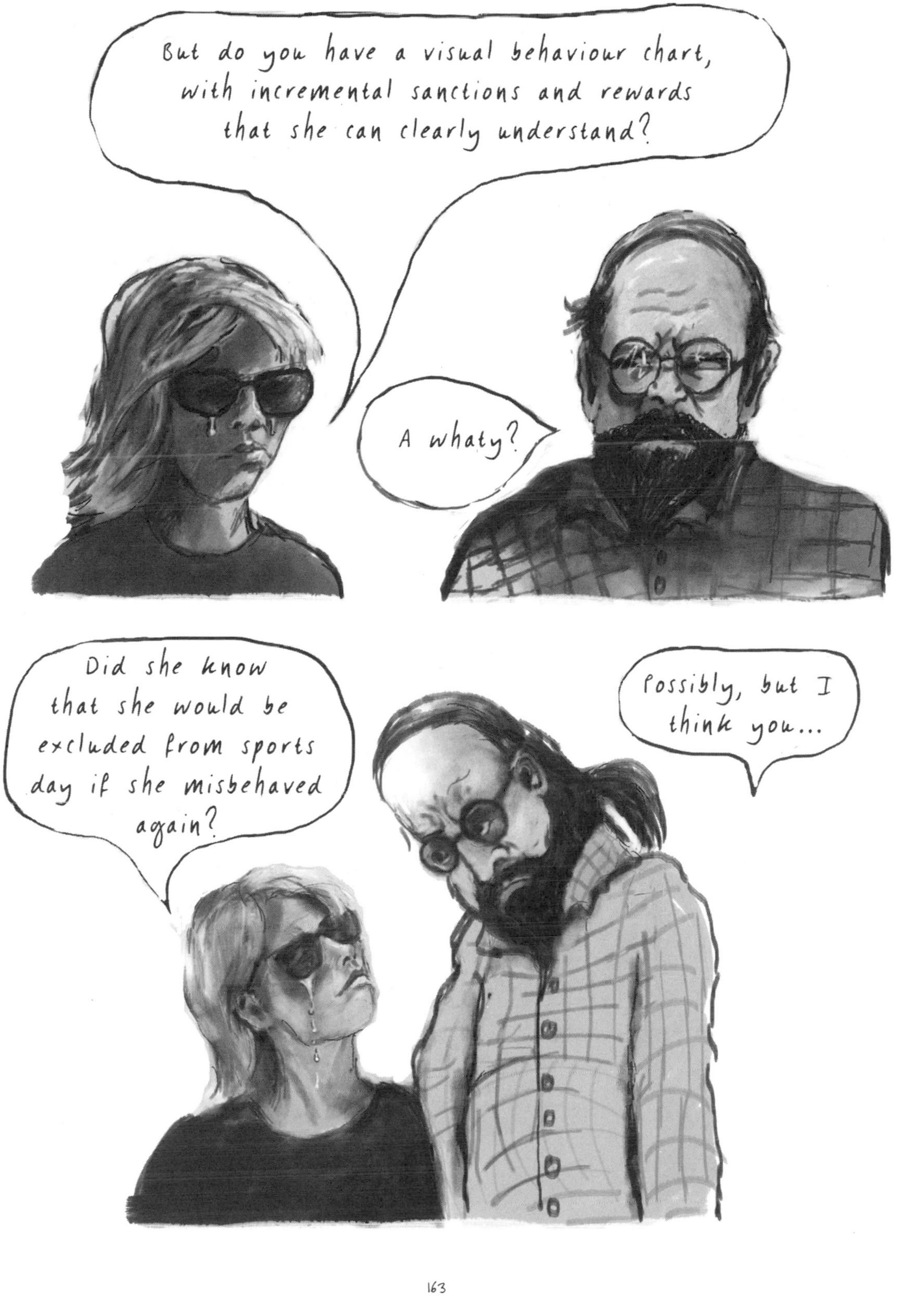
But do you have a visual behaviour chart, with incremental sanctions and rewards that she can clearly understand?
A whaty?
Did she know that she would be excluded from sports day if she misbehaved again?
Possibly, but I think you...

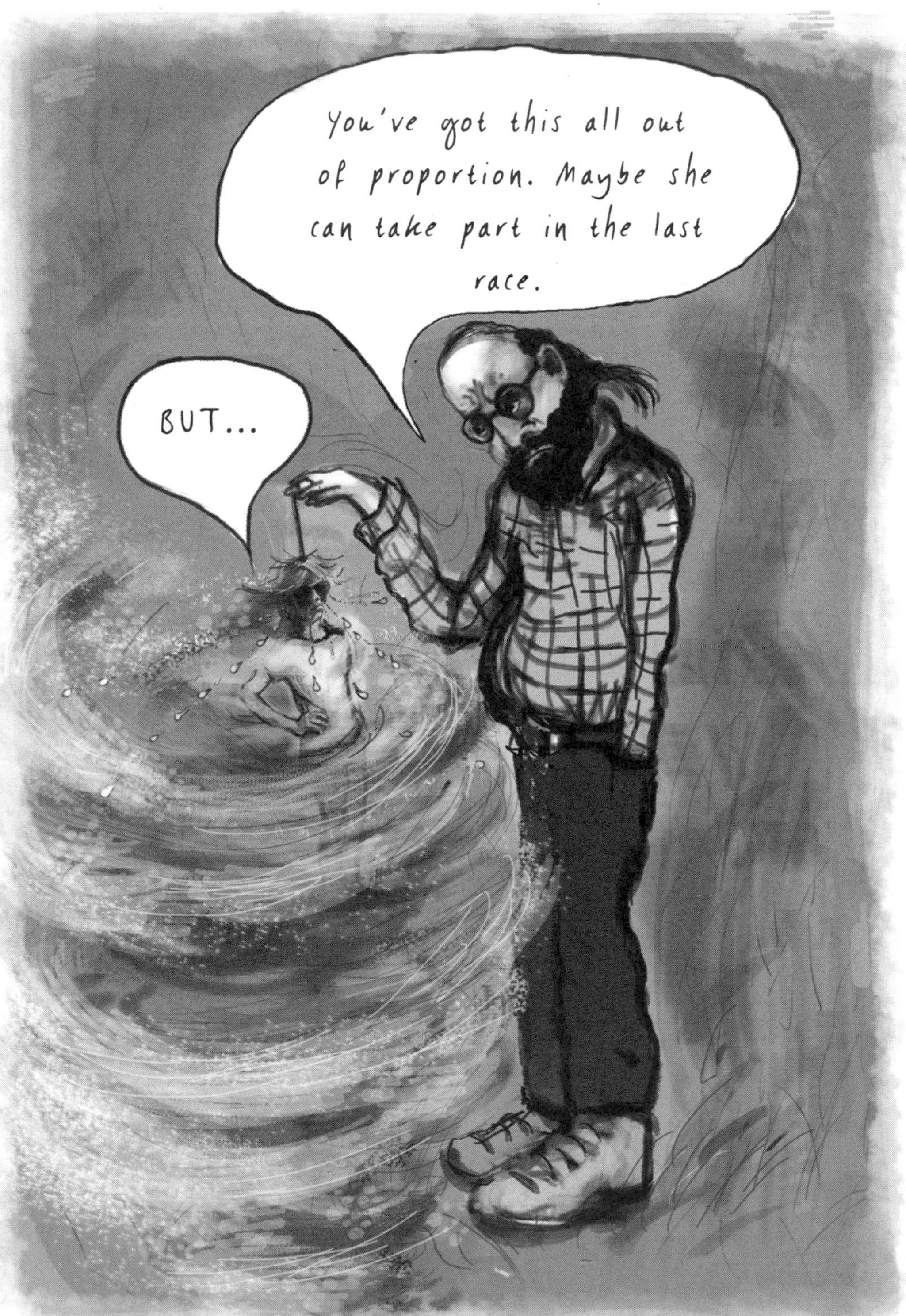
You've got this all out of proportion. Maybe she can take part in the last race.
BUT...

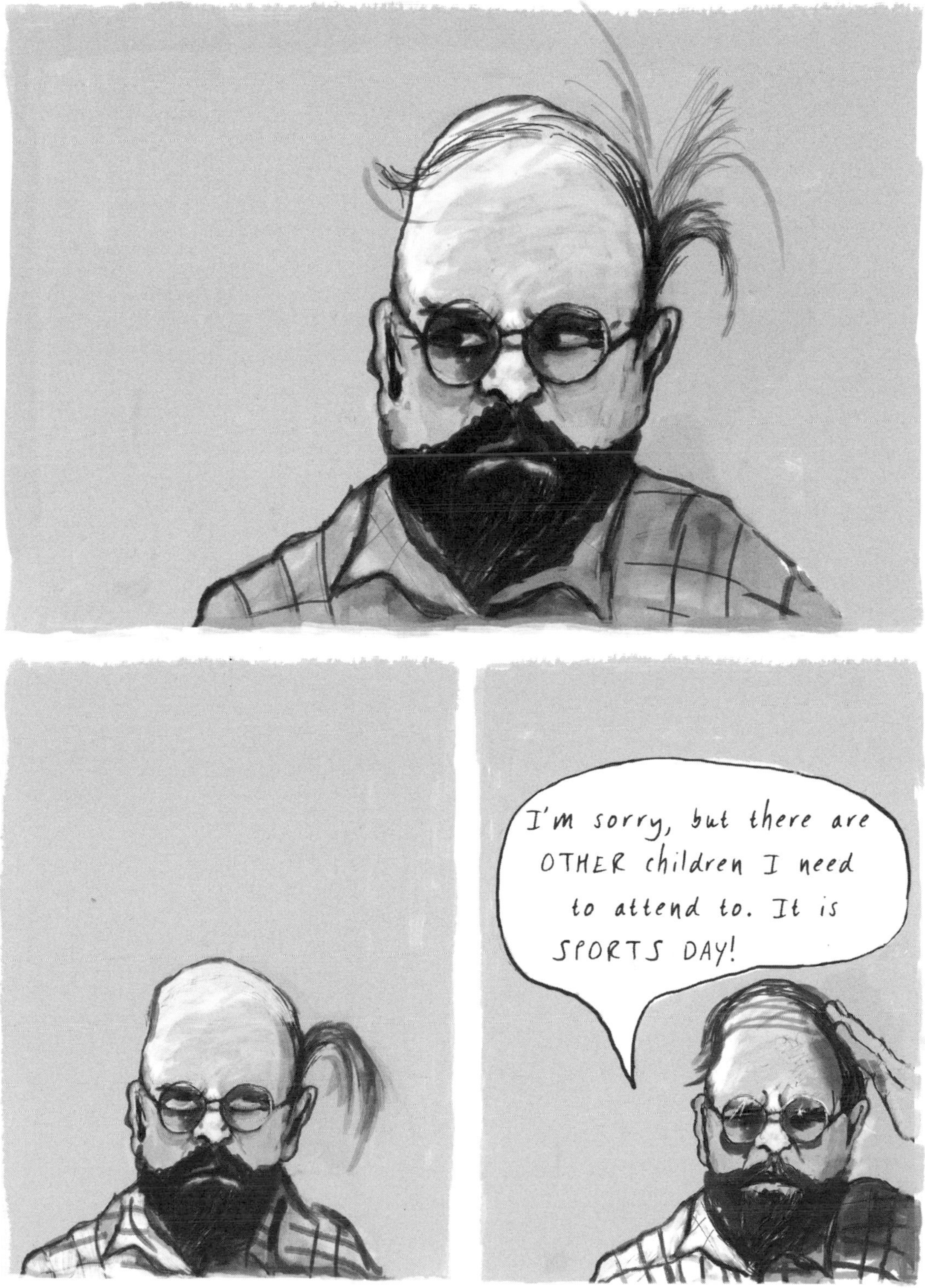
I'm sorry, but there are OTHER children I need to attend to. It is SPORTS DAY!

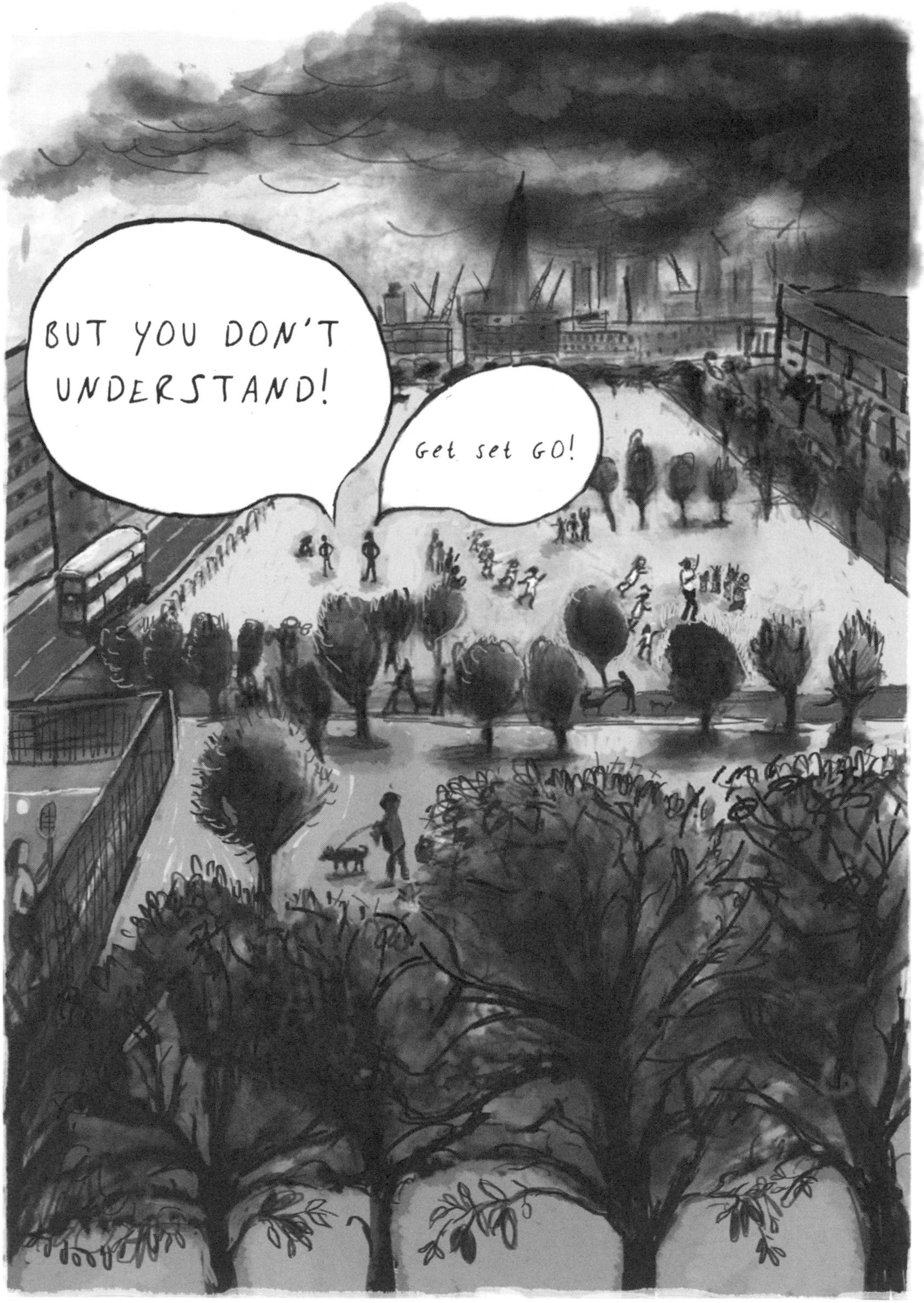
BUT YOU DON'T UNDERSTAND!
Get set GO!

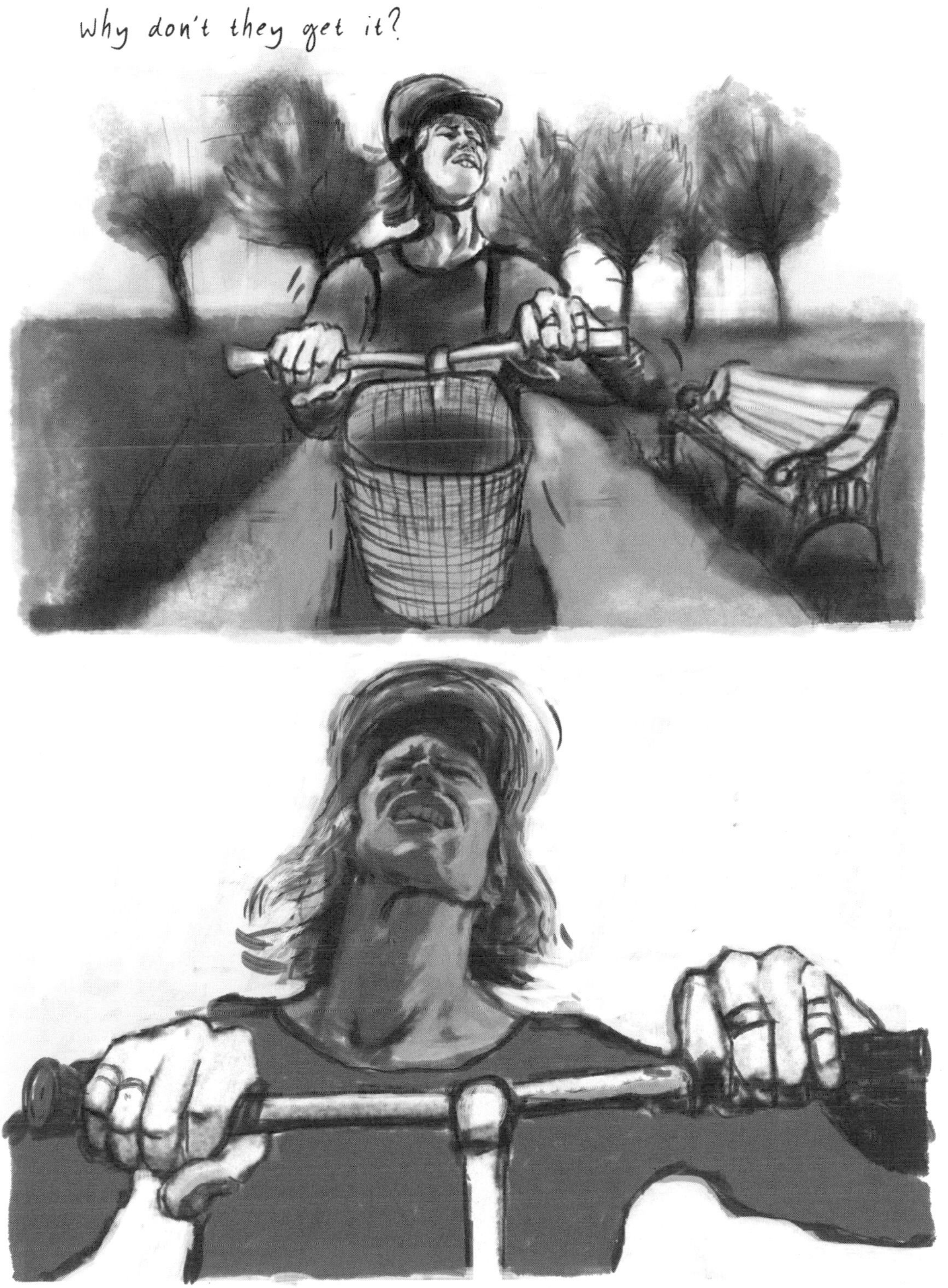
why don't they get it?

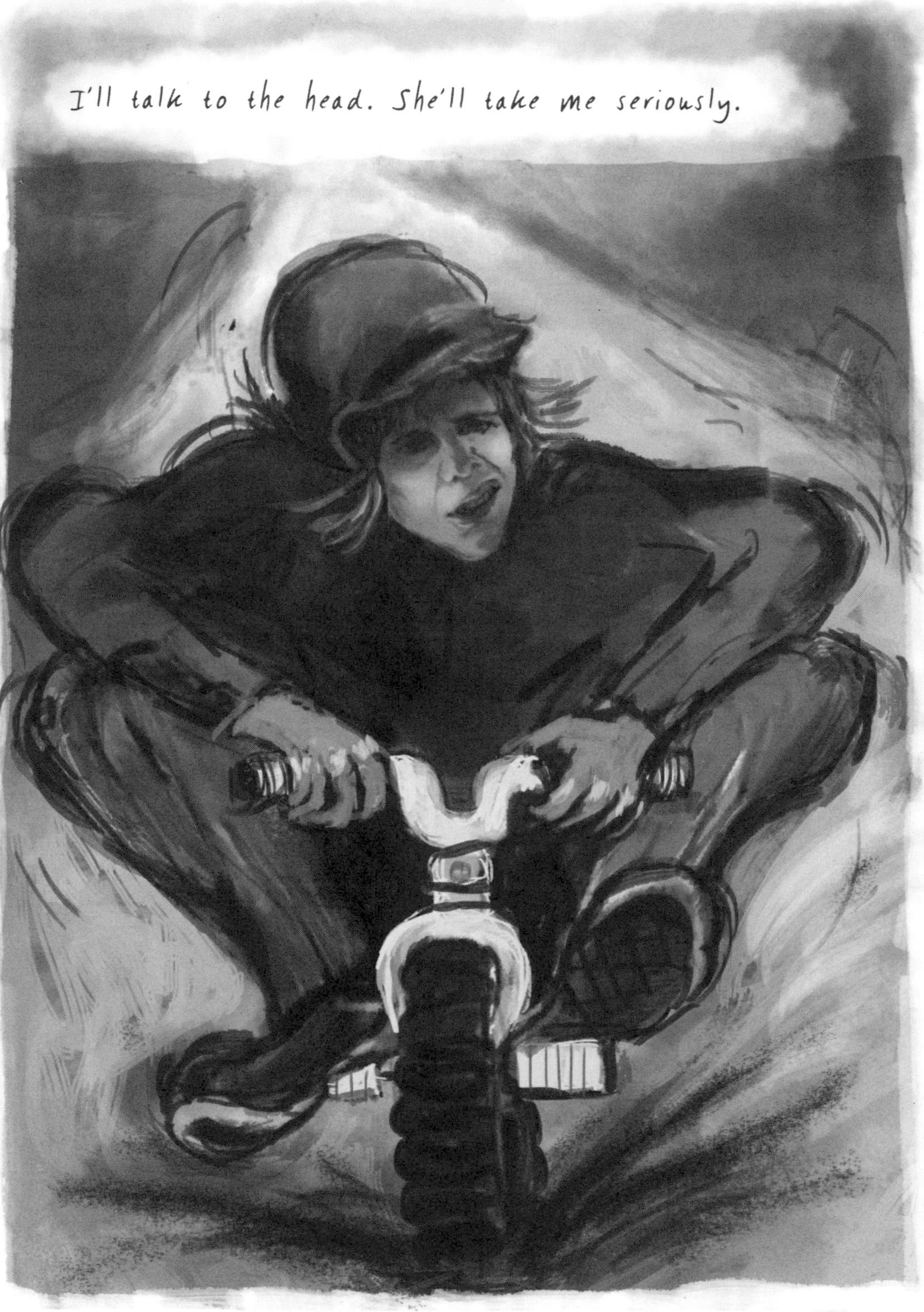
I'll talk to the head. She'll take me seriously.

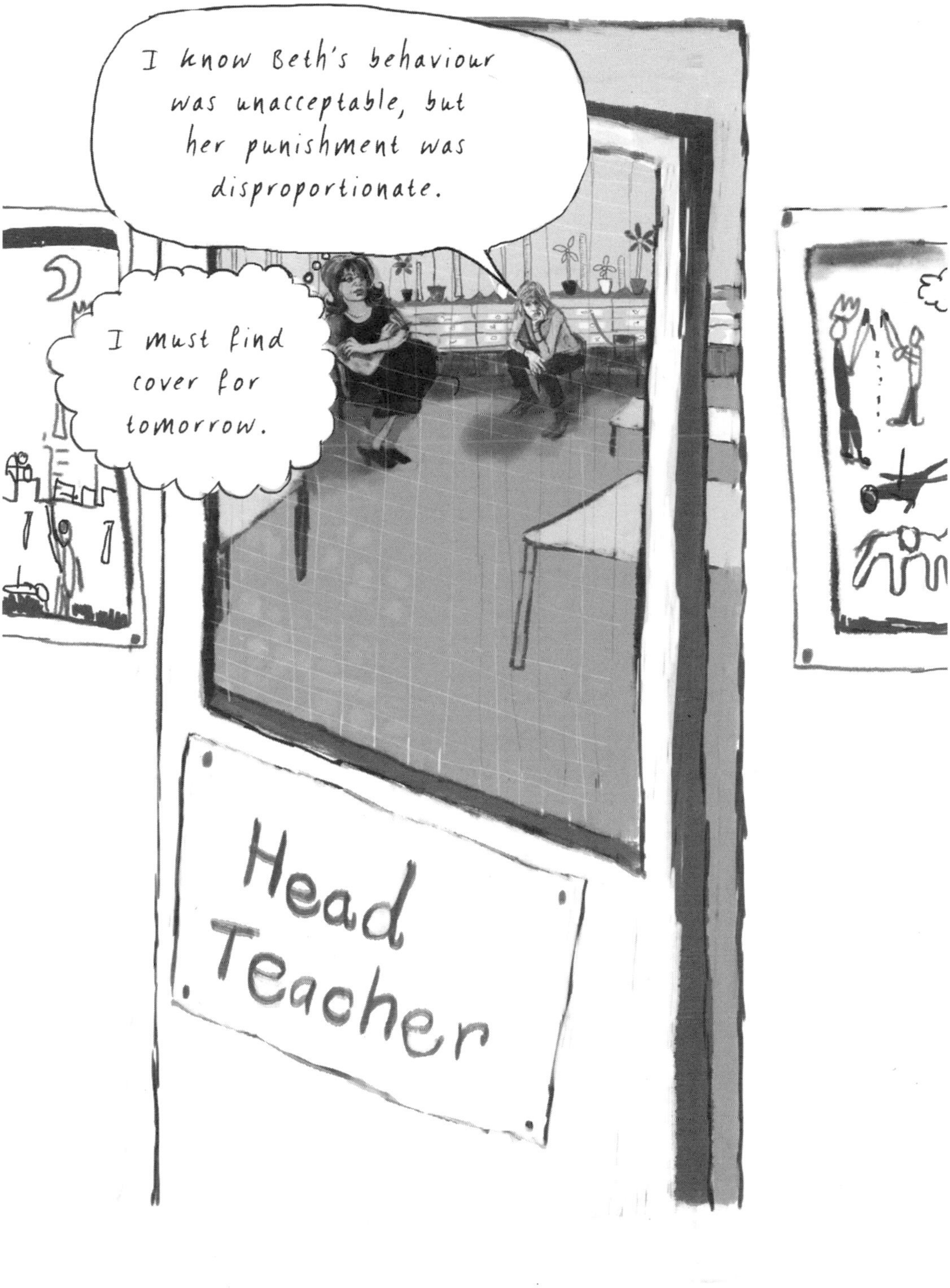
I know Beth's behaviour was unacceptable, but her punishment was disproportionate.
I must find cover for tomorrow.
Head Teacher

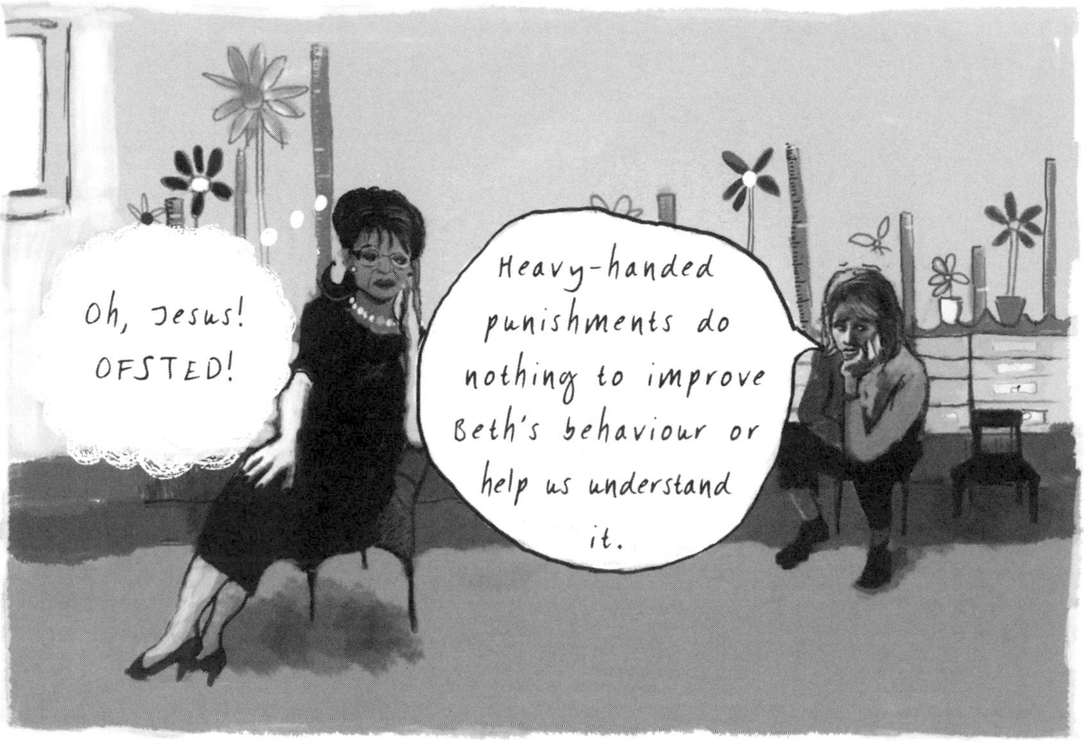
Oh, Jesus! OFSTED!
Heavy-handed punishments do nothing to improve Beth's behaviour or help us understand it.

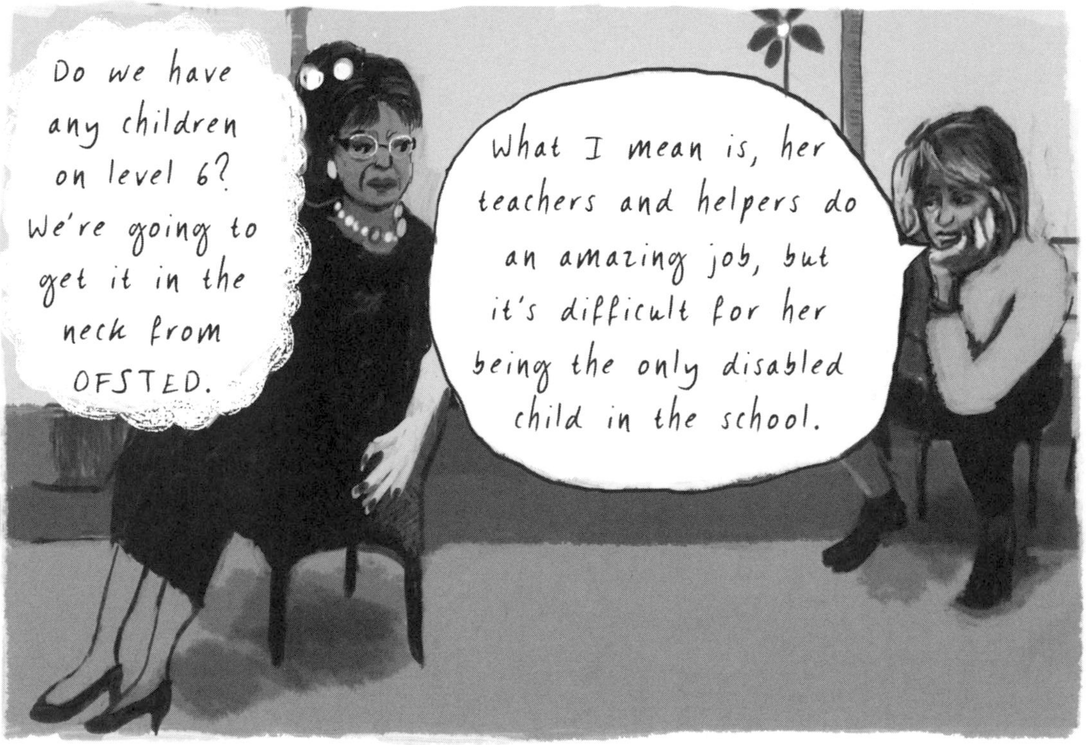
Do we have any children on level 6? We're going to get it in the neck from OFSTED.
What I mean is, her teachers and helpers do an amazing job, but it's difficult for her being the only disabled child in the school.

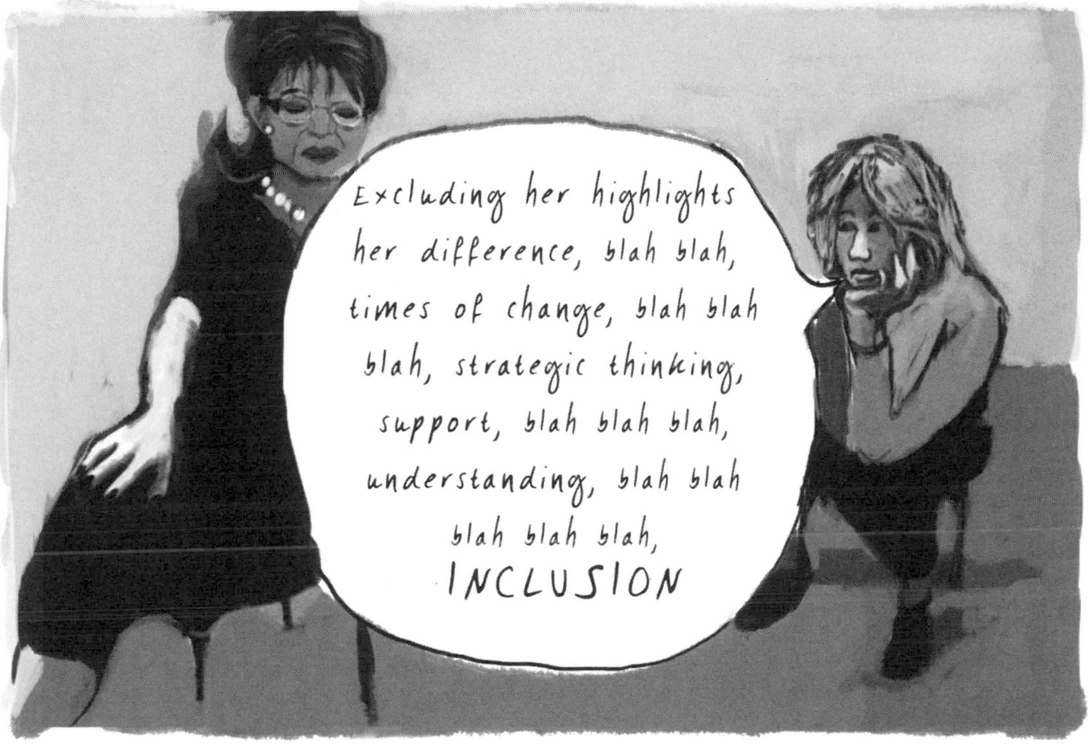
Excluding her highlights her difference, blah blah, times of change, blah blah blah, strategic thinking, support, blah blah blah, understanding, blah blah blah blah blah,
INCLUSION

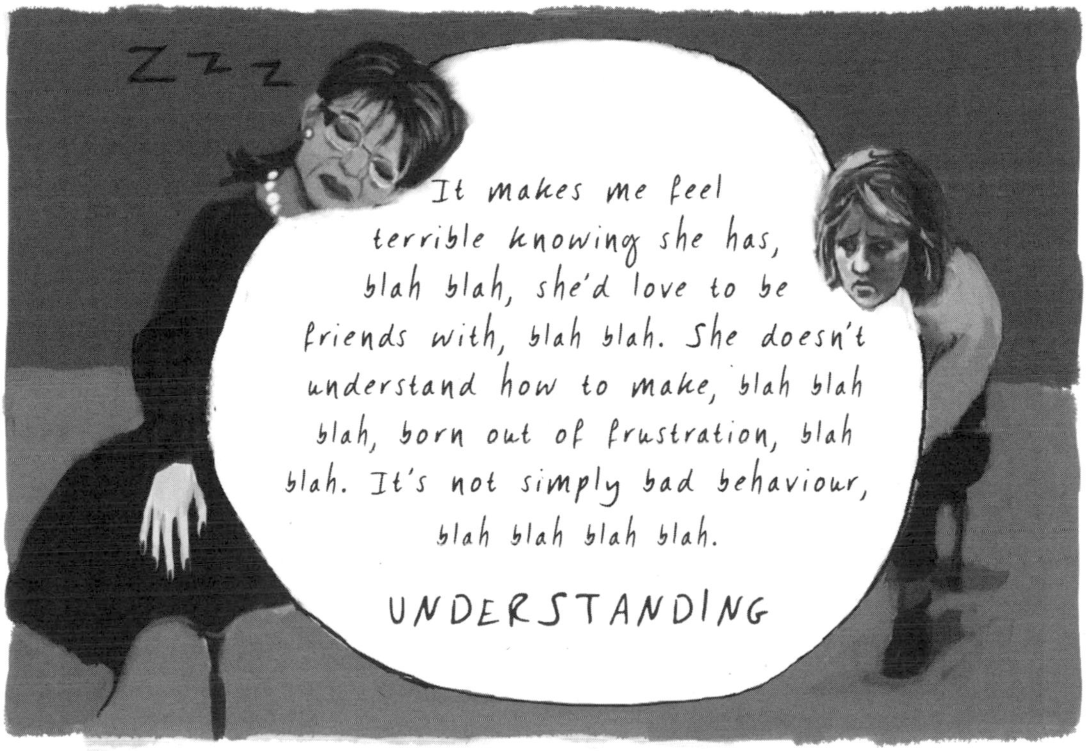
ZZZ
It makes me feel terrible knowing she has, blah blah, she'd love to be friends with, blah blah. She doesn't understand how to make, blah blah blah, born out of frustration, blah blah. It's not simply bad behaviour, blah blah blah blah.
UNDERSTANDING

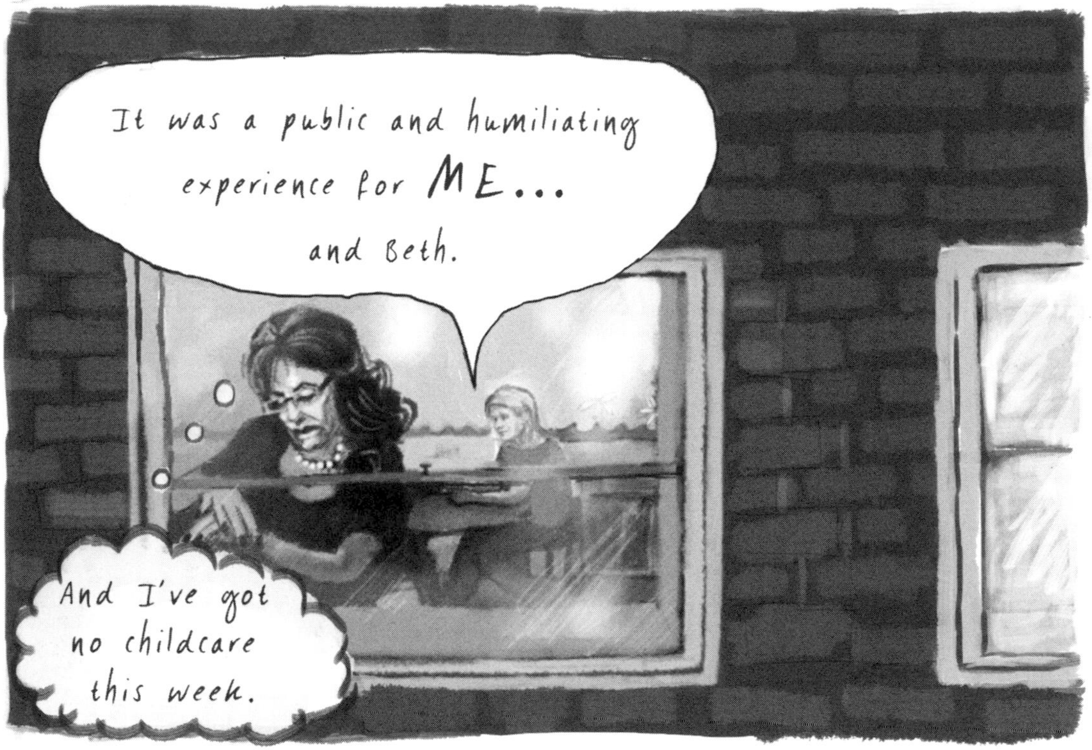
It was a public and humiliating experience for ME... and Beth.
And I've got no childcare this week.

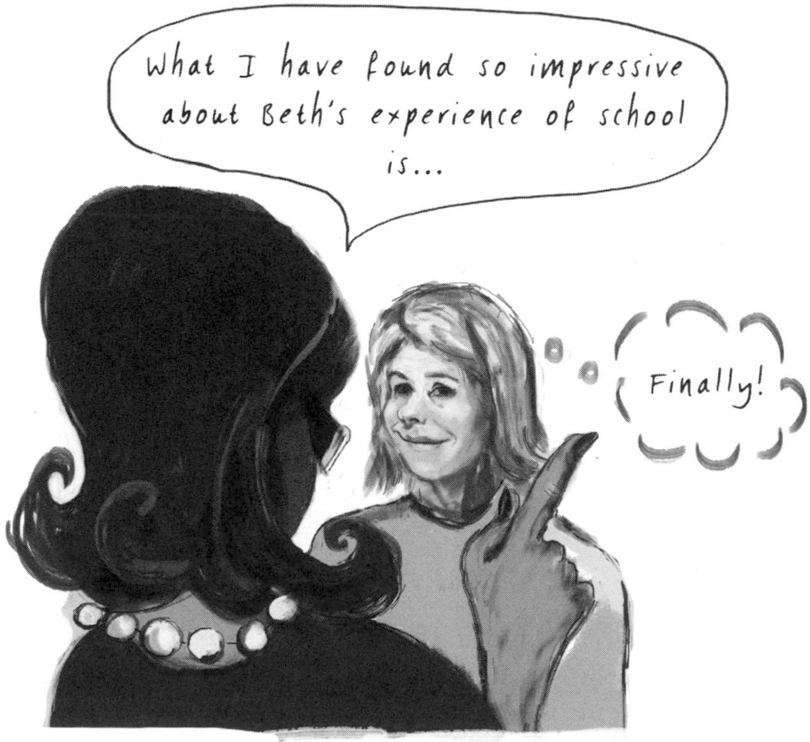
What I have found so impressive about Beth's experience of school is...
Finally!

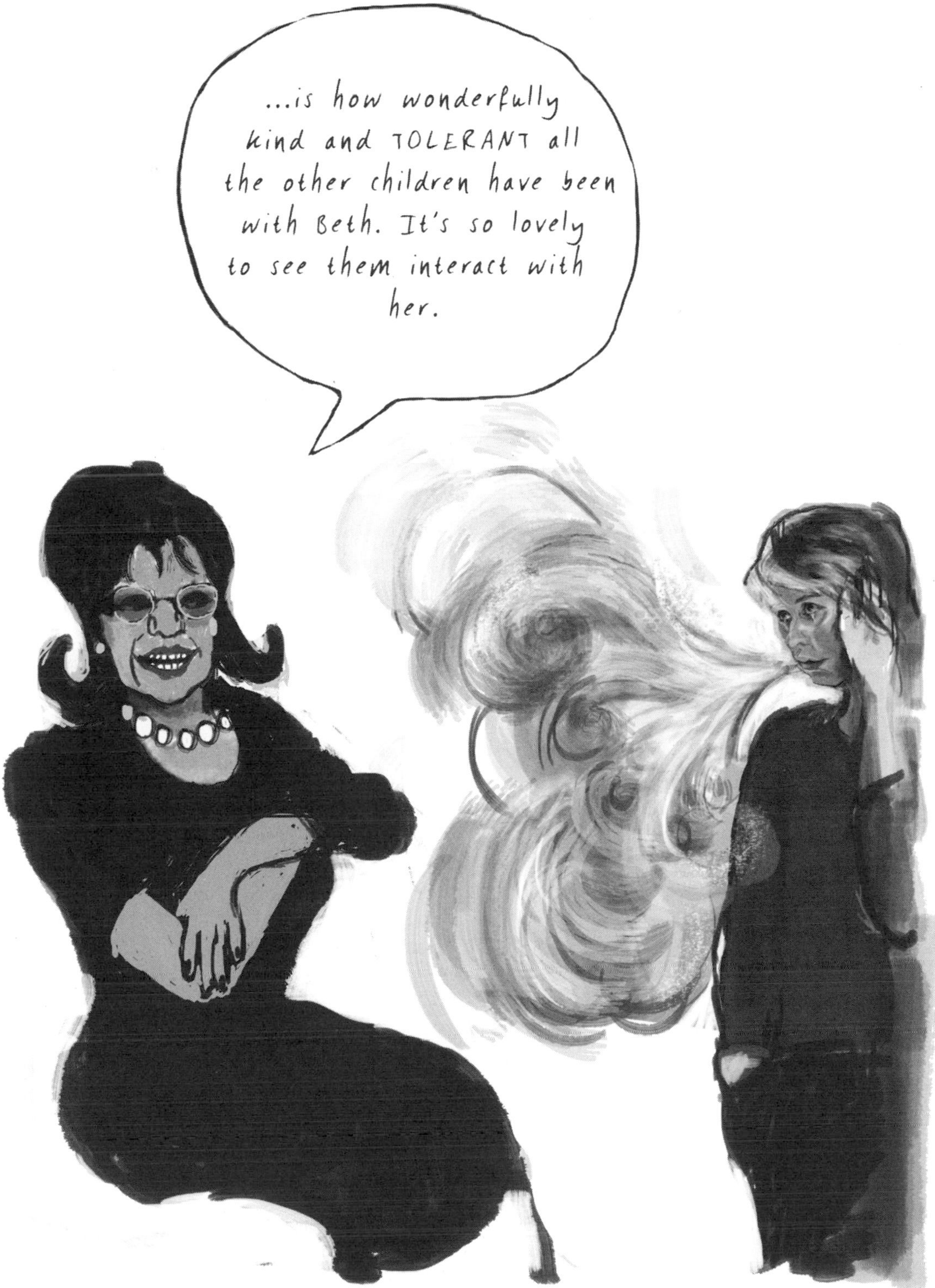
...is how wonderfully kind and TOLERANT all the other children have been with Beth. It's so lovely to see them interact with her.

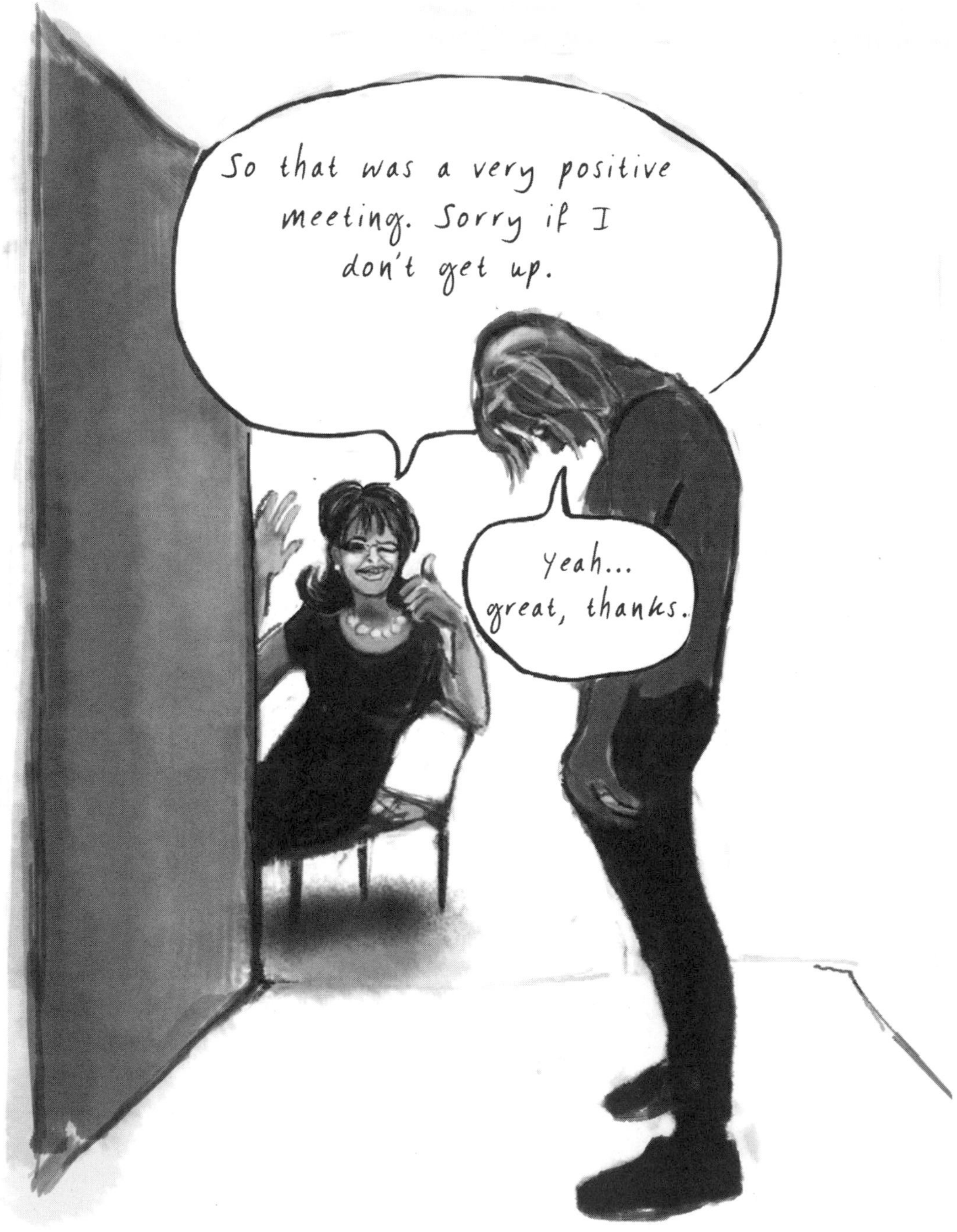
So that was a very positive meeting. Sorry if I don't get up.
yeah... great, thanks.

Part Four

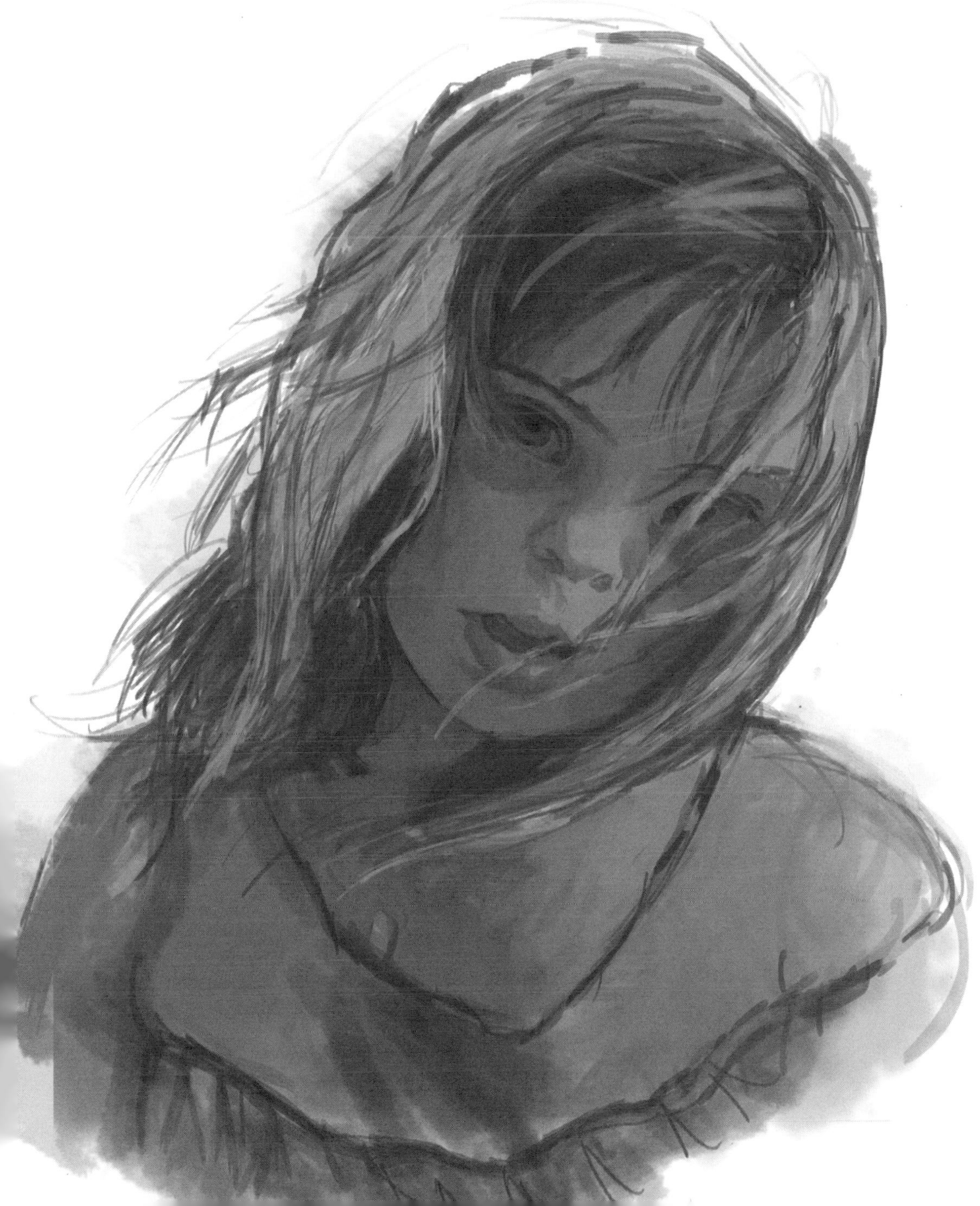

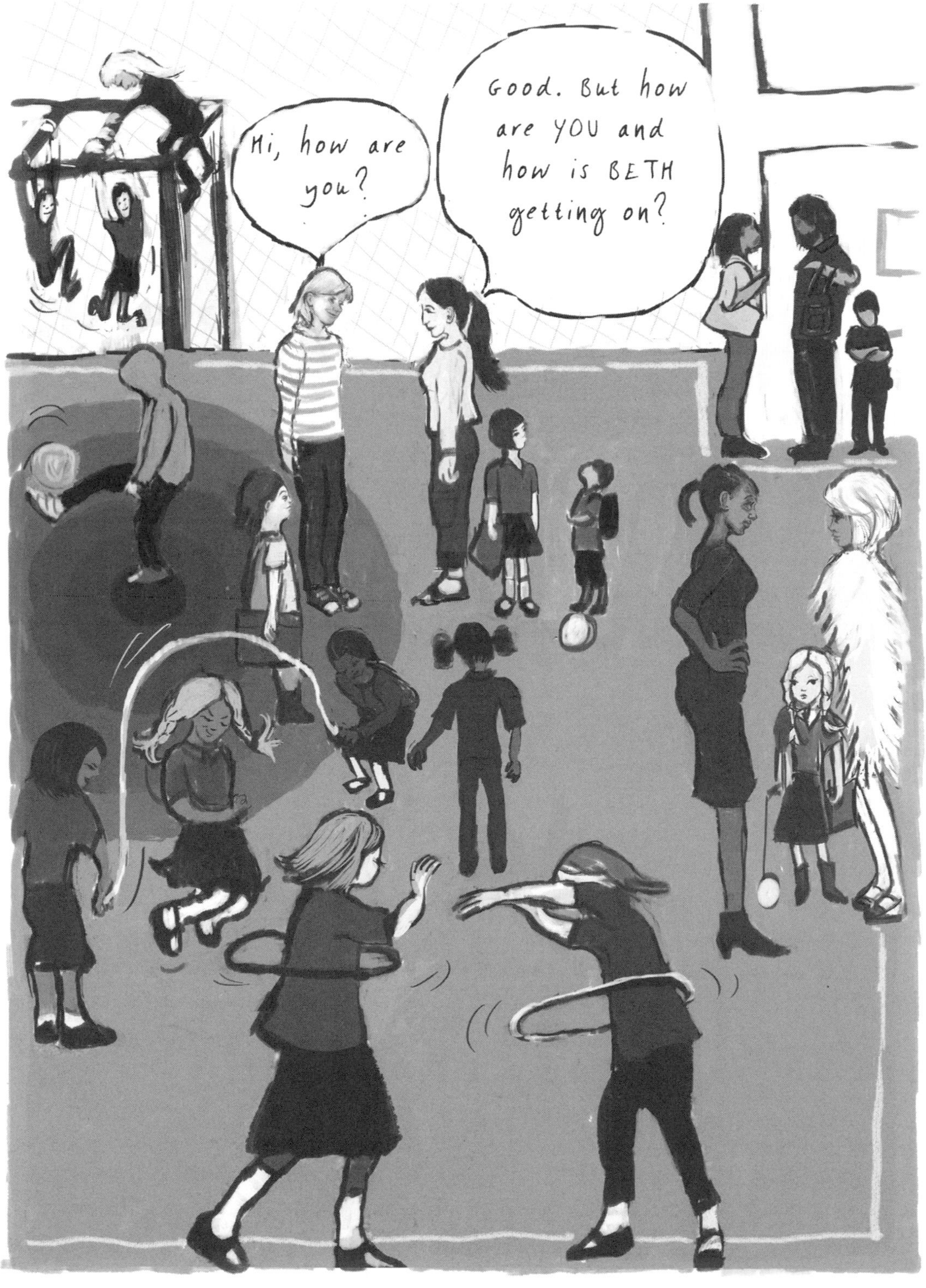
Hi, how are you?
Good. But how are YOU and how is BETH getting on?

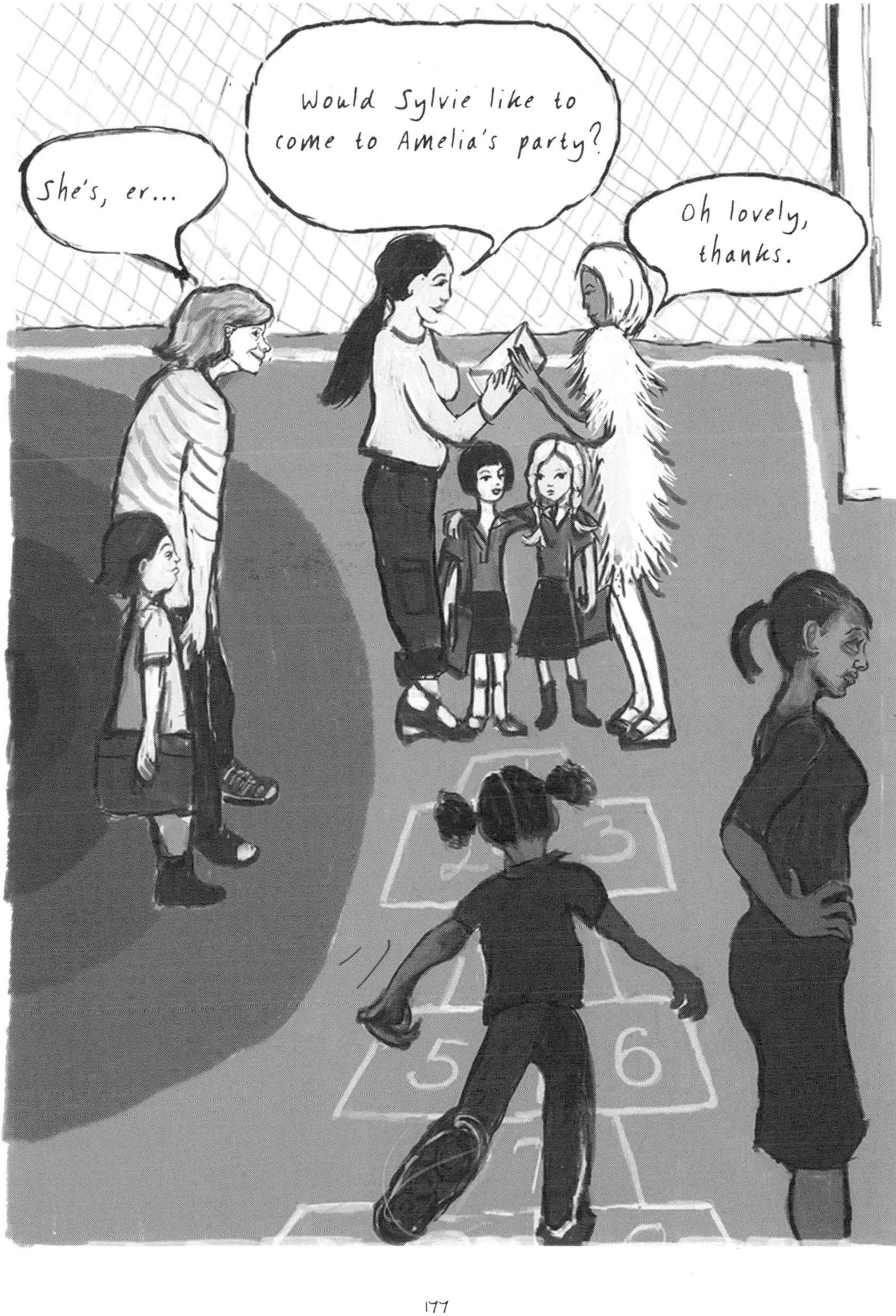
She's, er...
Would Sylvie like to come to Amelia's party?
Oh lovely, thanks.
3
5
6
7

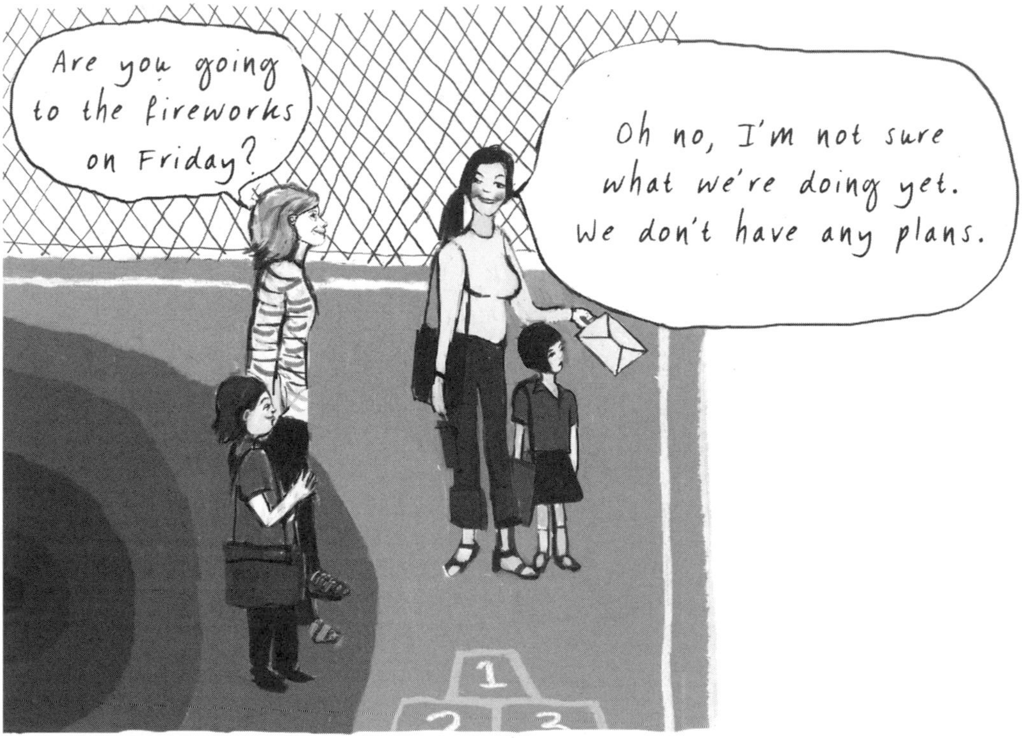
Are you going to the fireworks on Friday?
Oh no, I'm not sure what we're doing yet. We don't have any plans.
1
2
3

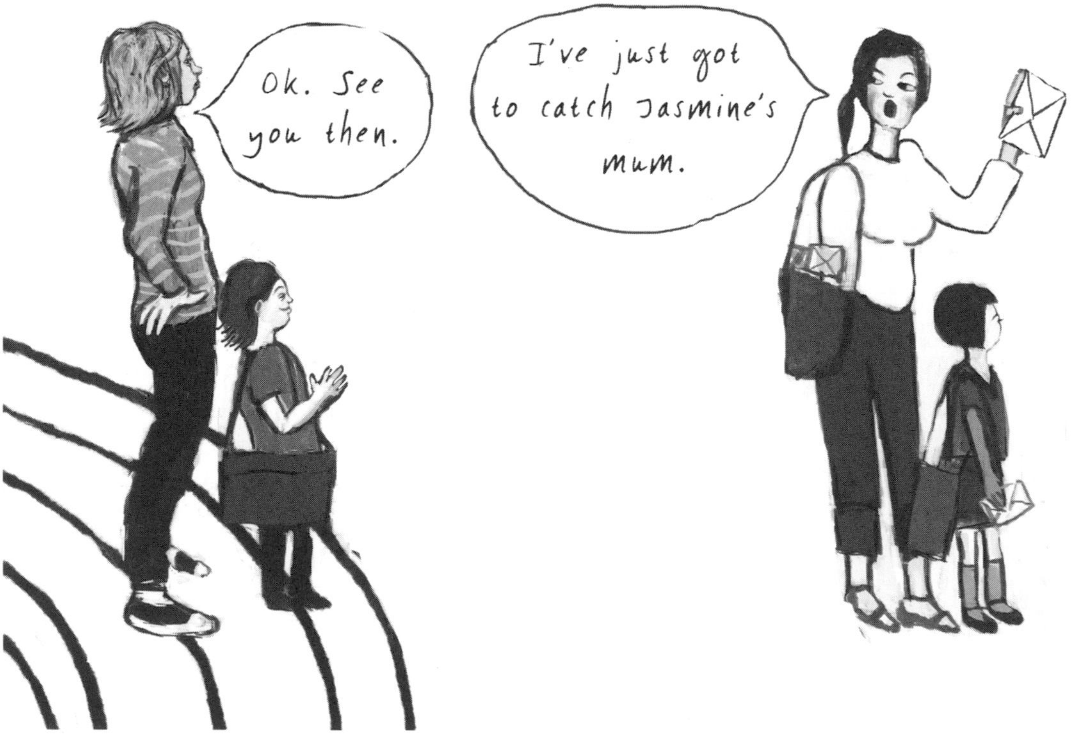
Ok. See you then.
I've just got to catch Jasmine's mum.

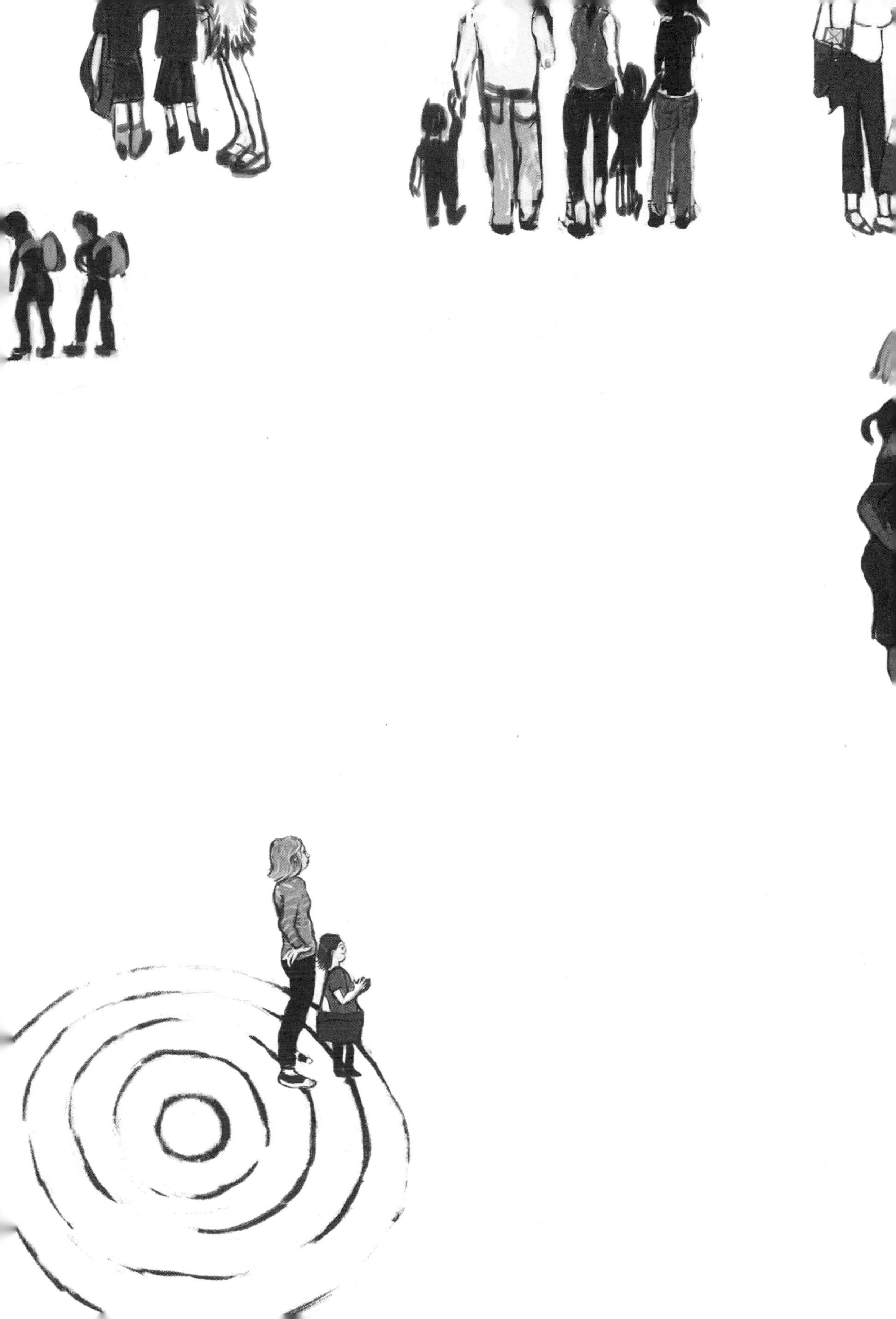

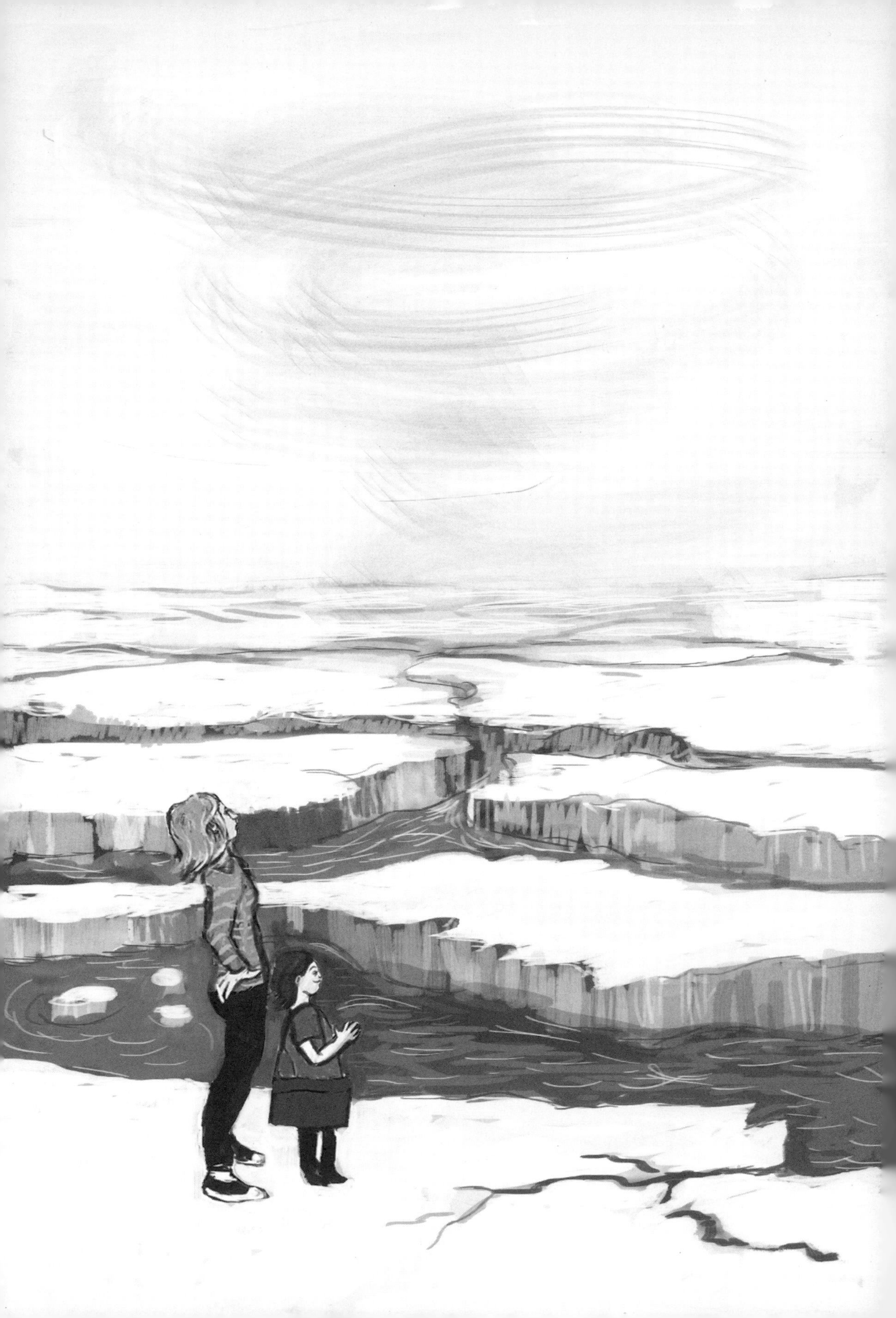

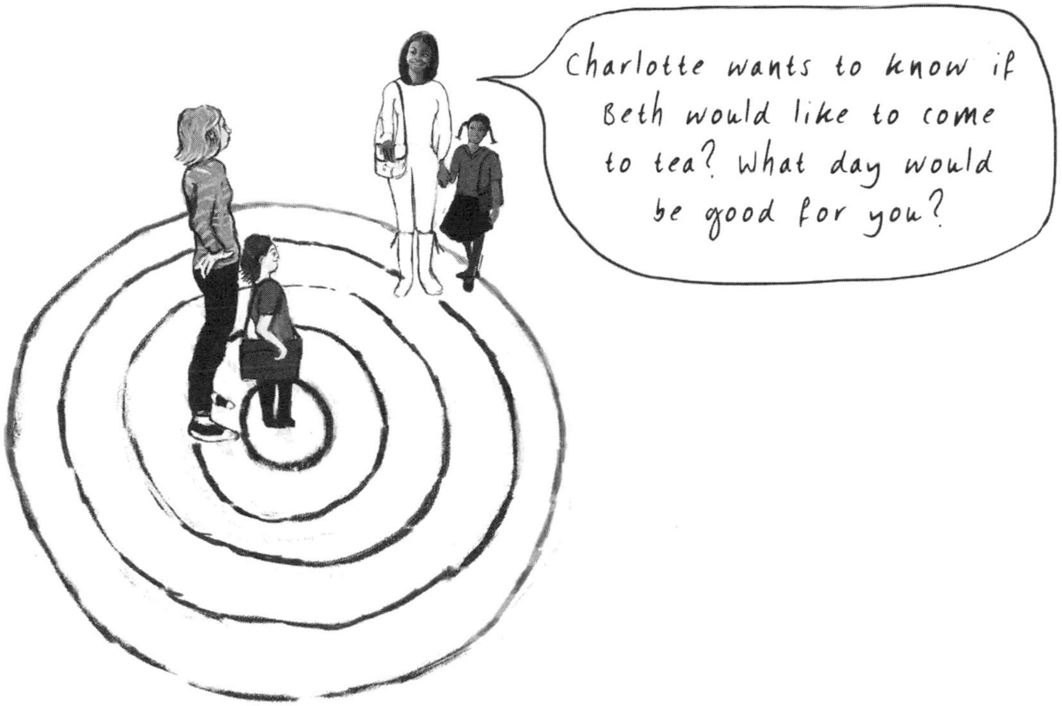
Charlotte wants to know if Beth would like to come to tea? What day would be good for you?

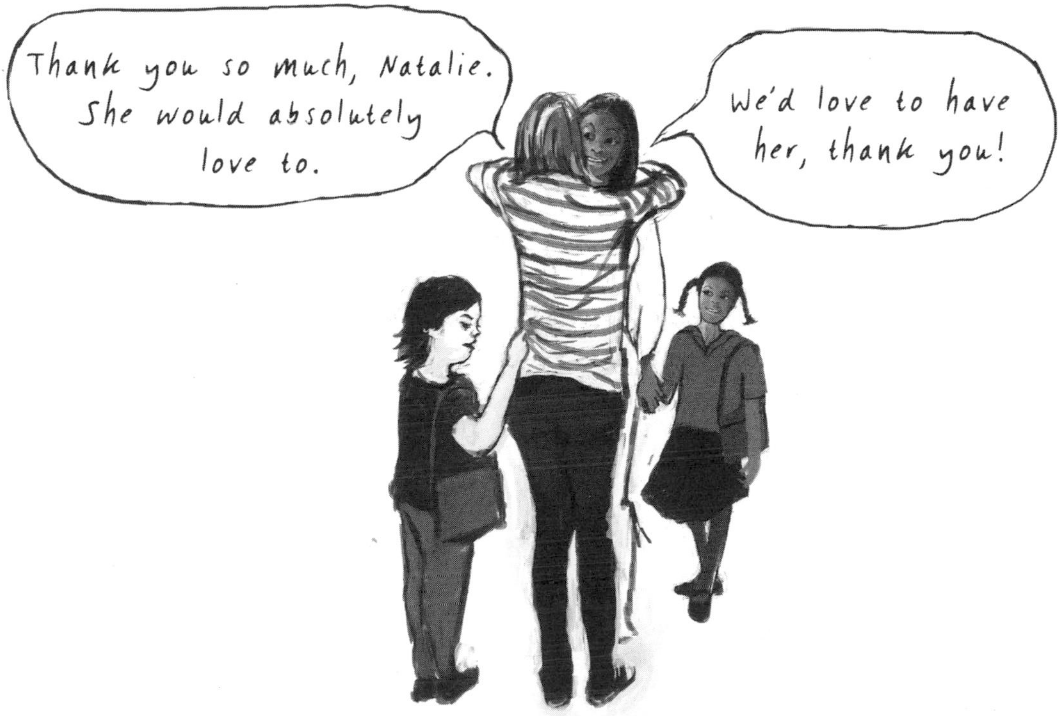
Thank you so much, Natalie. She would absolutely love to.
We'd love to have her, thank you!

November 2011

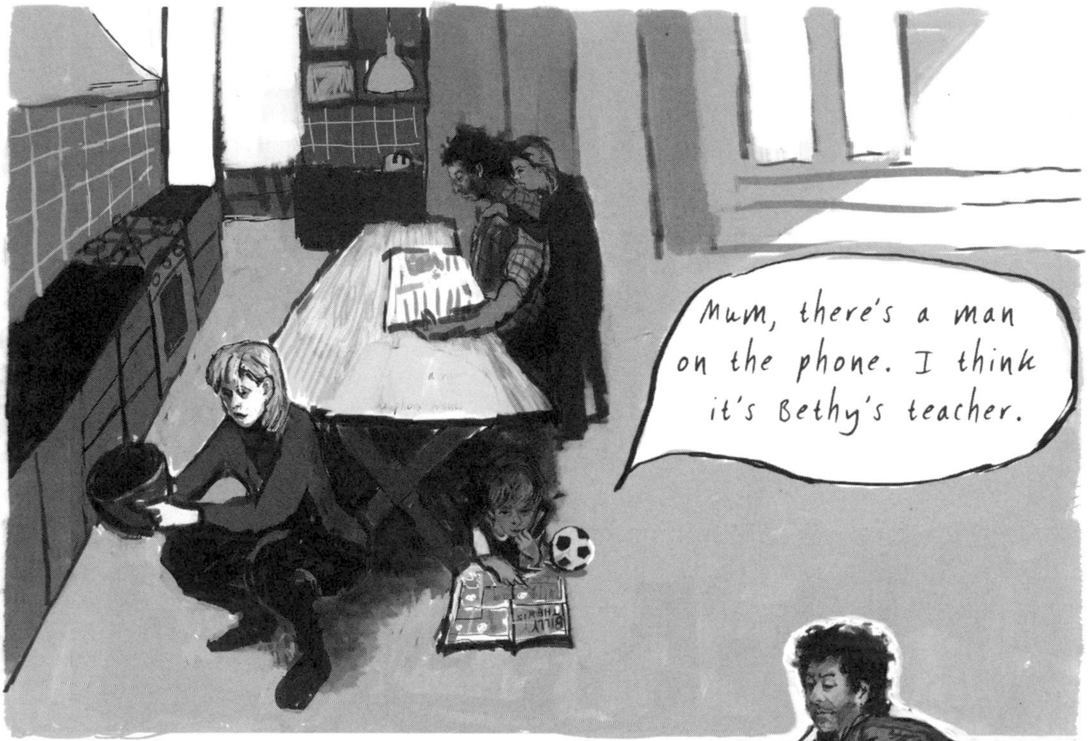
Mum, there's a man on the phone. I think it's Bethy's teacher.

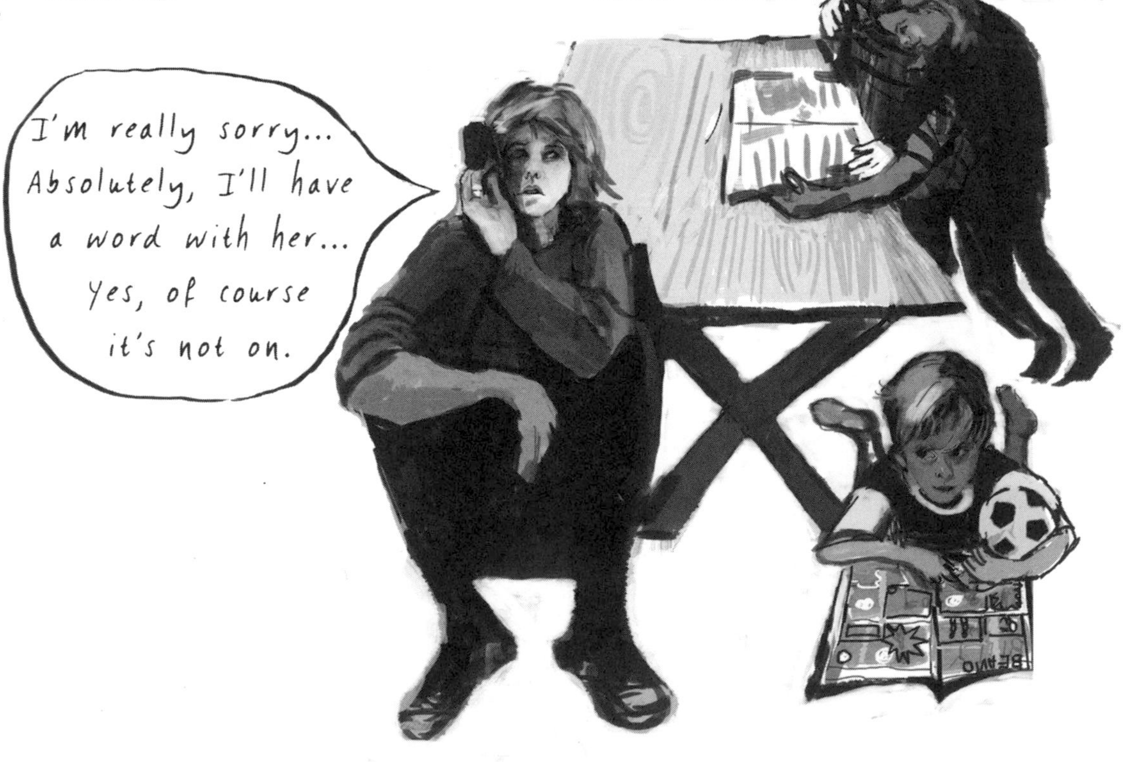
I'm really sorry... Absolutely, I'll have a word with her... Yes, of course it's not on.

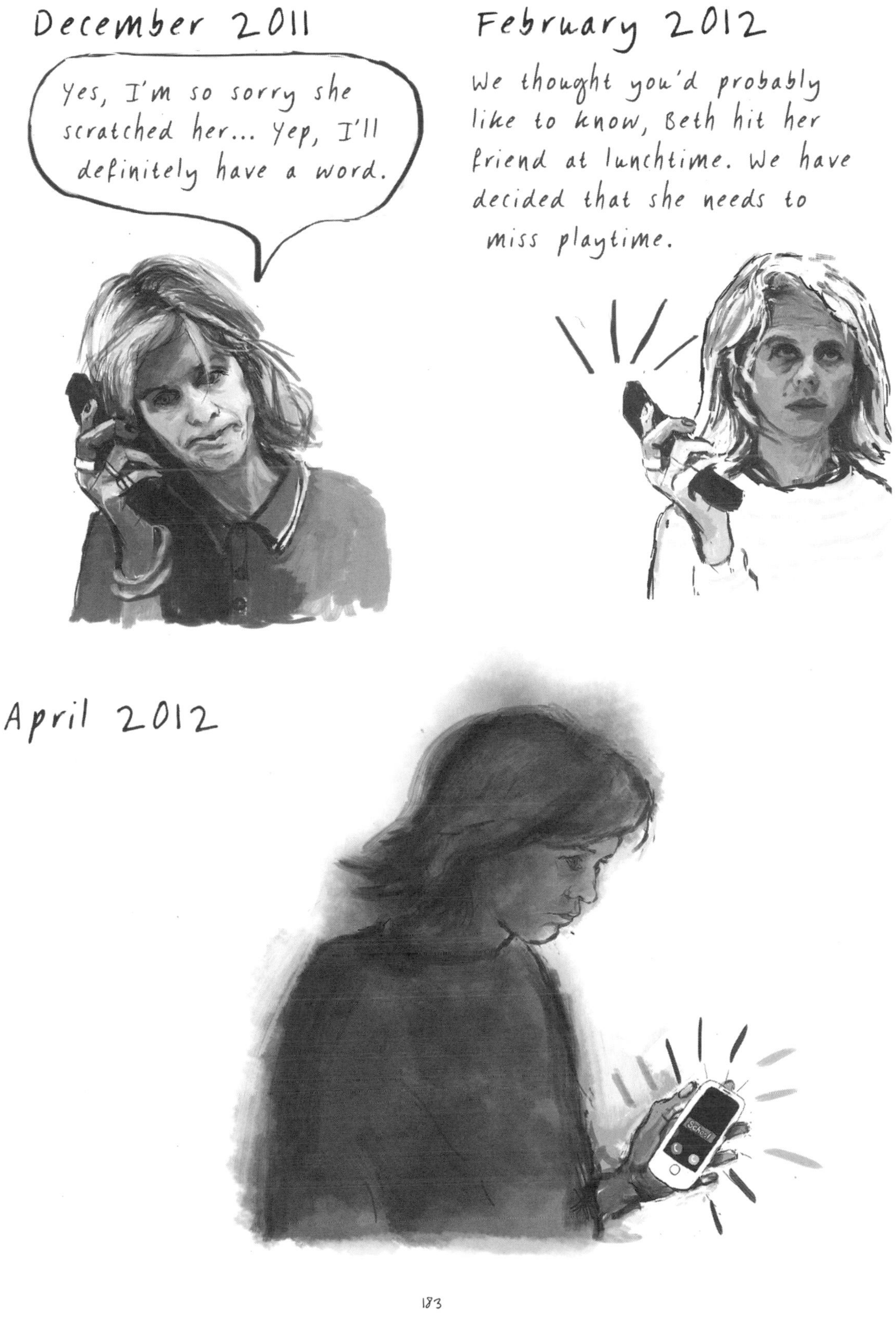
December 2011
Yes, I'm so sorry she scratched her... Yep, I'll definitely have a word.
February 2012
We thought you'd probably like to know, Beth hit her friend at lunchtime. We have decided that she needs to miss playtime.
April 2012

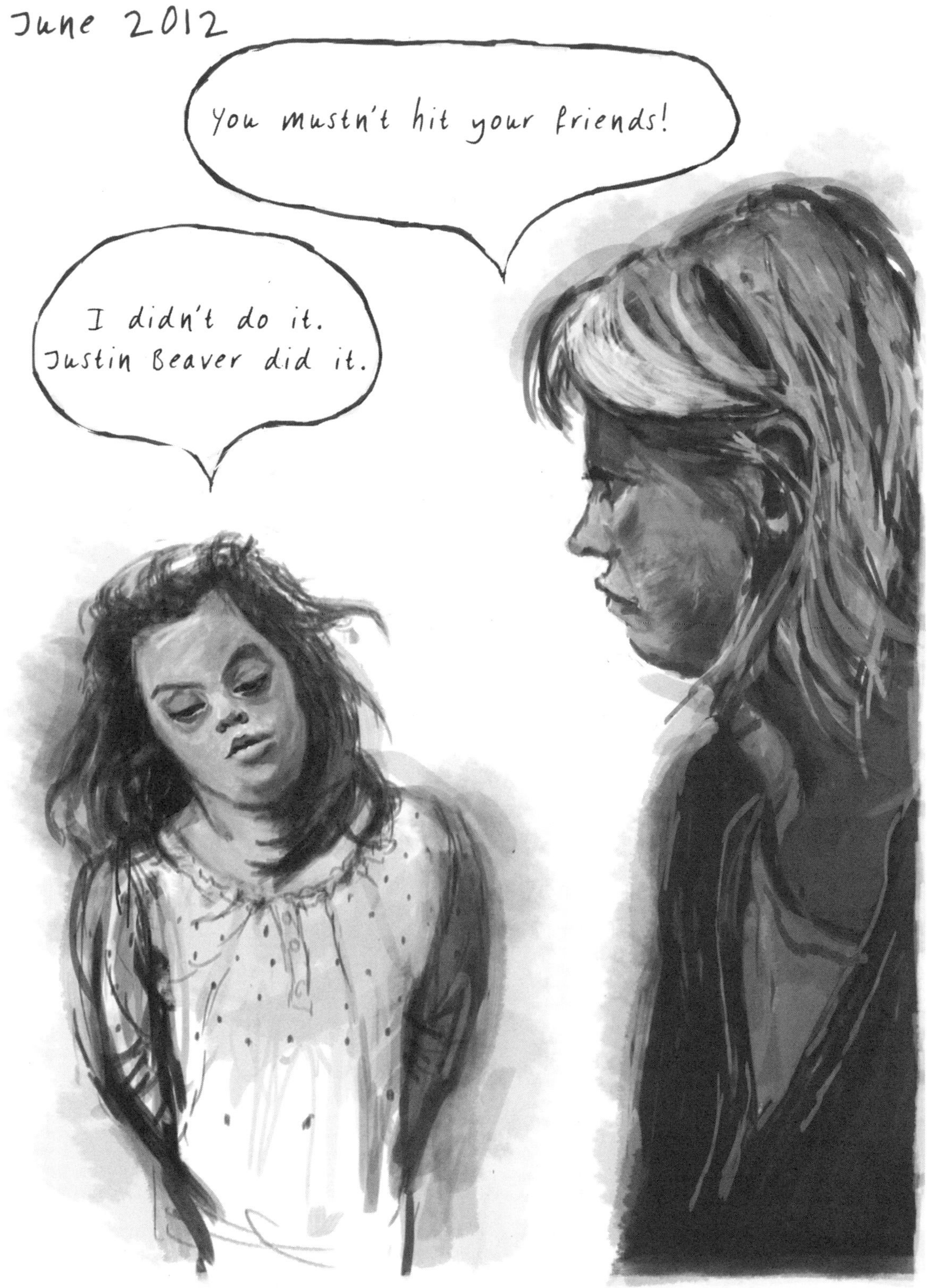
June 2012
You mustn't hit your friends!
I didn't do it. Justin Beaver did it.

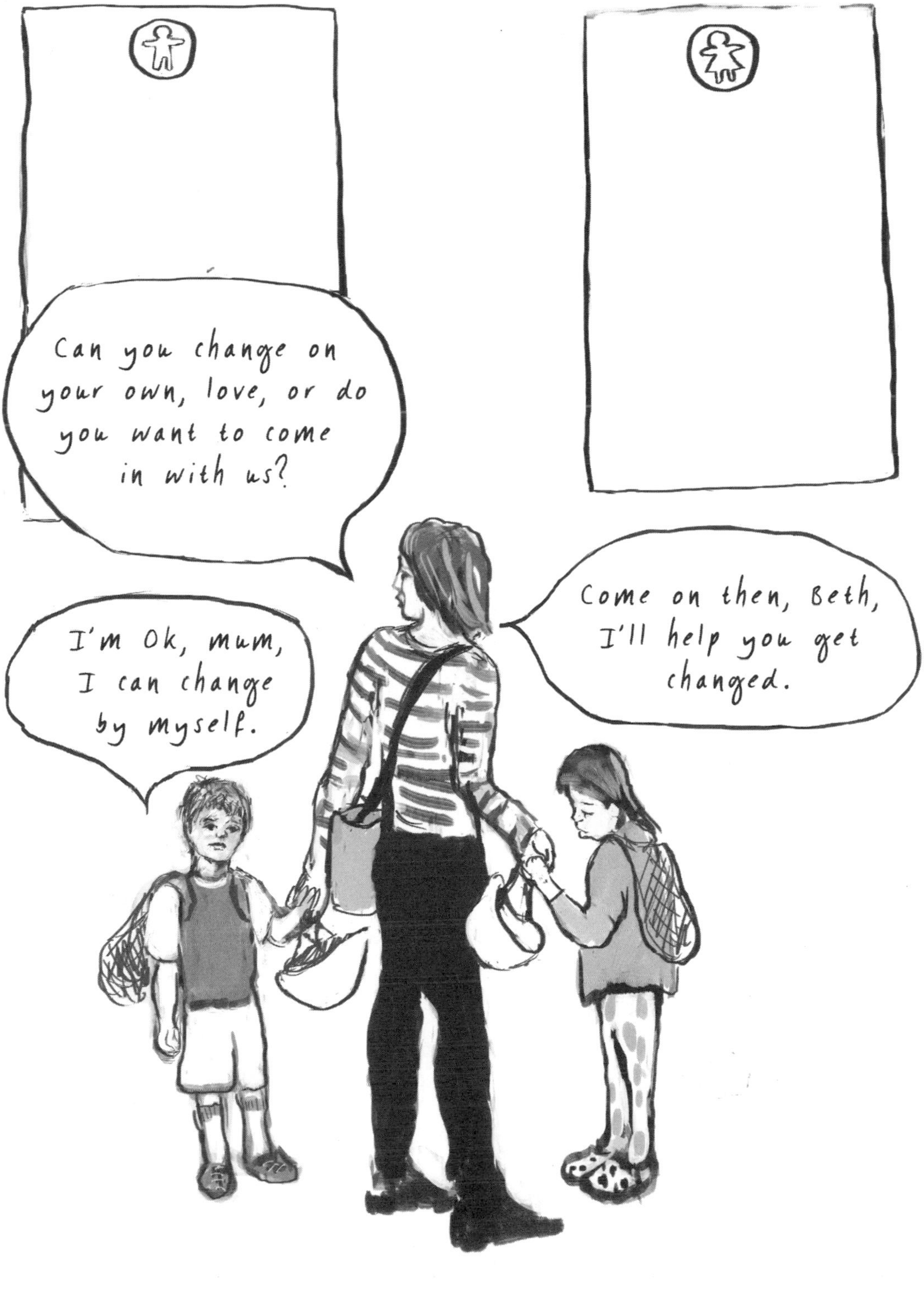
Can you change on your own, love, or do you want to come in with us?
Come on then, Beth, I'll help you get changed.
I'm Ok, mum, I can change by myself.

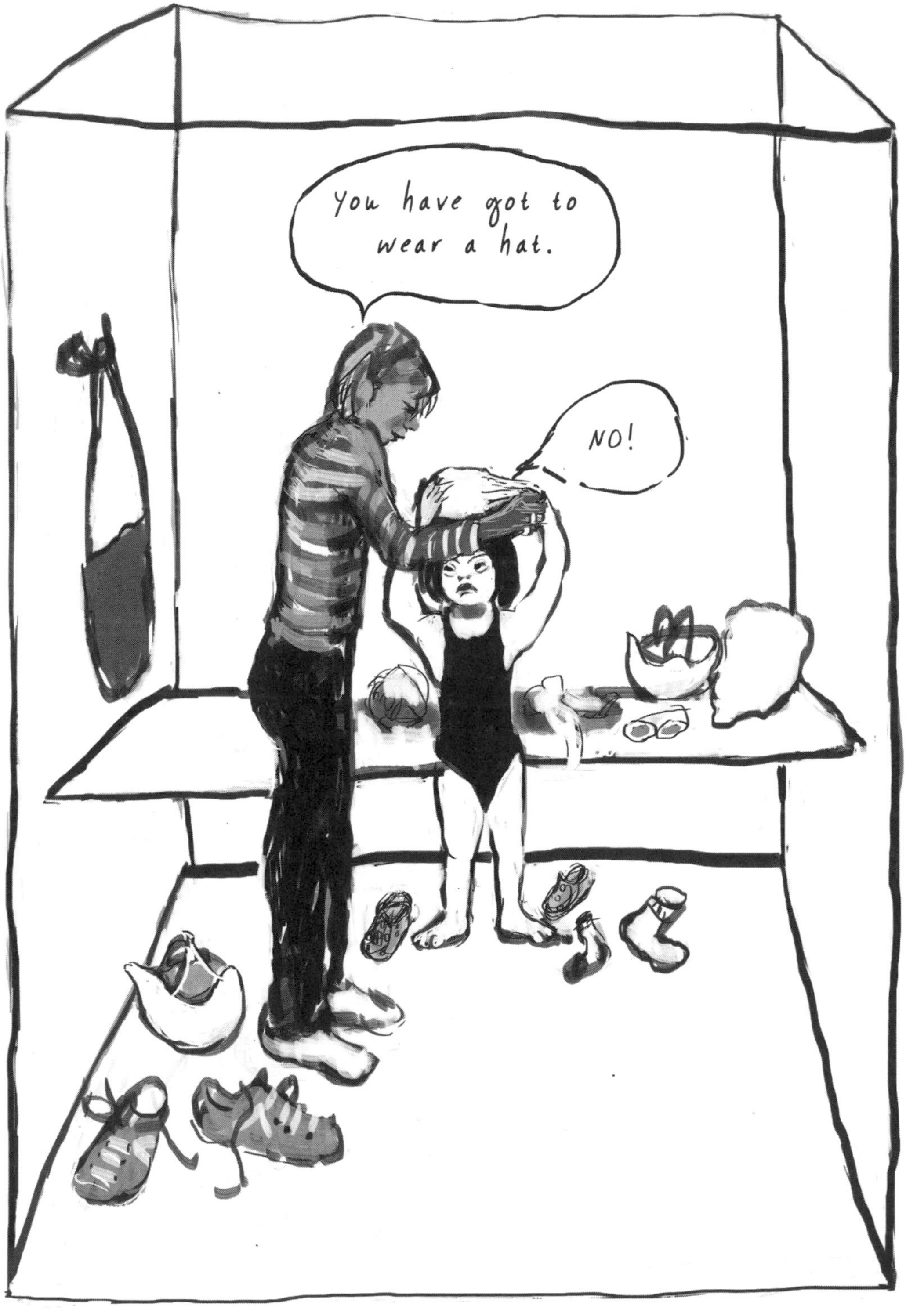
You have got to wear a hat.
NO!

NO!

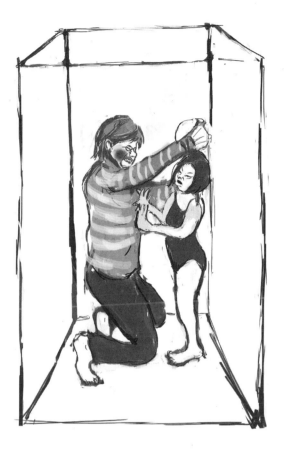

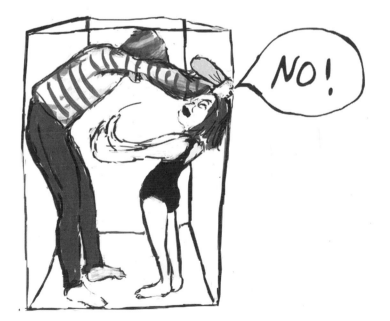

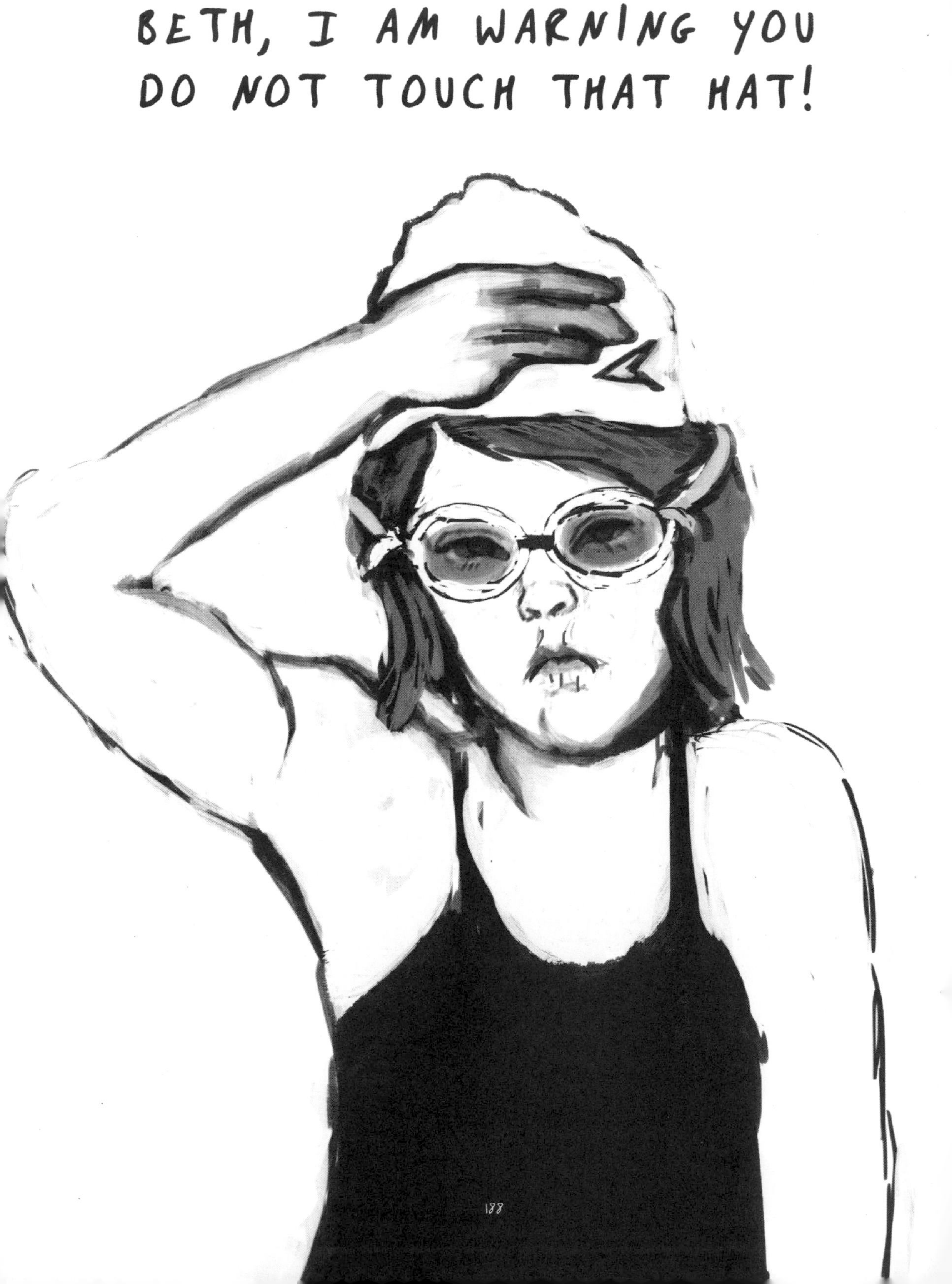
BETH, I AM WARNING YOU
DO NOT TOUCH THAT HAT!

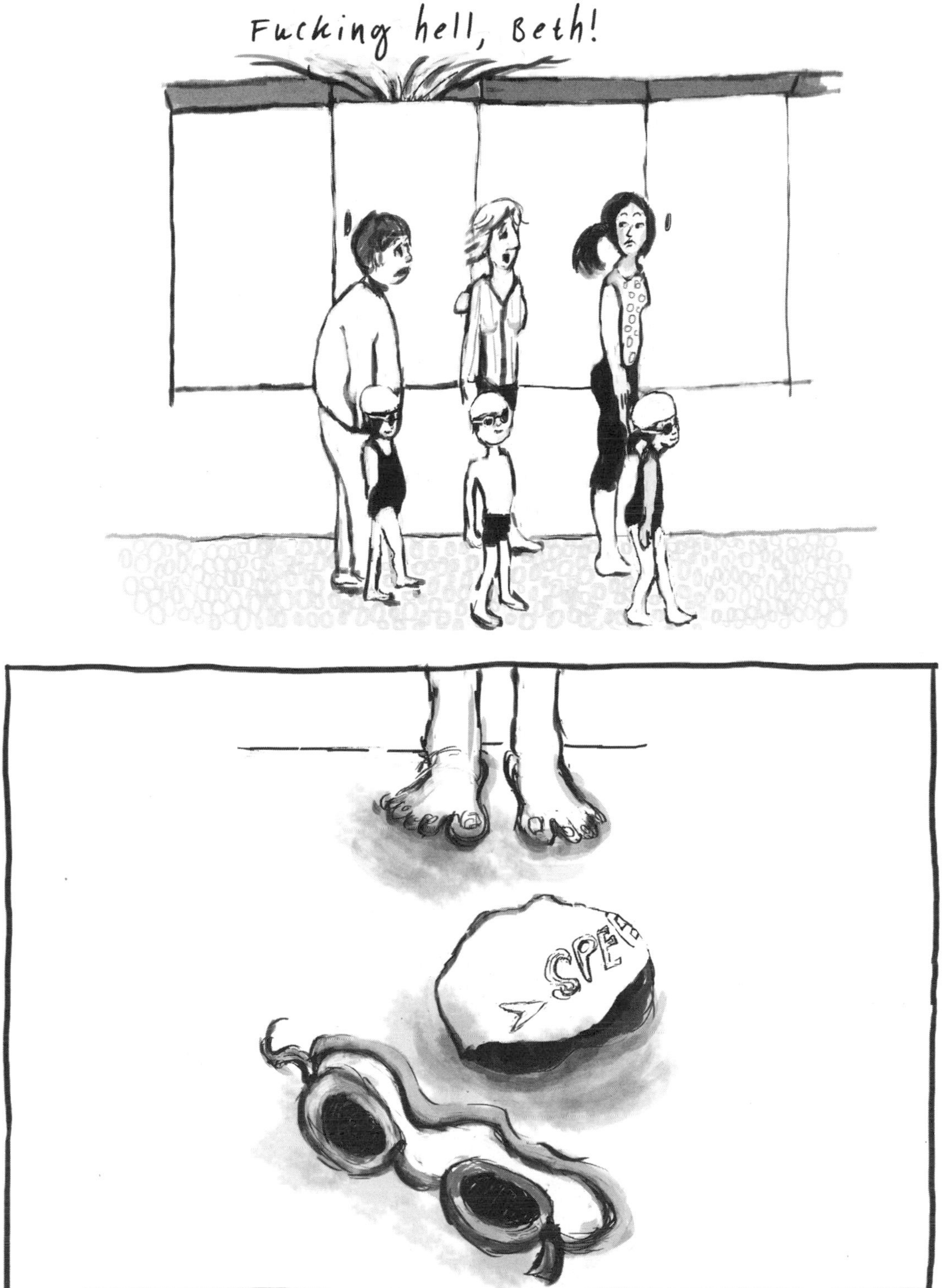
Fucking hell, Beth!

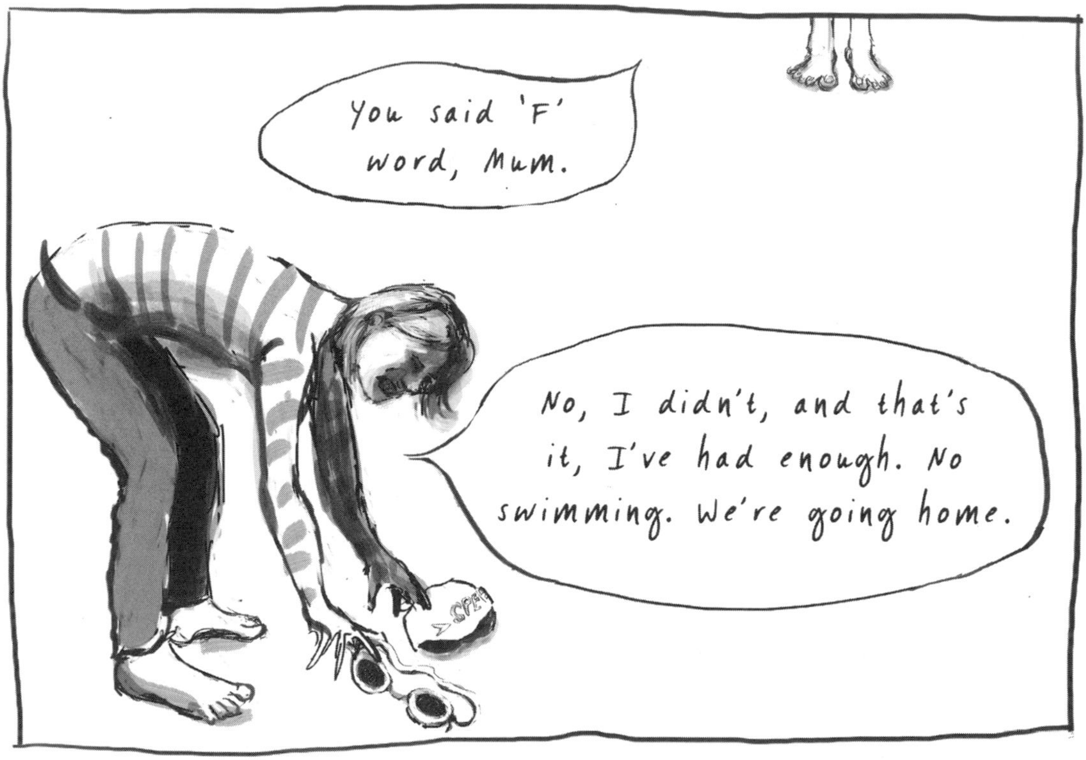
You said 'F' word, Mum.
No, I didn't, and that's it, I've had enough. No swimming. We're going home.

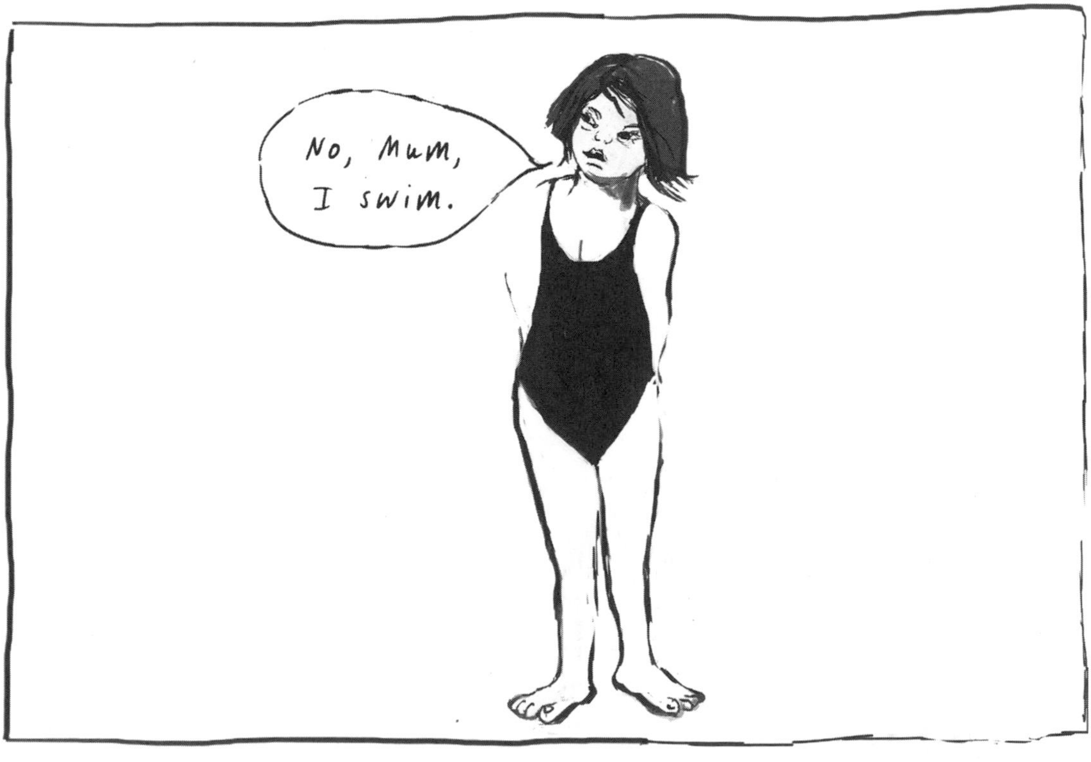
No, Mum, I swim.

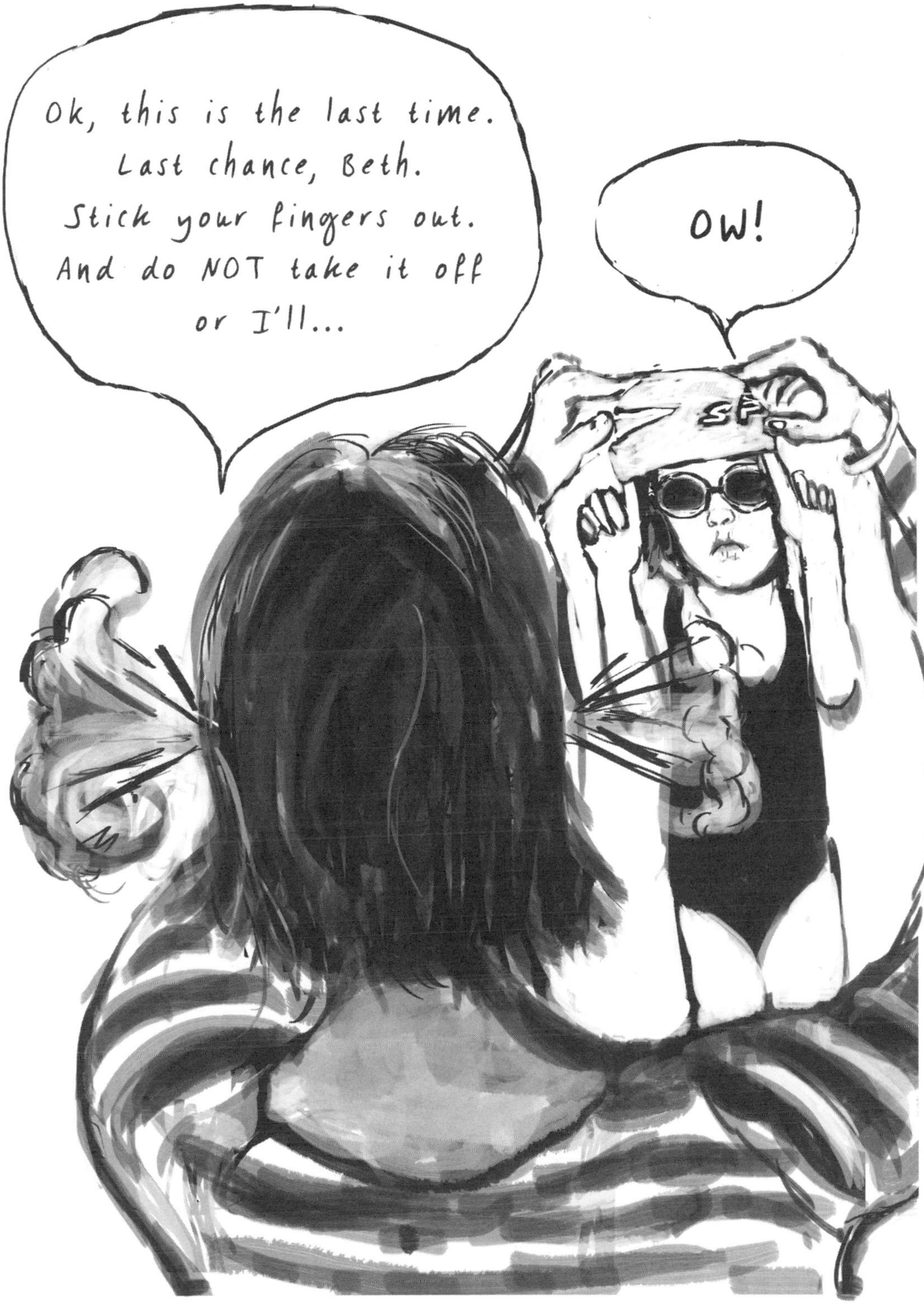
Ok, this is the last time. Last chance, Beth. Stick your fingers out. And do NOT take it off or I'll...
OW!

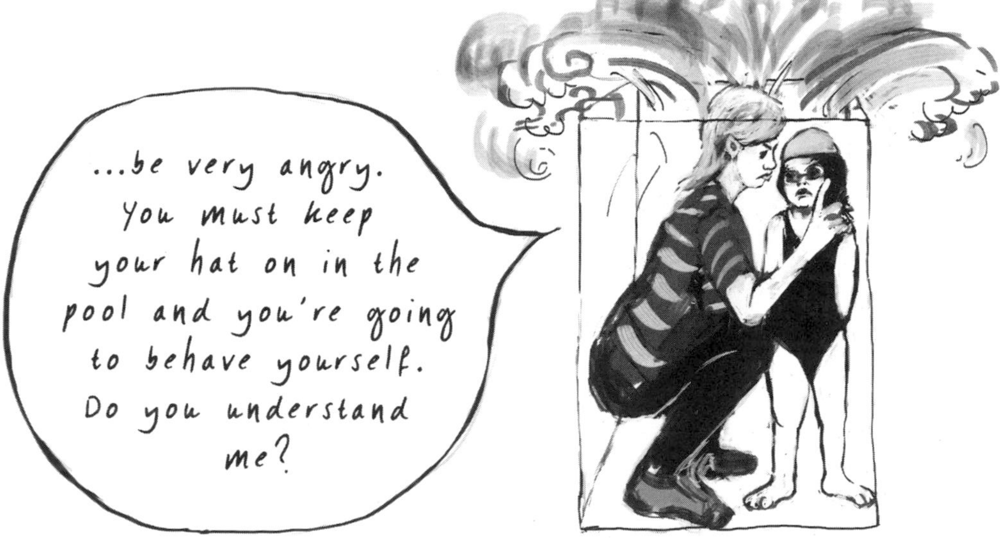
...be very angry. You must keep your hat on in the pool and you're going to behave yourself. Do you understand me?

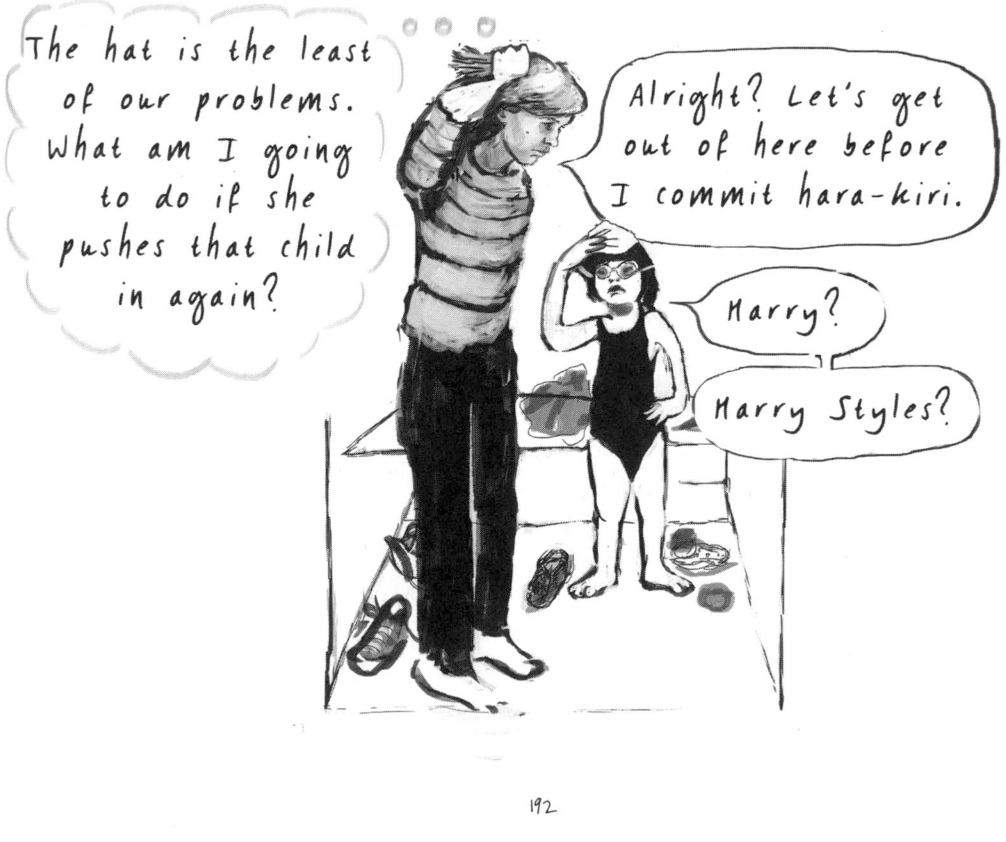
The hat is the least of our problems. What am I going to do if she pushes that child in again?
Alright? Let's get out of here before I commit hara-kiri.
Harry?
Harry Styles?

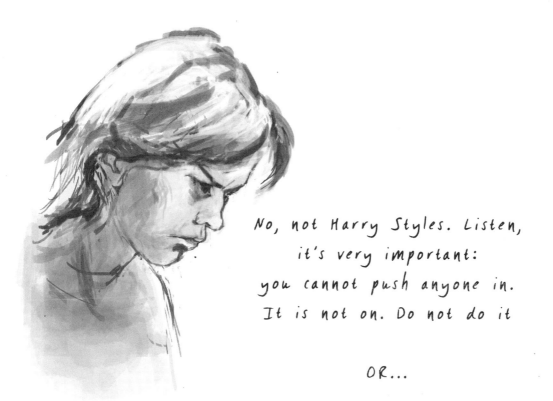

No, not Harry Styles. Listen,
it's very important:
you cannot push anyone in.
It is not on. Do not do it

OR...

THERE WILL BE BIG TROUBLE.

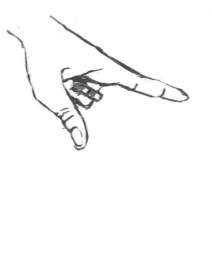

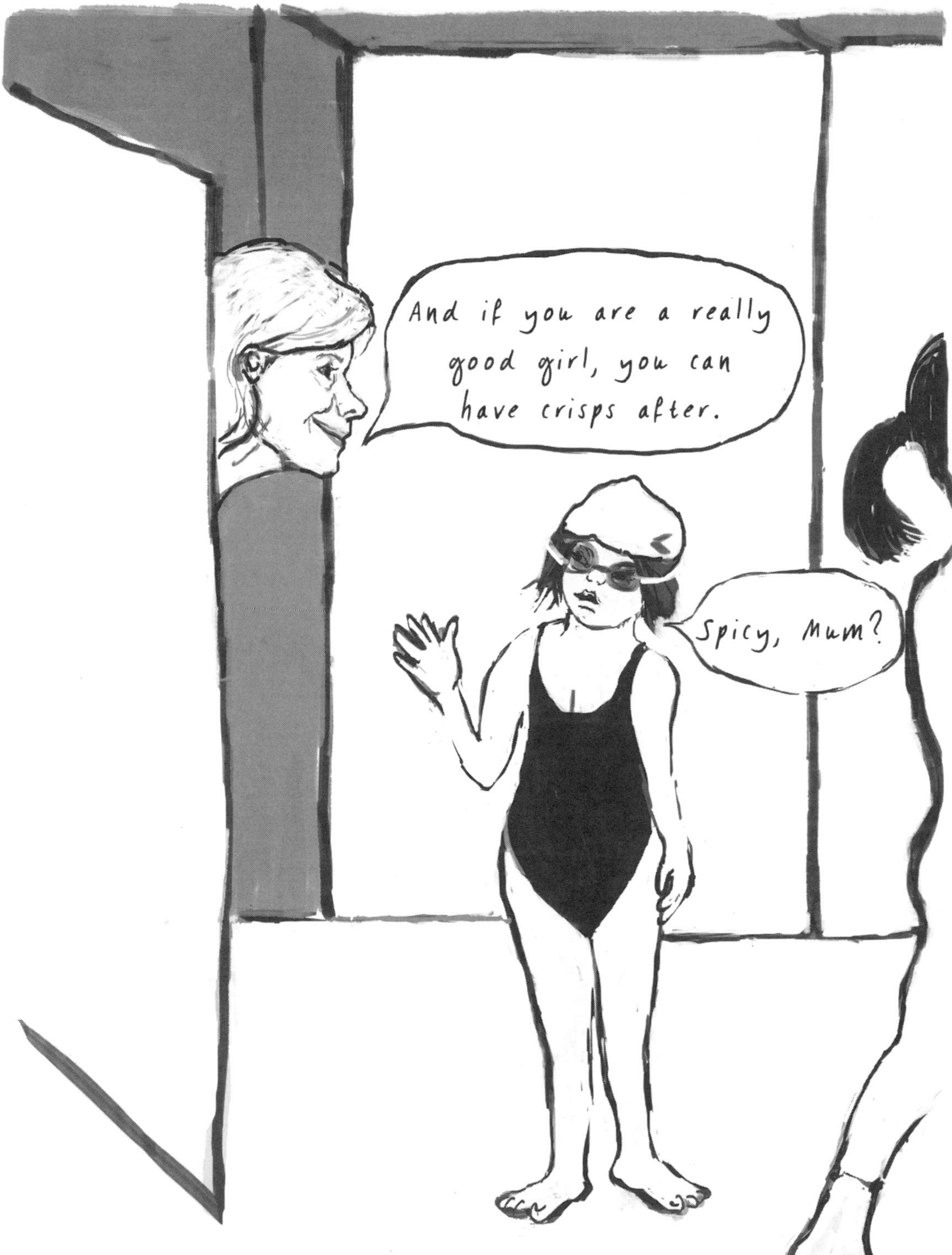
And if you are a really good girl, you can have crisps after.
Spicy, Mum?

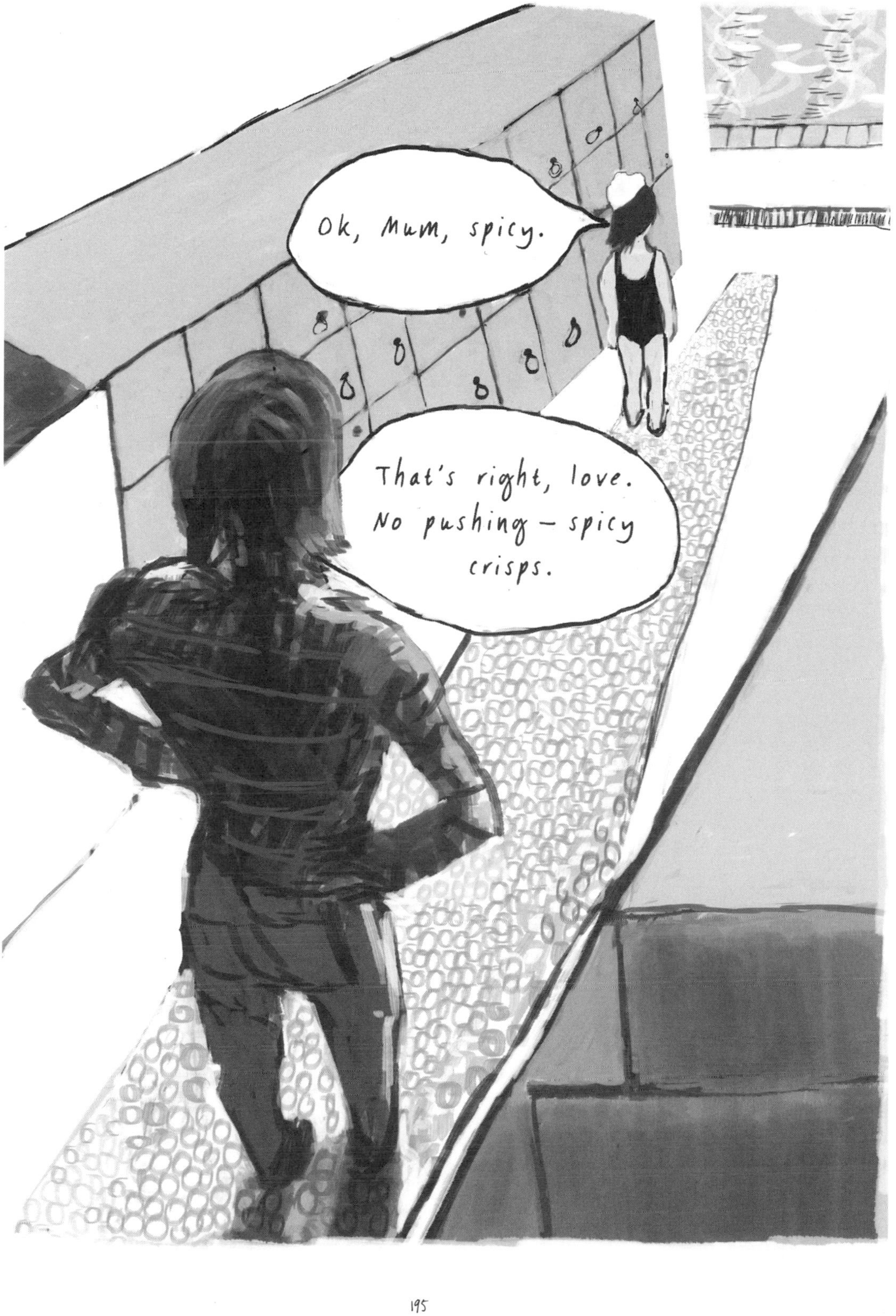
Ok, Mum, spicy.
That's right, love. No pushing – spicy crisps.

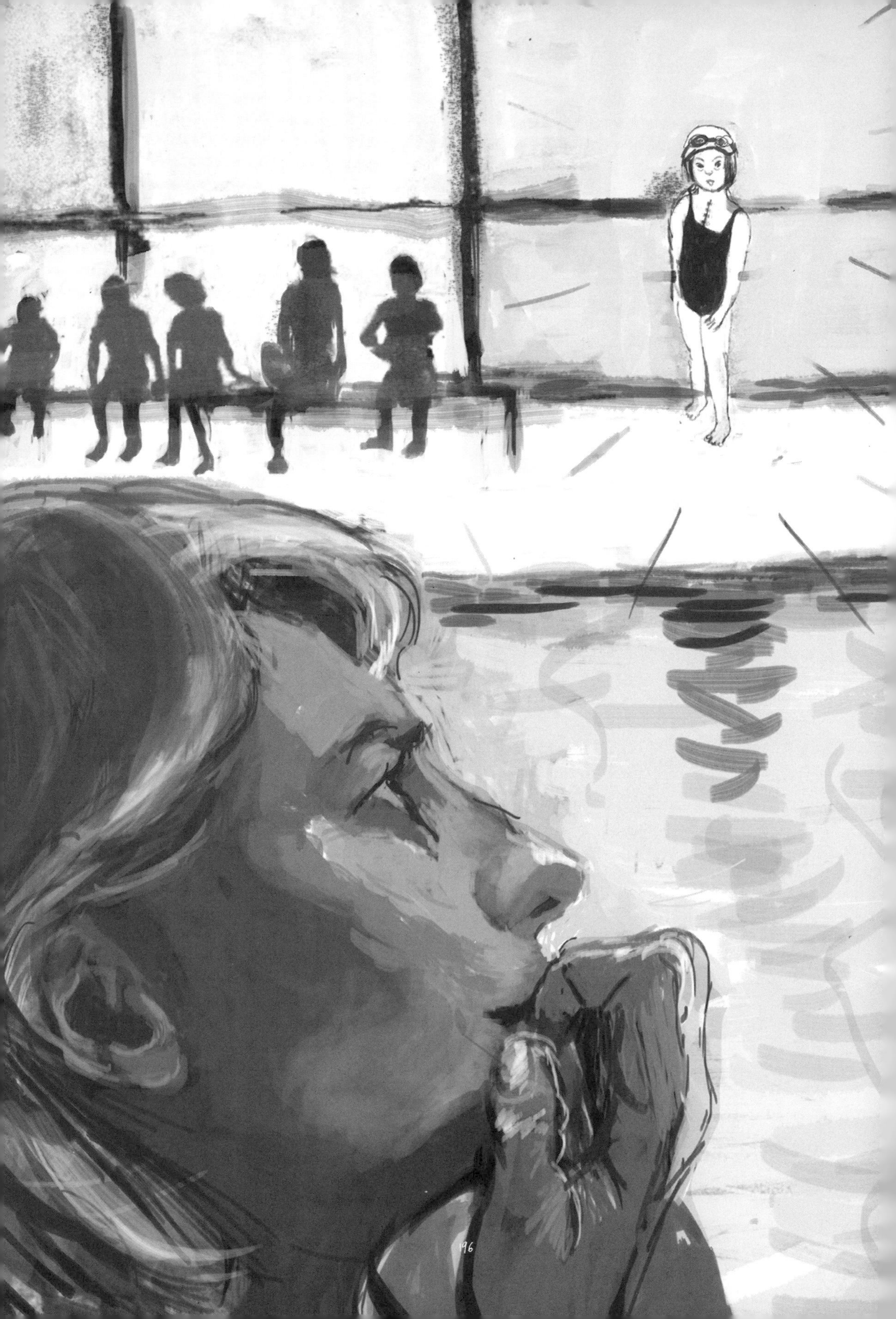

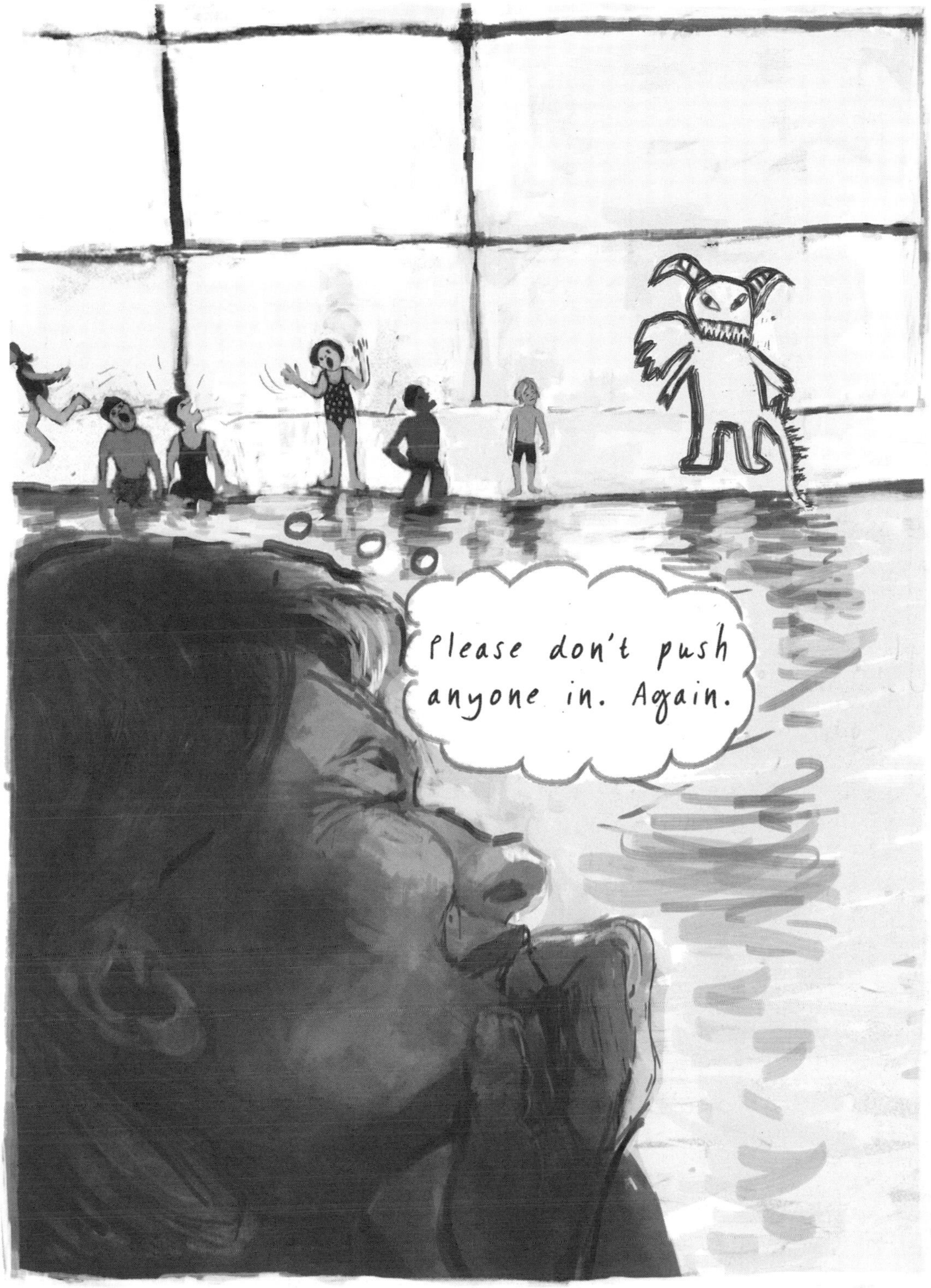
Please don't push anyone in. Again.

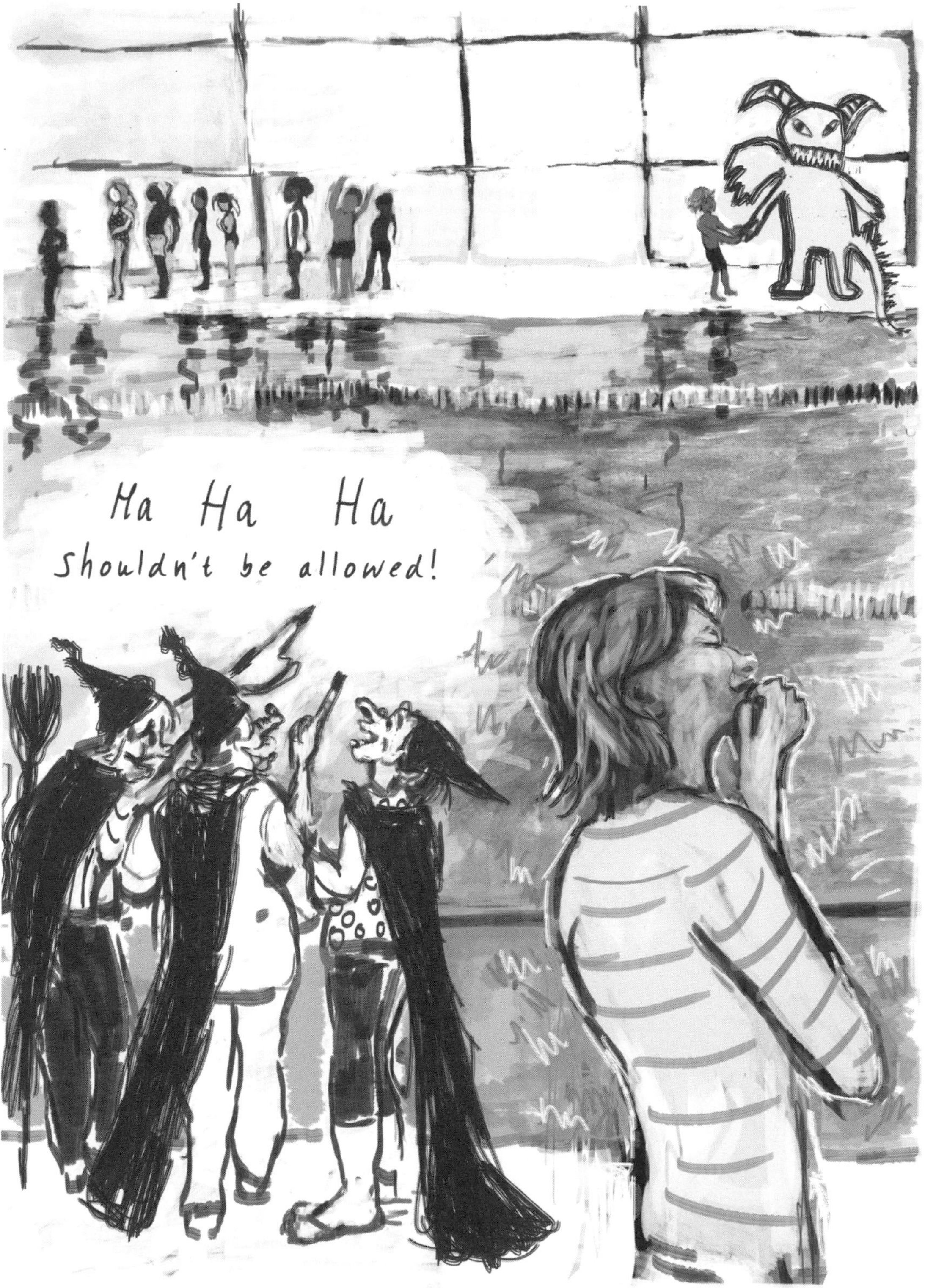
Ha Ha Ha
Shouldn't be allowed!

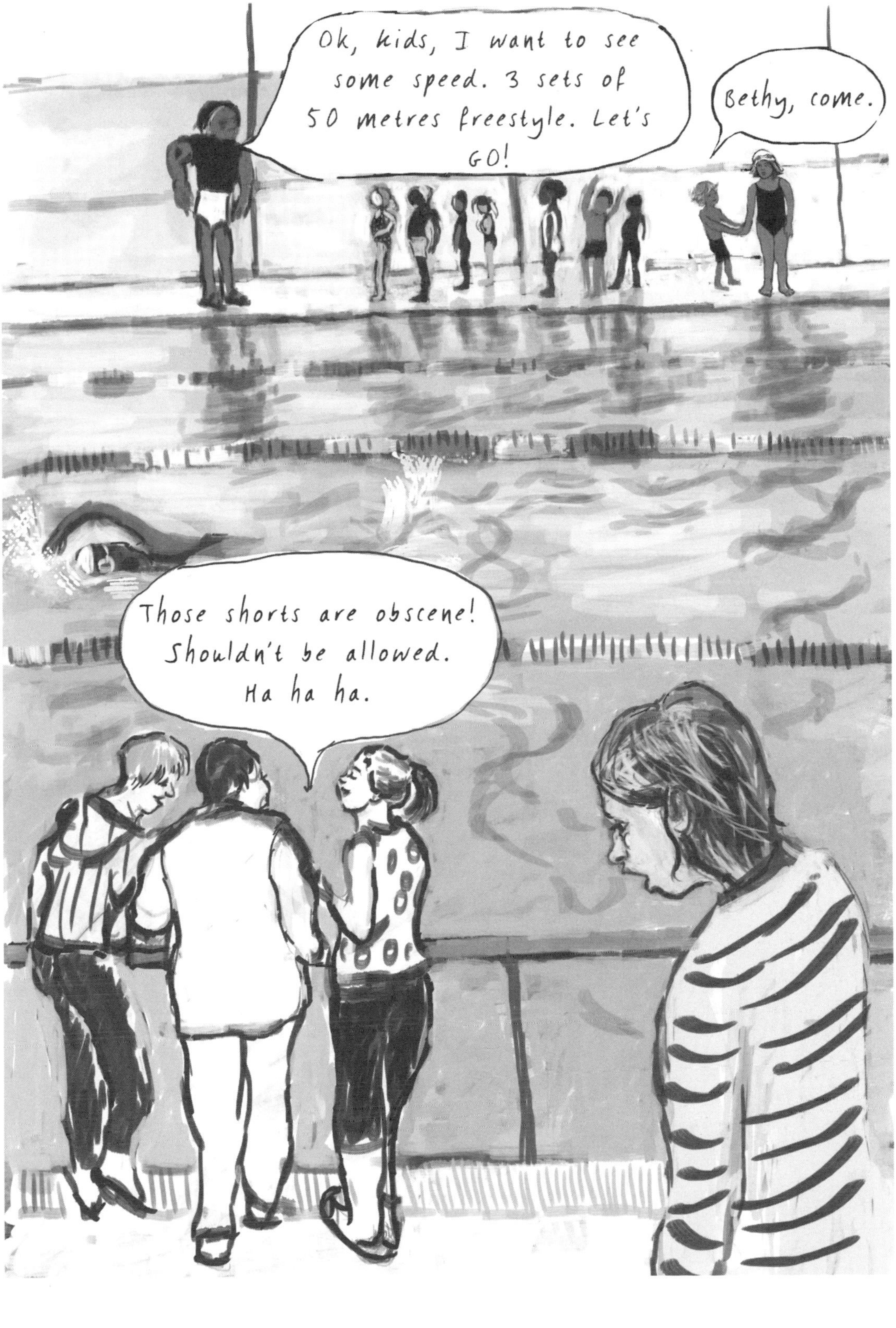
Ok, kids, I want to see some speed. 3 sets of 50 metres freestyle. Let's GO!
Bethy, come.
Those shorts are obscene! Shouldn't be allowed. Ha ha ha.

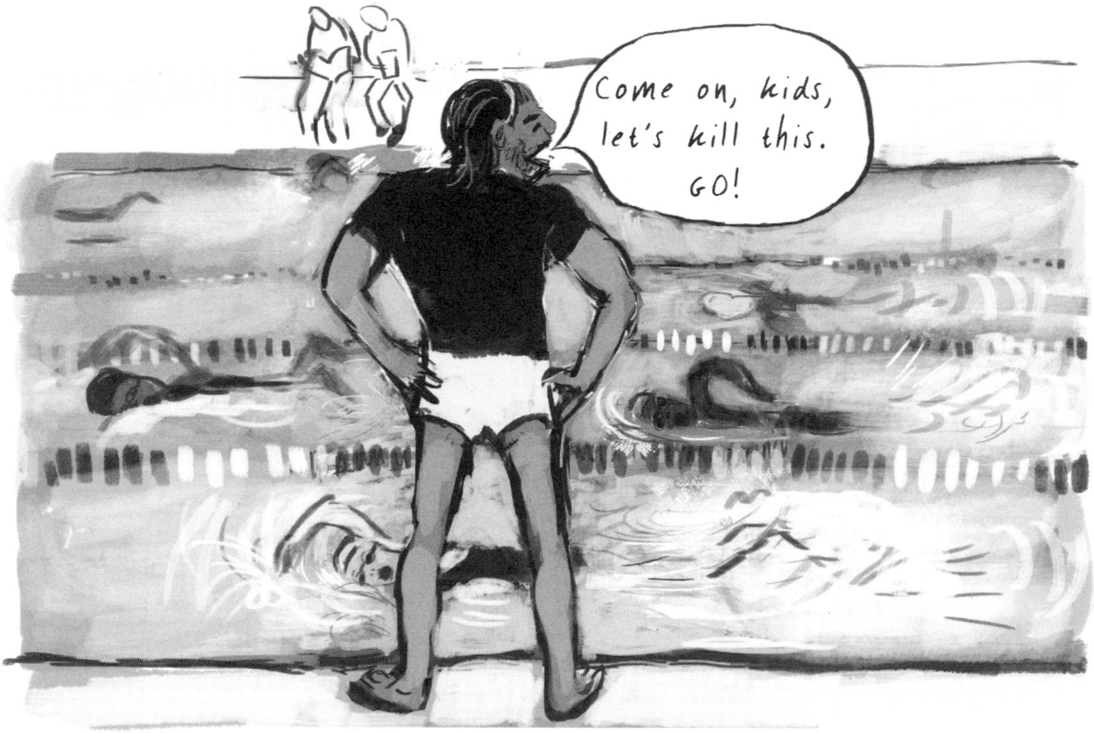
Come on, kids, let's kill this. GO!

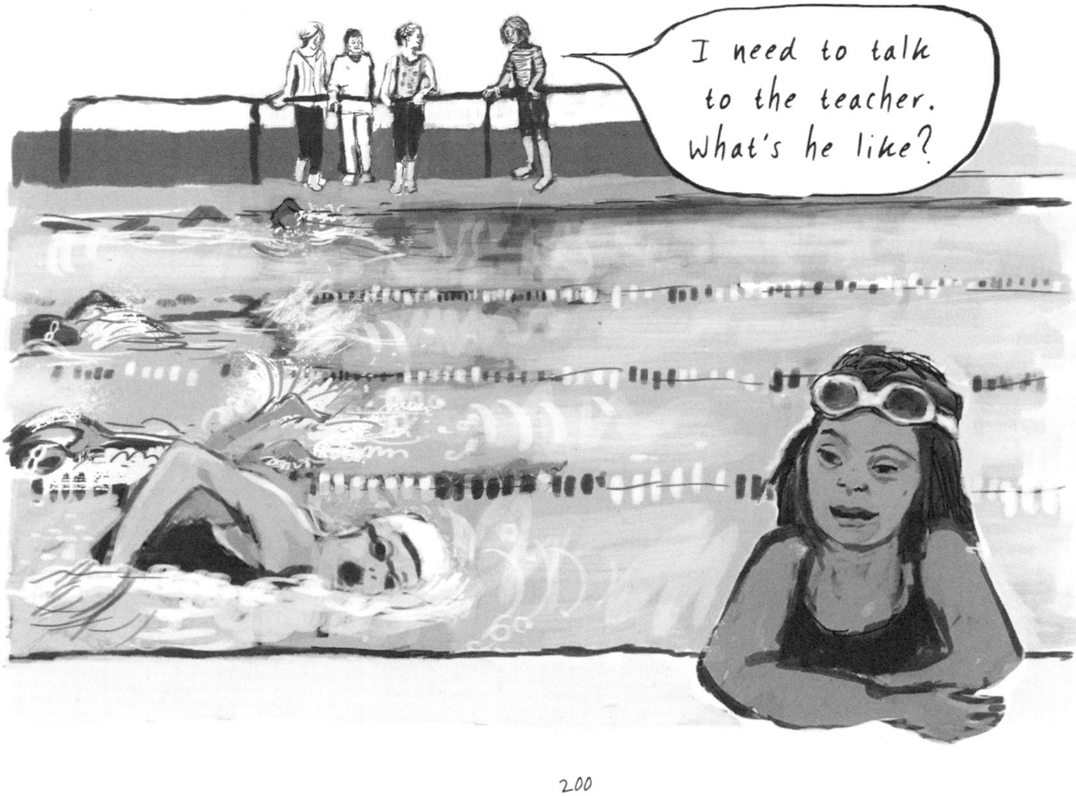
I need to talk to the teacher. What's he like?

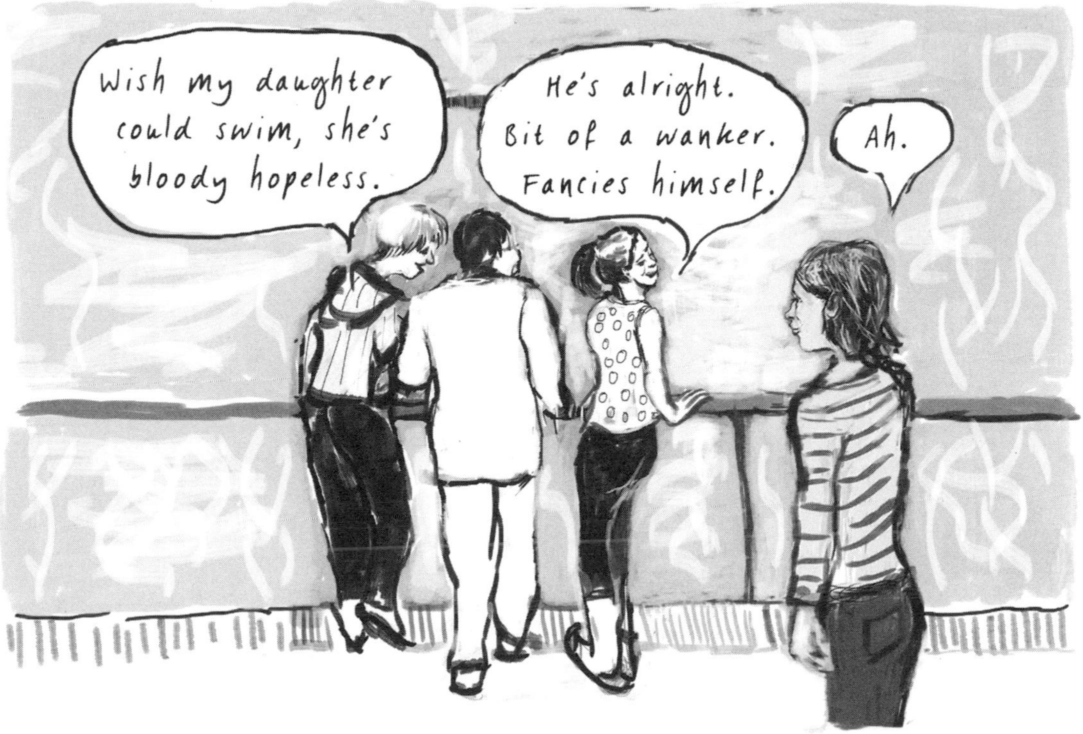
Wish my daughter could swim, she's bloody hopeless.
He's alright. Bit of a wanker. Fancies himself.
Ah.

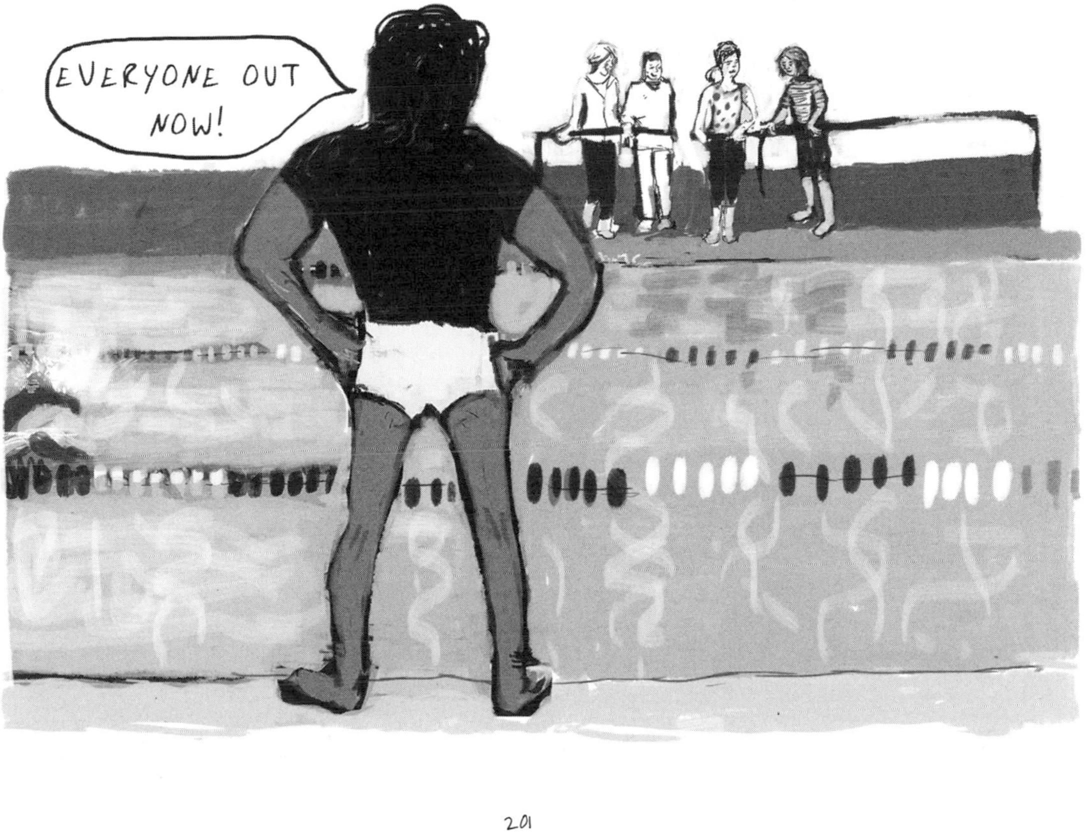
EVERYONE OUT NOW!

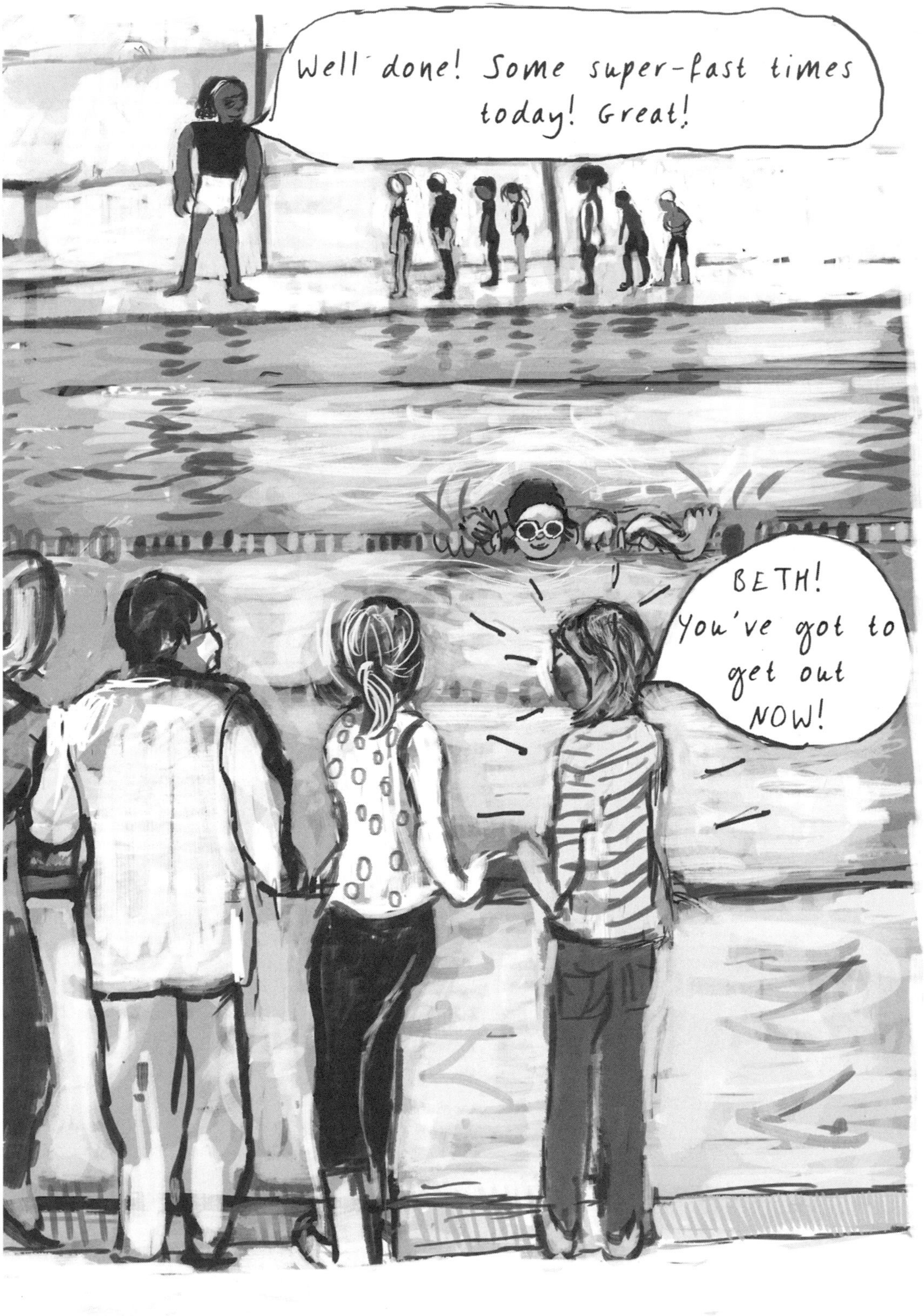
Well done! Some super-fast times today! Great!
BETH! You've got to get out NOW!

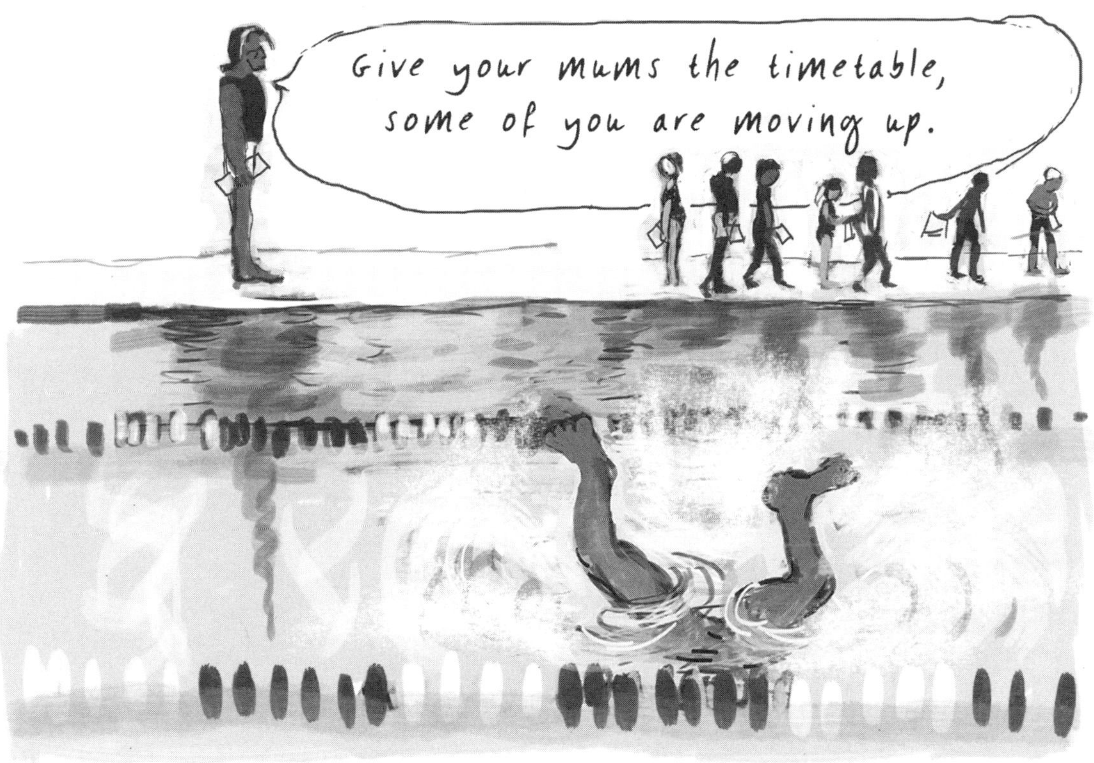
Give your mums the timetable, some of you are moving up.

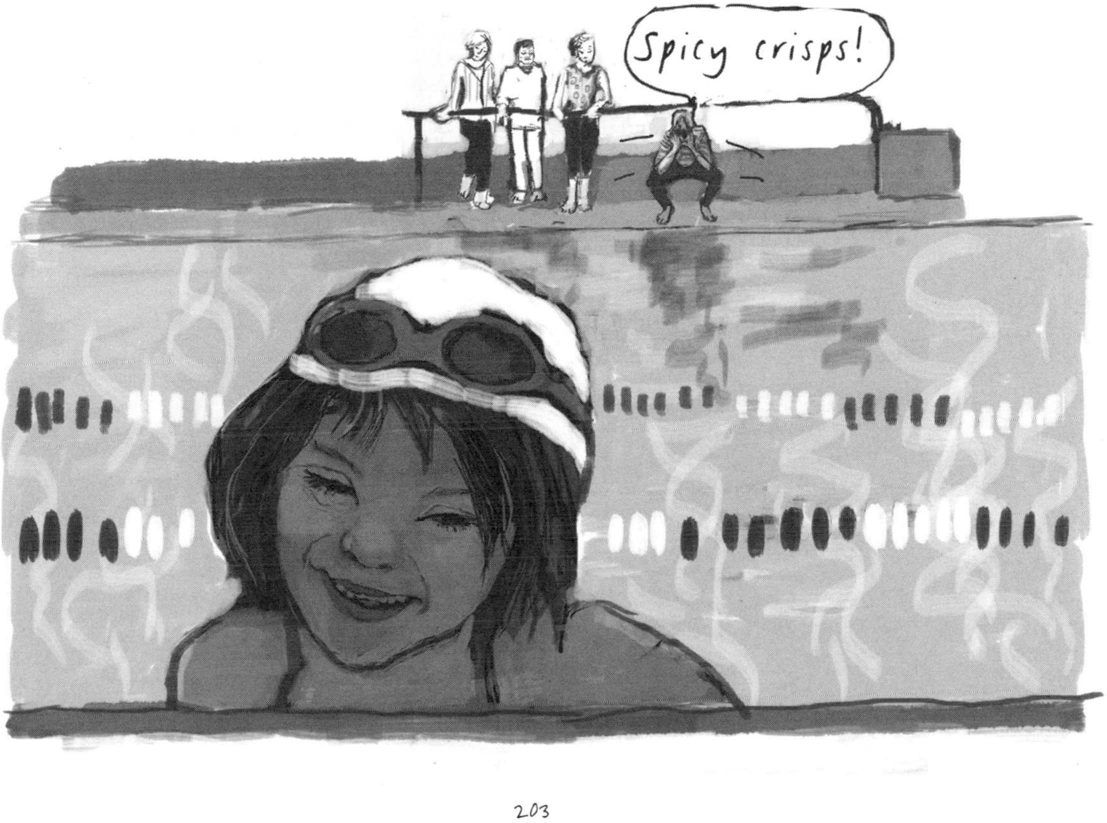
Spicy crisps!

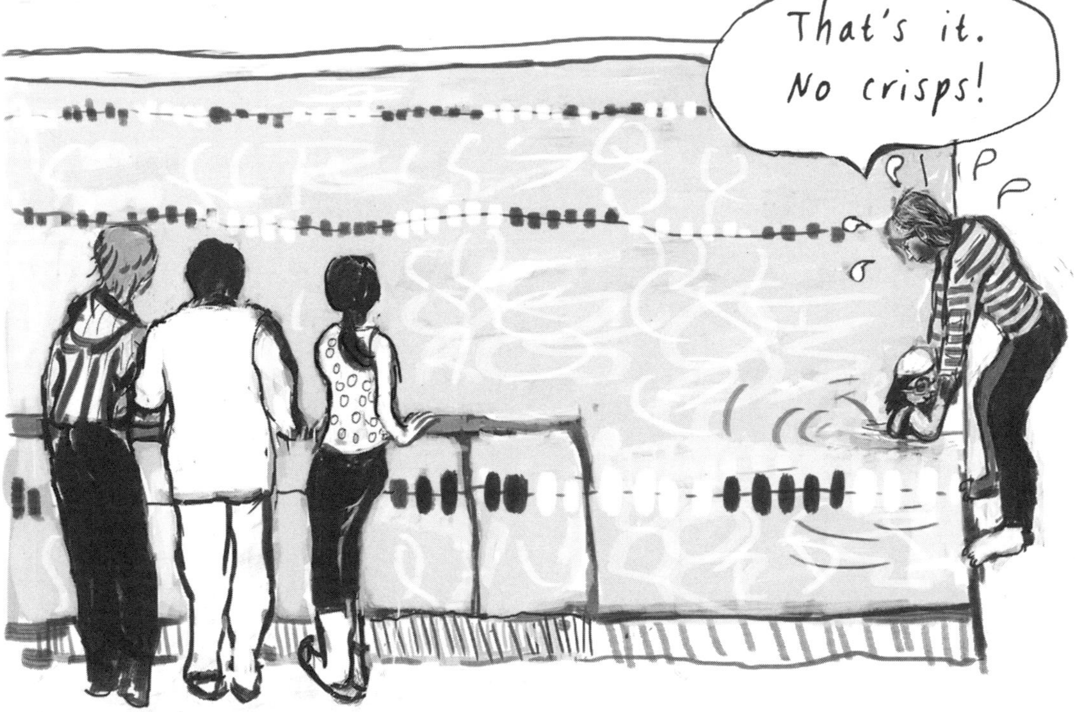
That's it.
No crisps!

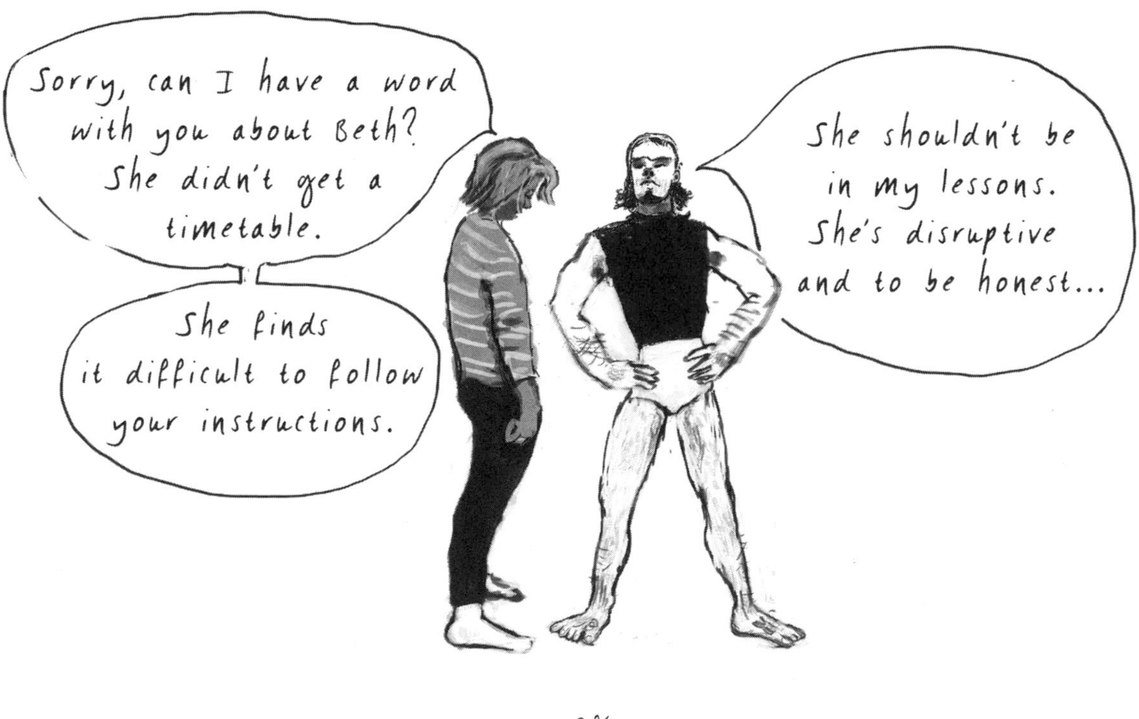
Sorry, can I have a word with you about Beth? She didn't get a timetable.
She finds it difficult to follow your instructions.
She shouldn't be in my lessons. She's disruptive and to be honest...

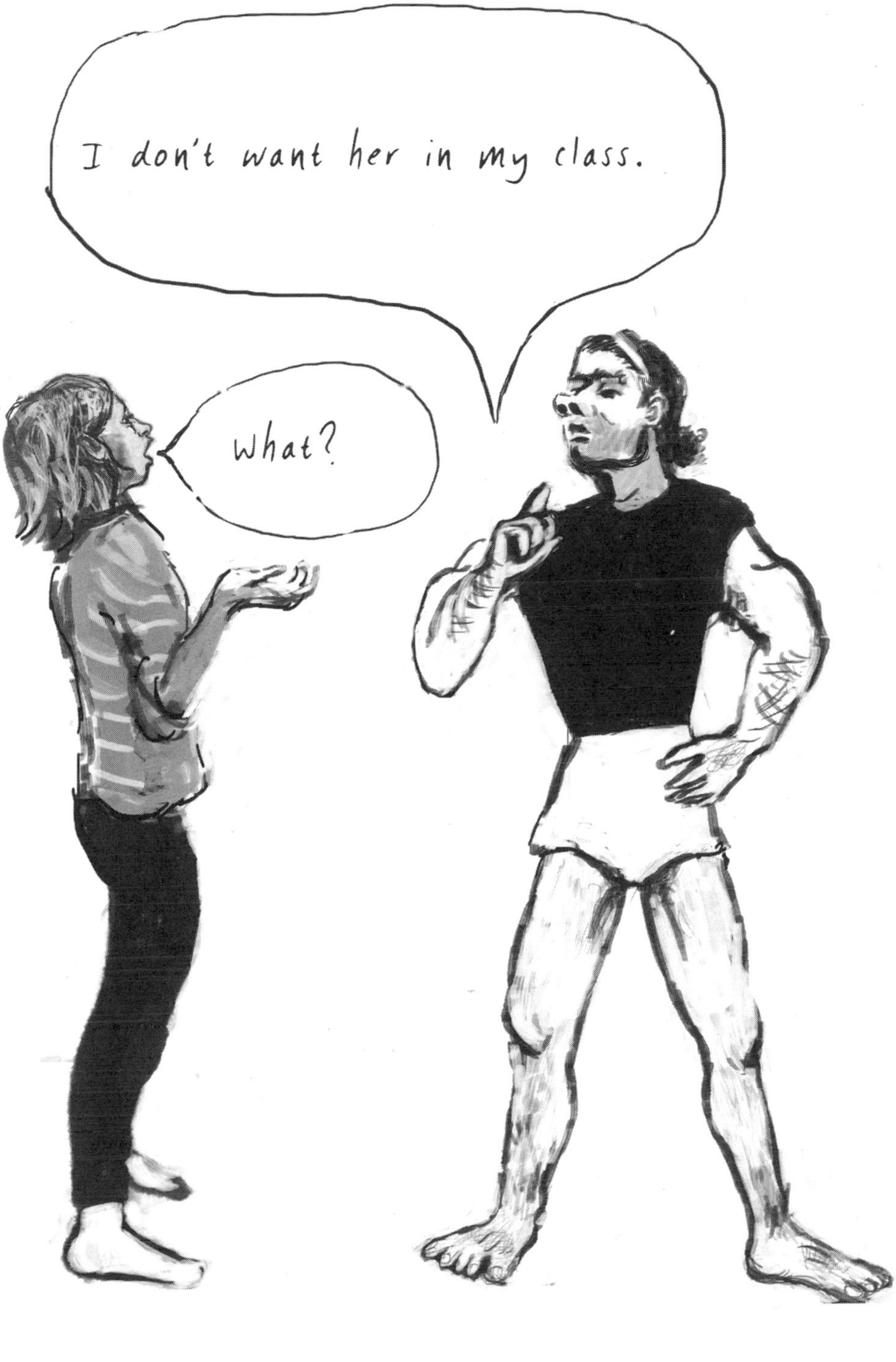
I don't want her in my class.
what?

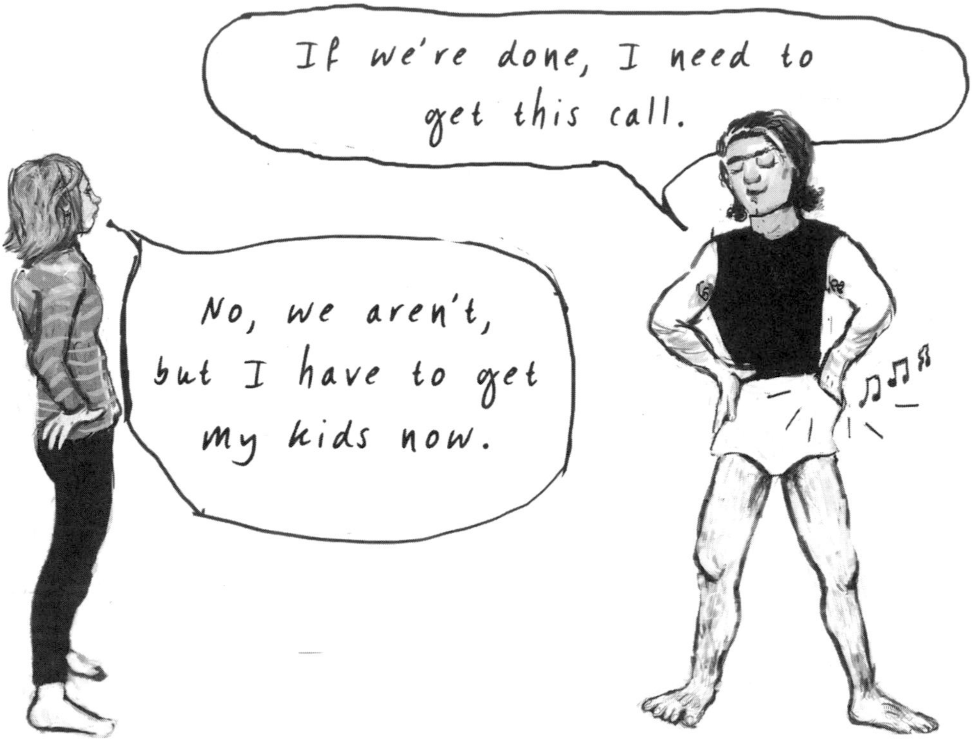
If we're done, I need to get this call.
No, we aren't, but I have to get my kids now.

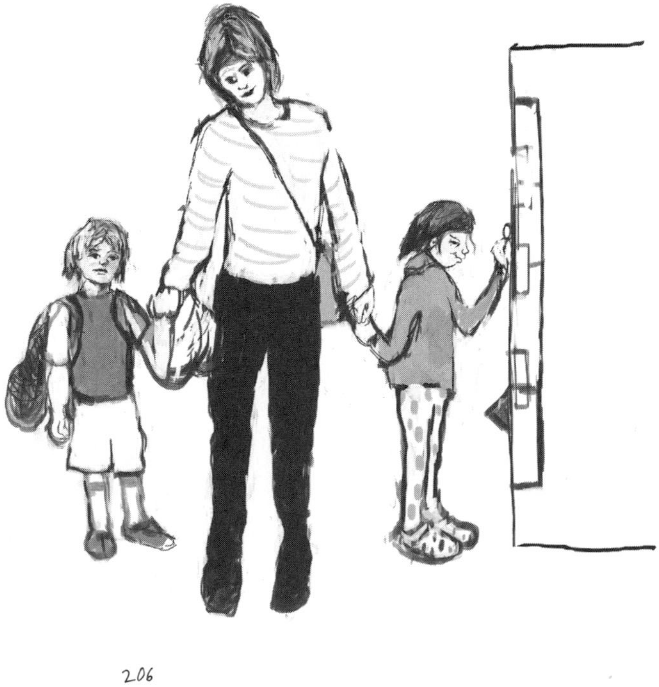

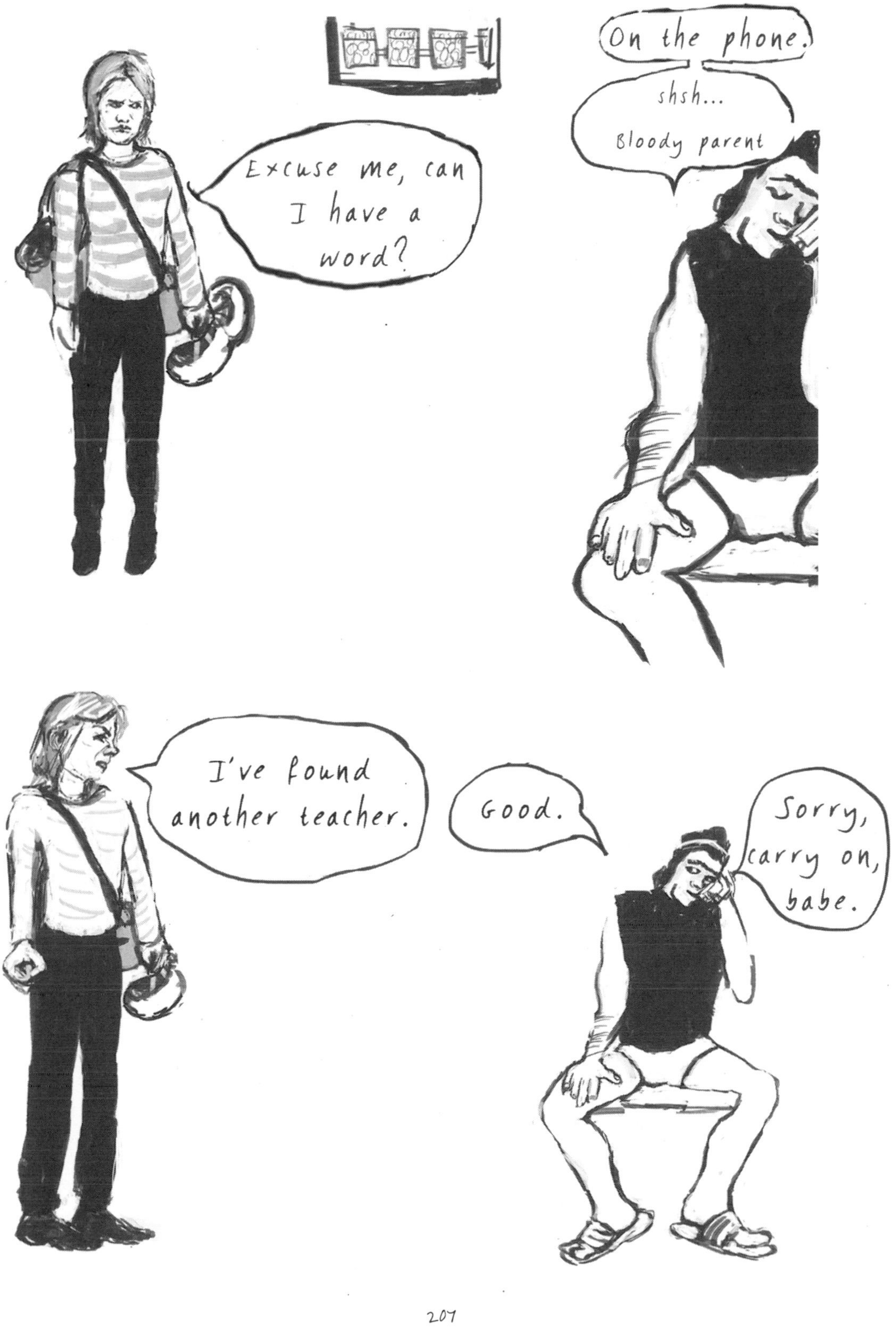
Excuse me, can I have a word?
On the phone.
shsh...
Bloody parent
I've found another teacher.
Good.
Sorry, carry on, babe.

SPICY
HOT
HOT

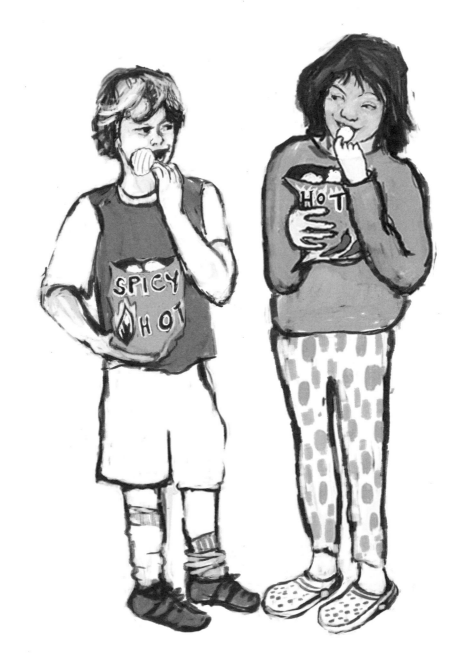

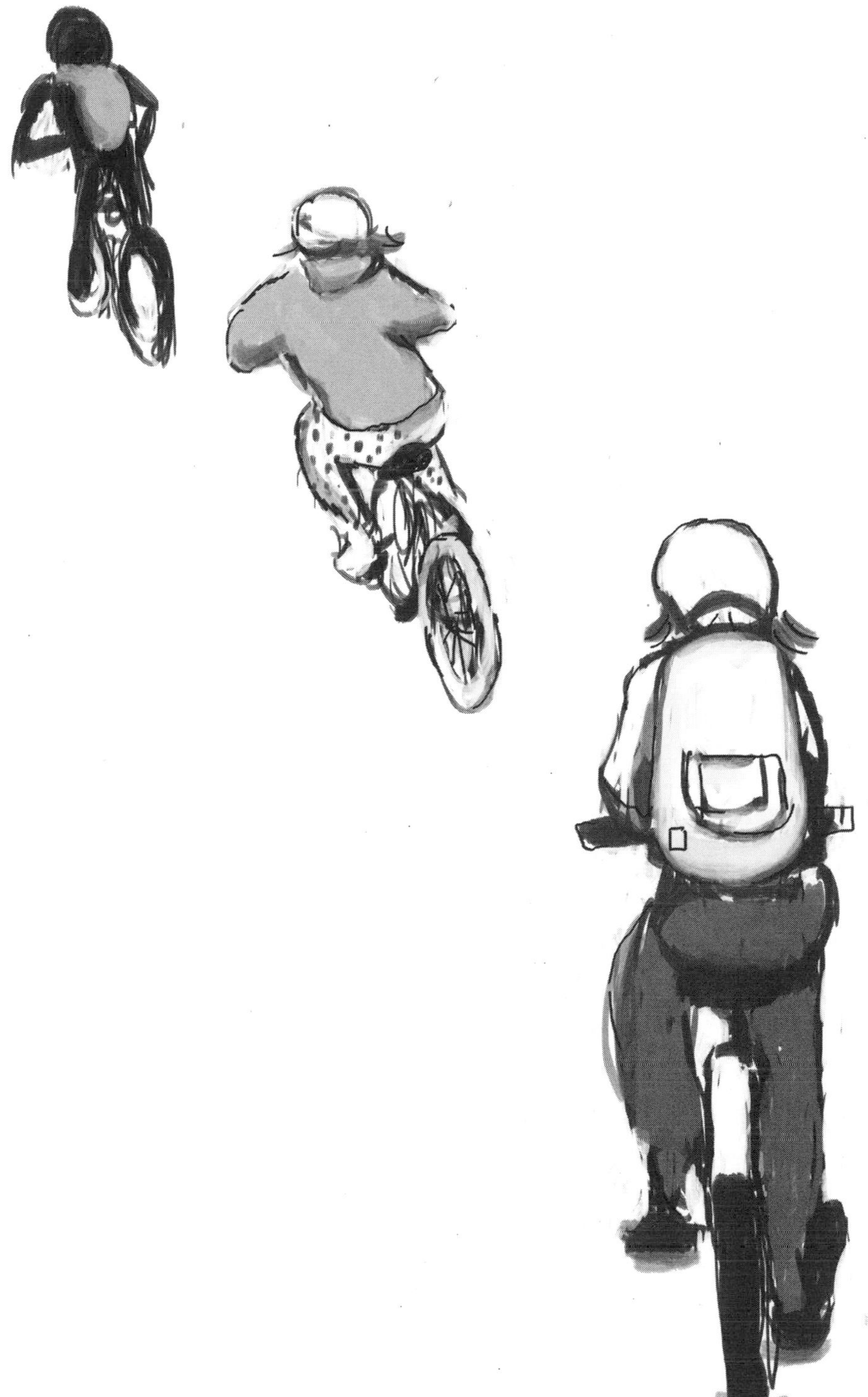

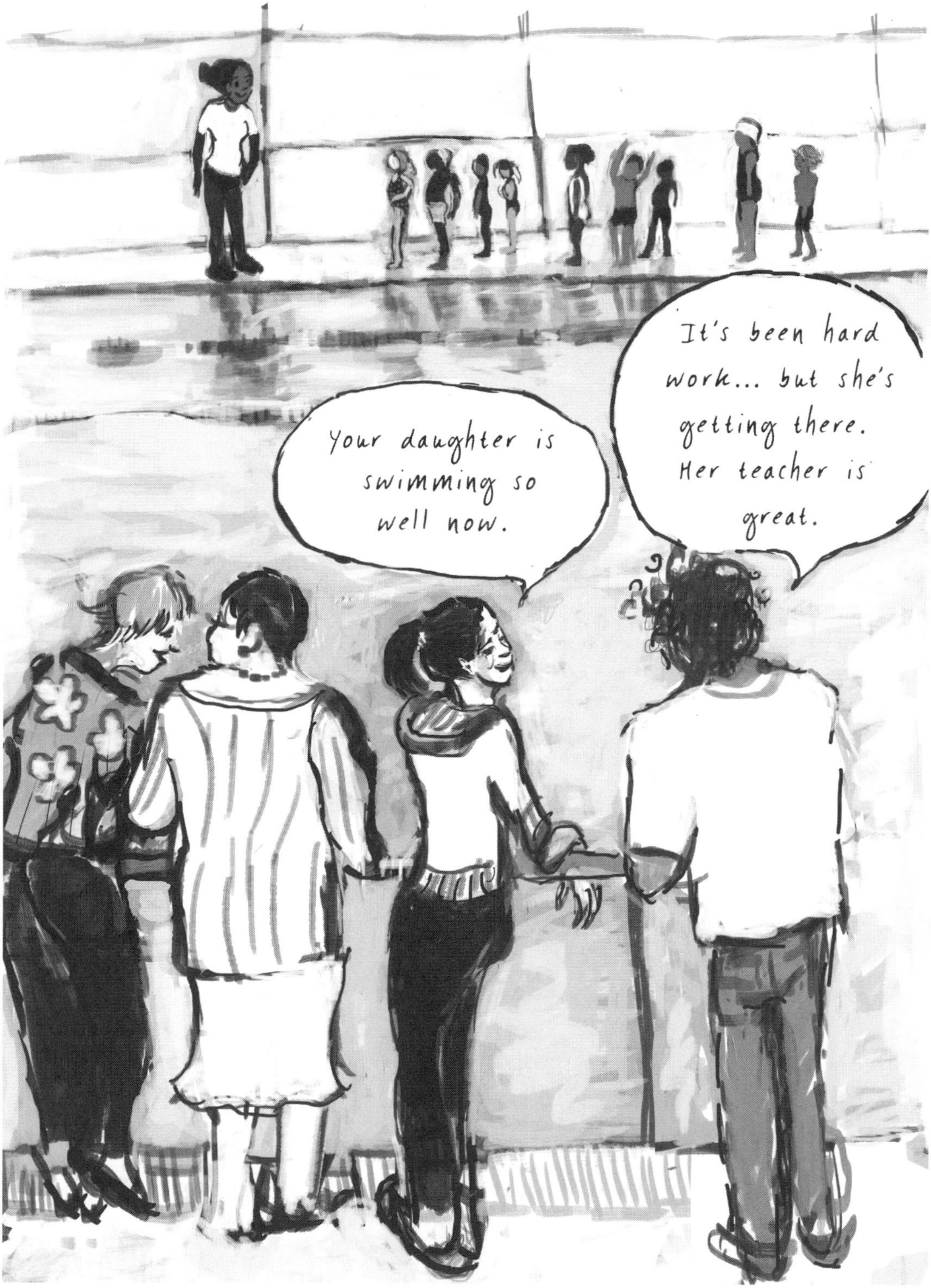
Your daughter is swimming so well now.
It's been hard work... but she's getting there. Her teacher is great.

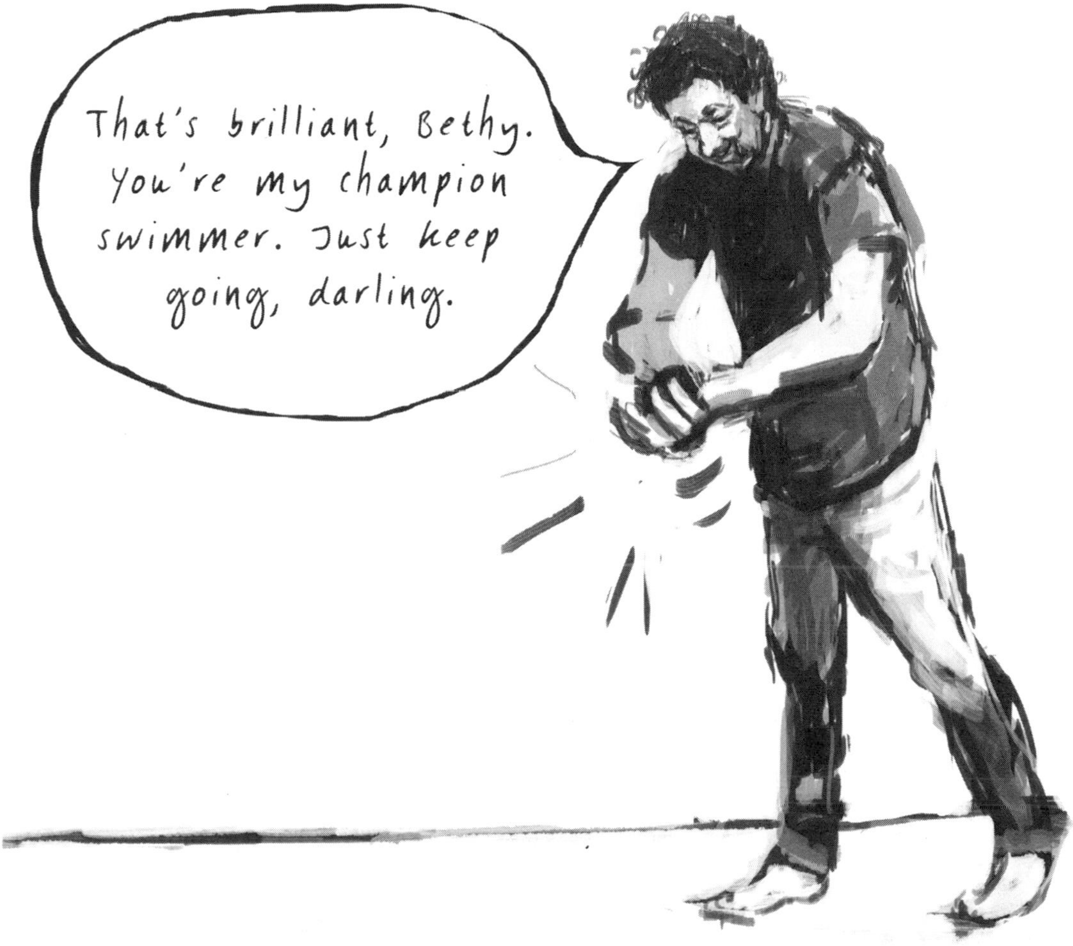
That's brilliant, Bethy. You're my champion swimmer. Just keep going, darling.

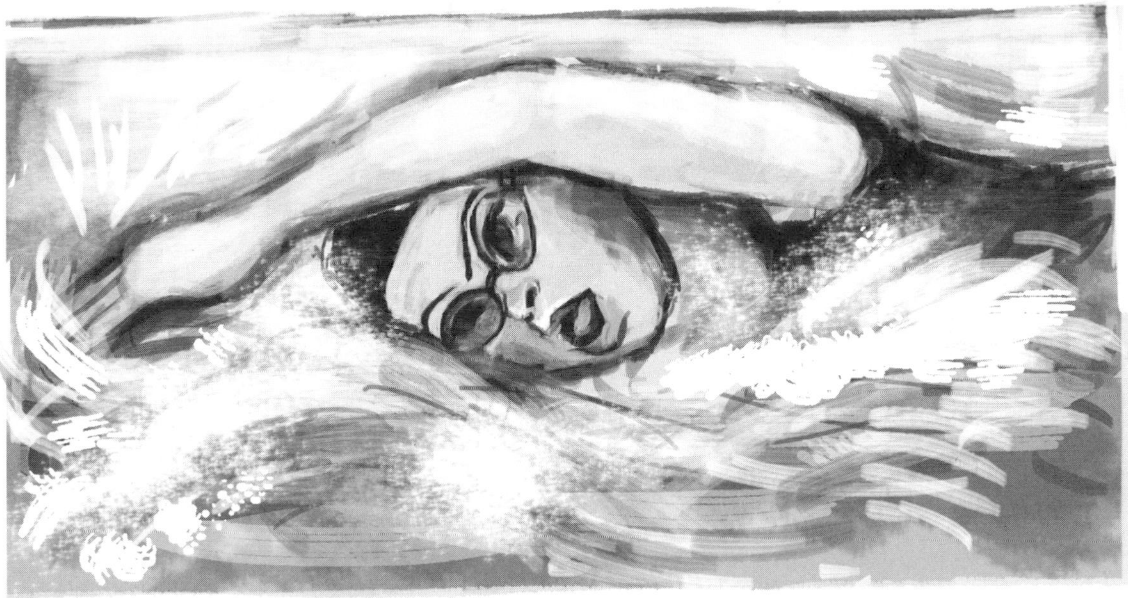

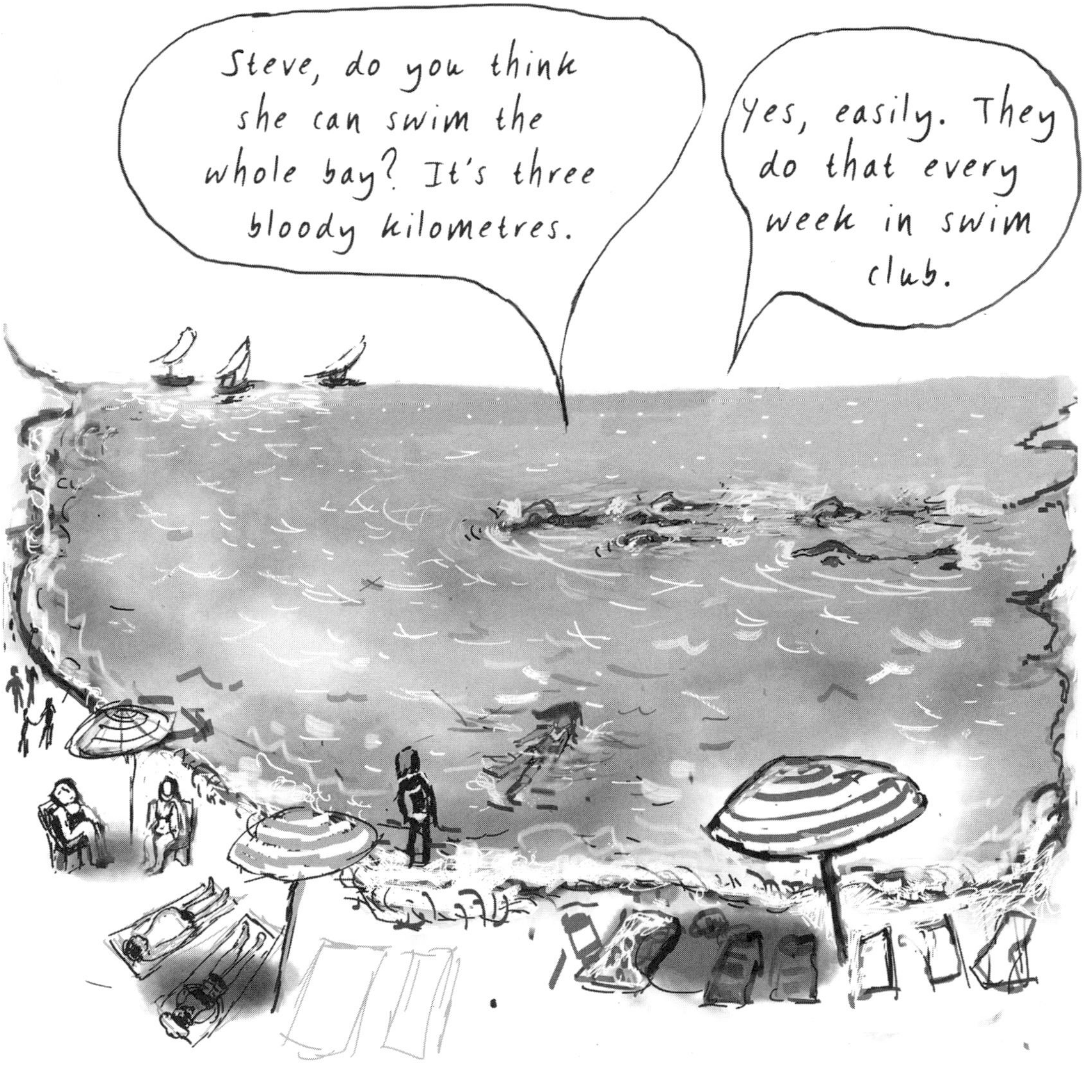
Steve, do you think she can swim the whole bay? It's three bloody kilometres.
Yes, easily. They do that every week in swim club.

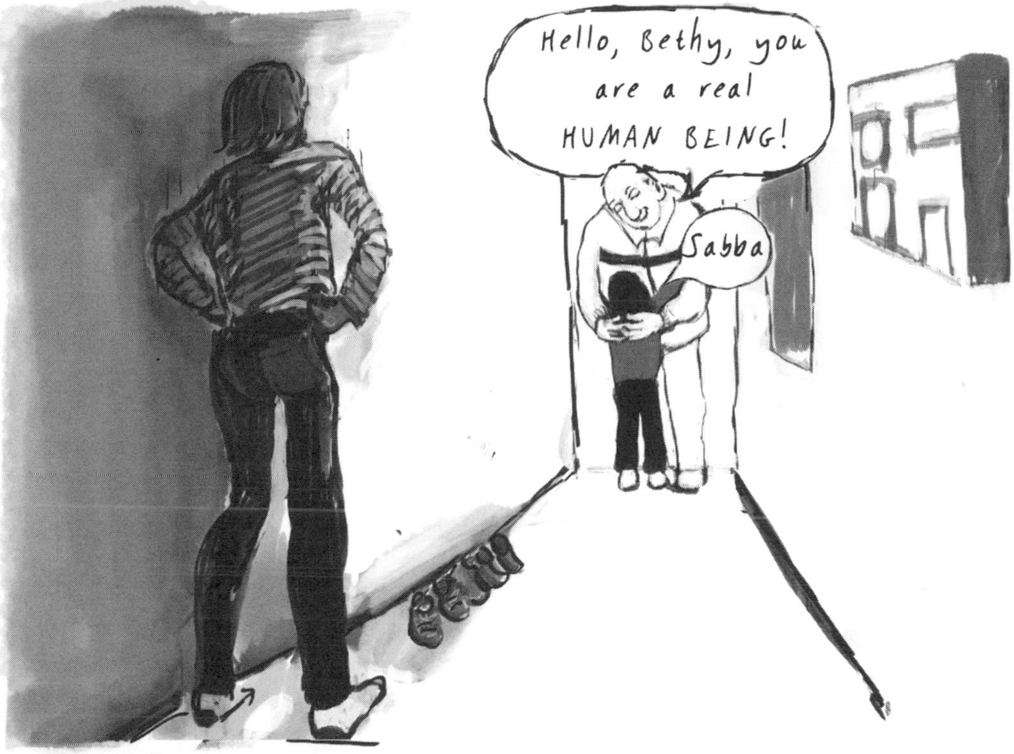
Hello, Bethy, you are a real HUMAN BEING!
Sabba

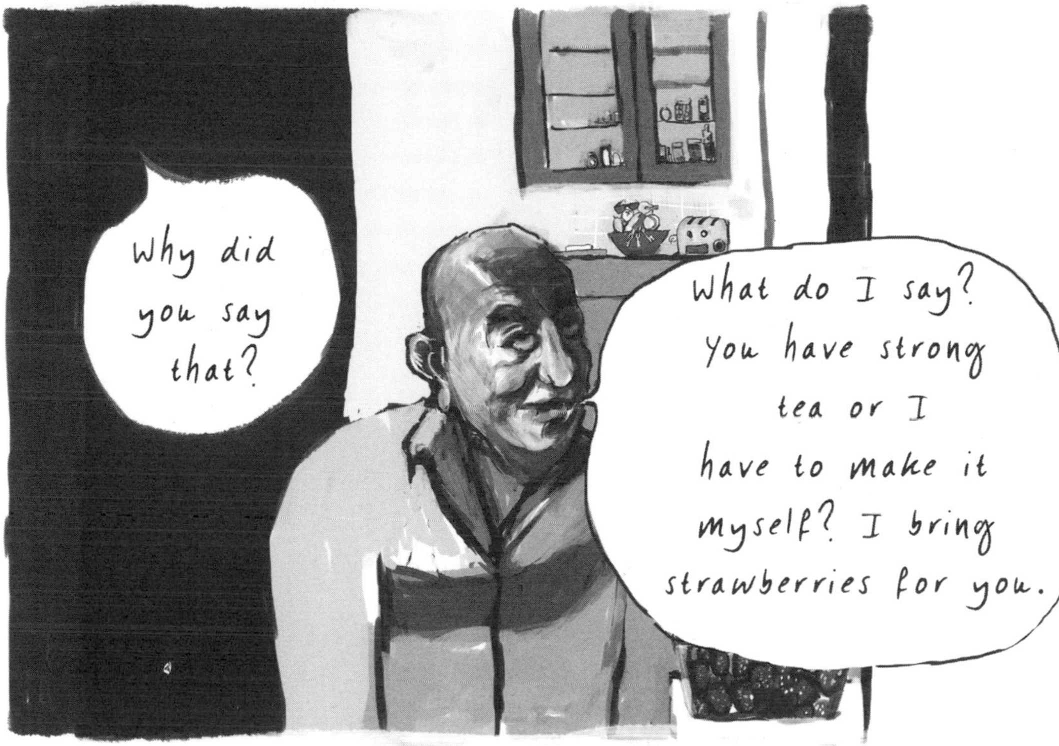
Why did you say that?
What do I say? You have strong tea or I have to make it myself? I bring strawberries for you.

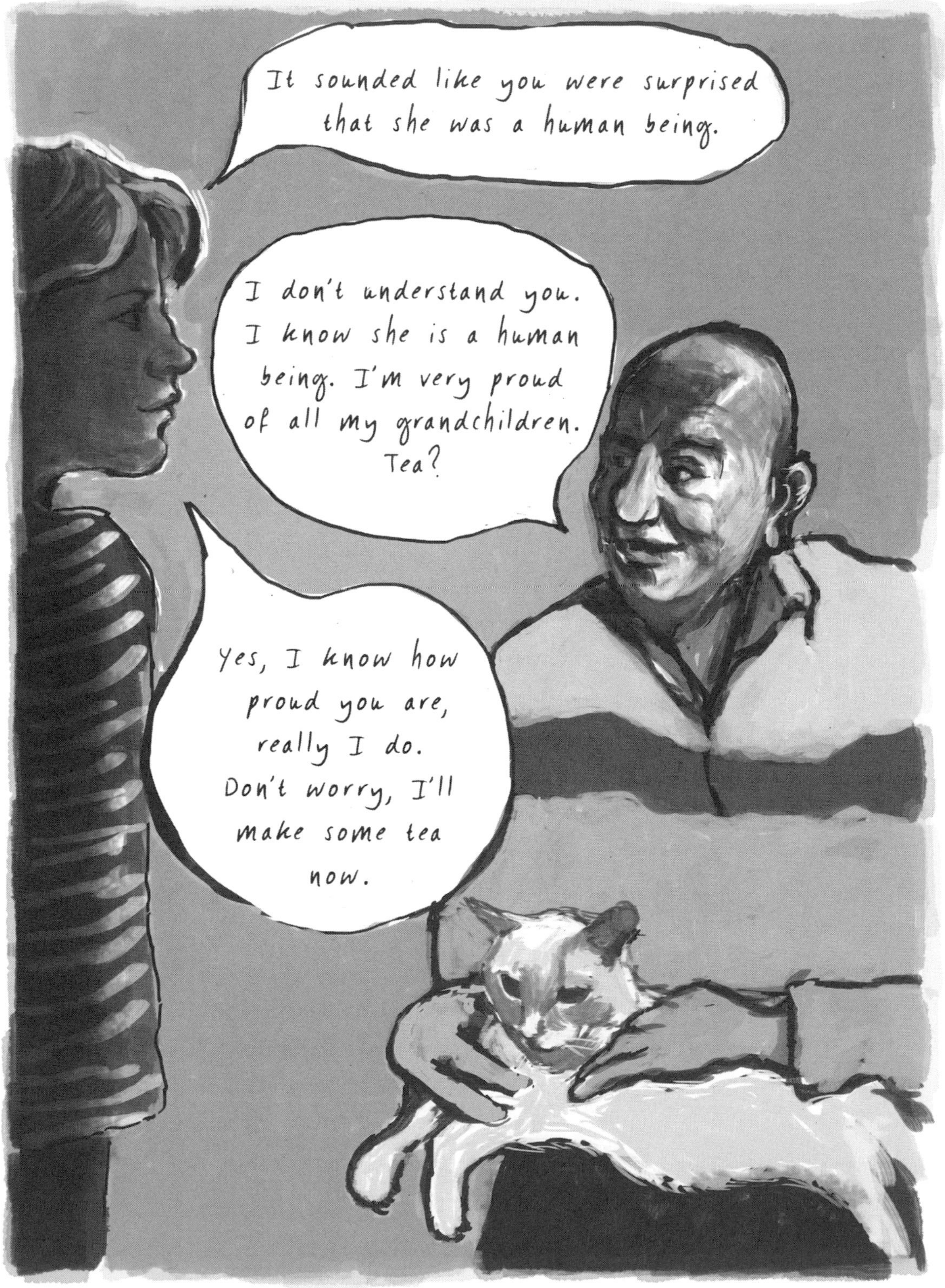
It sounded like you were surprised that she was a human being.
I don't understand you. I know she is a human being. I'm very proud of all my grandchildren. Tea?
Yes, I know how proud you are, really I do. Don't worry, I'll make some tea now.

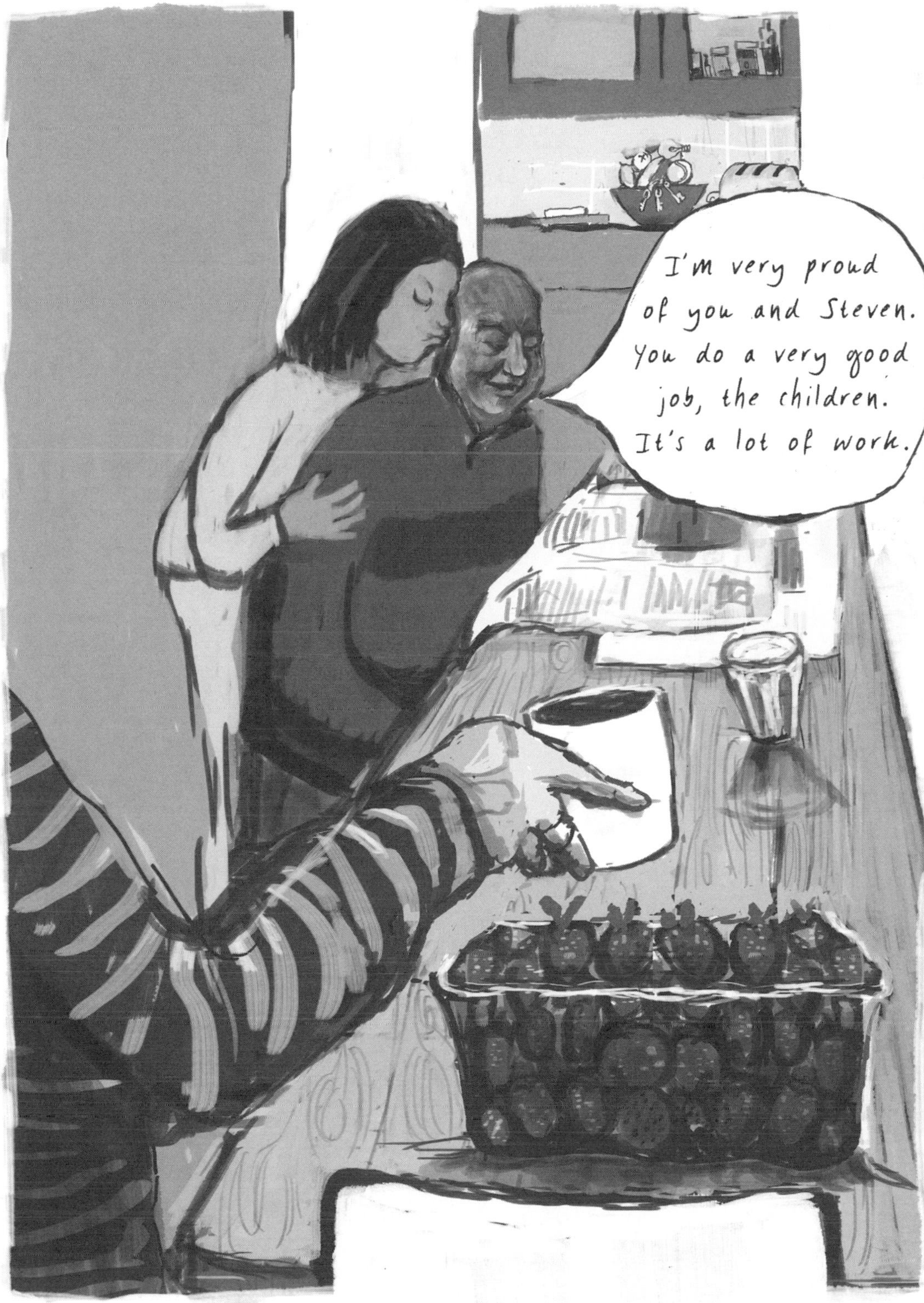
I'm very proud of you and Steven. You do a very good job, the children. It's a lot of work.

I love all my children, all my grandchildren. They're all human beings. Take a photo.

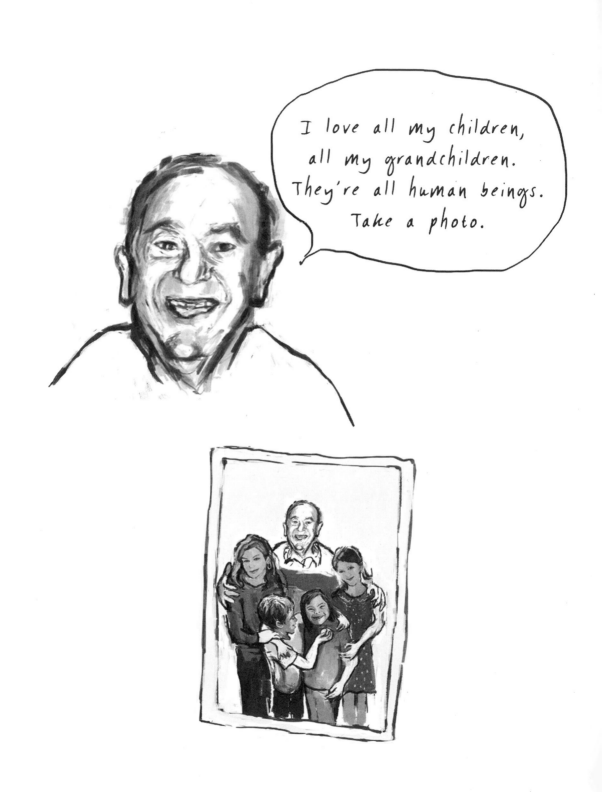

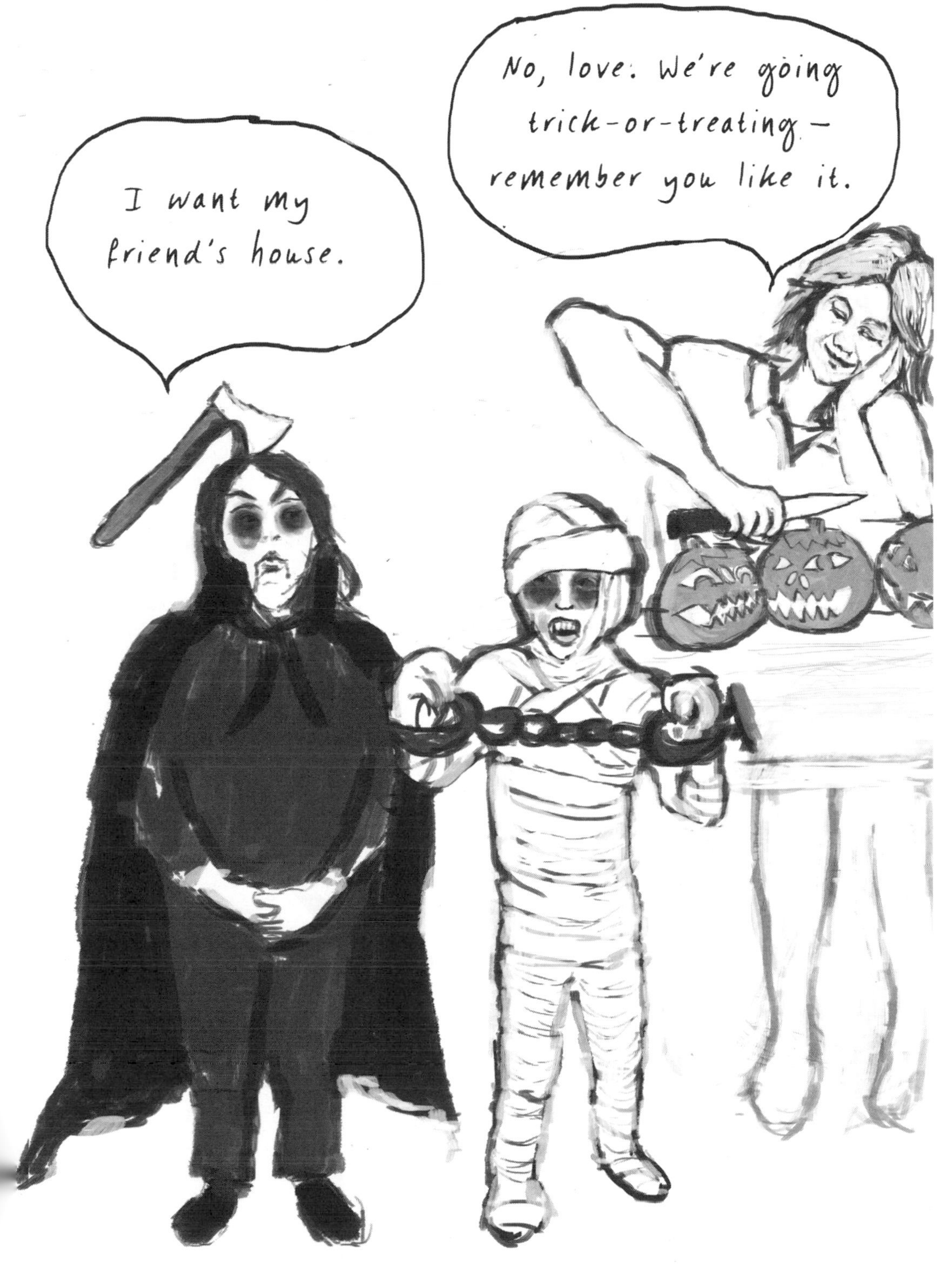
I want my friend's house.
No, love. We're going trick-or-treating – remember you like it.

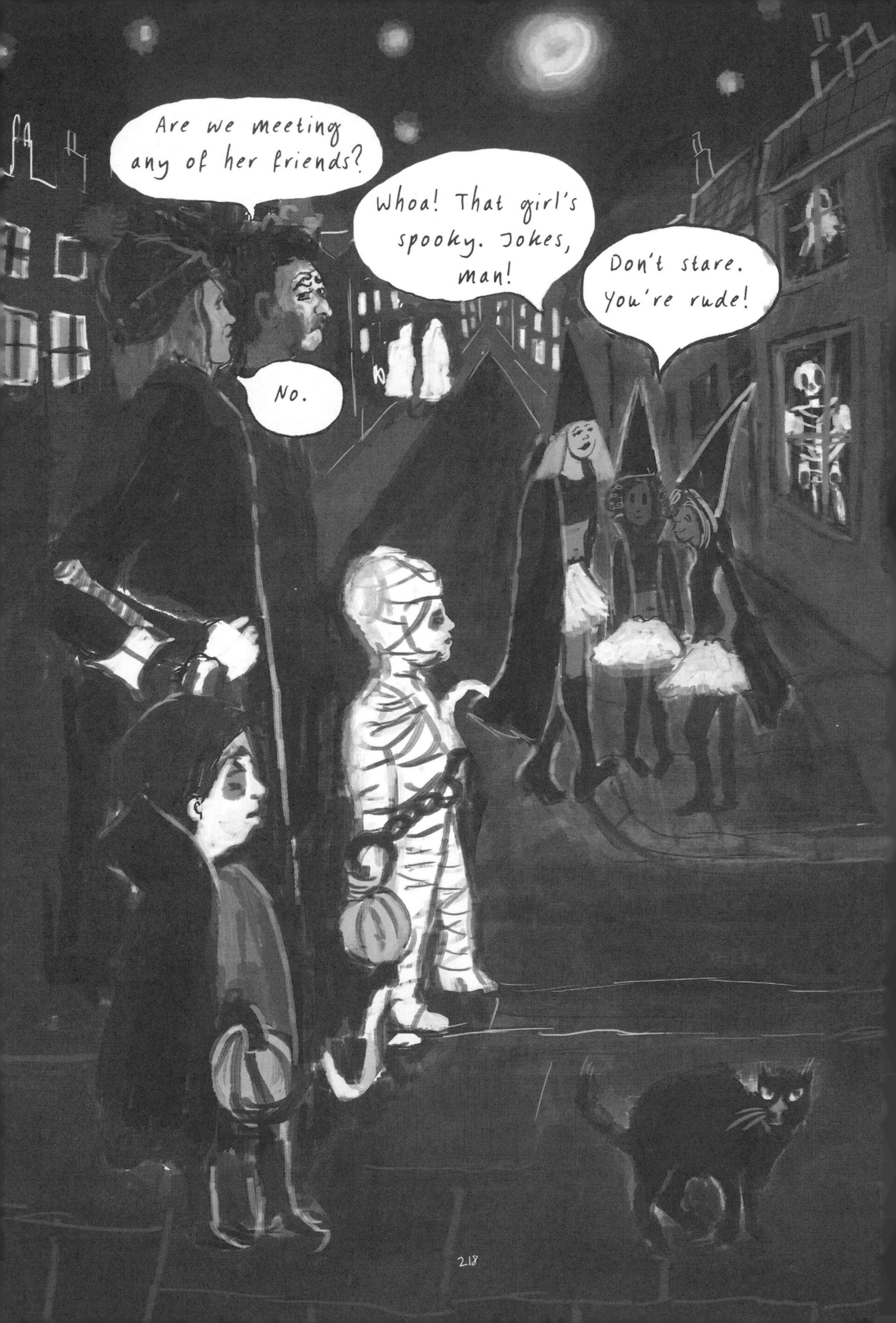
Are we meeting any of her friends?
No.
Whoa! That girl's spooky. Jokes, man!
Don't stare. You're rude!

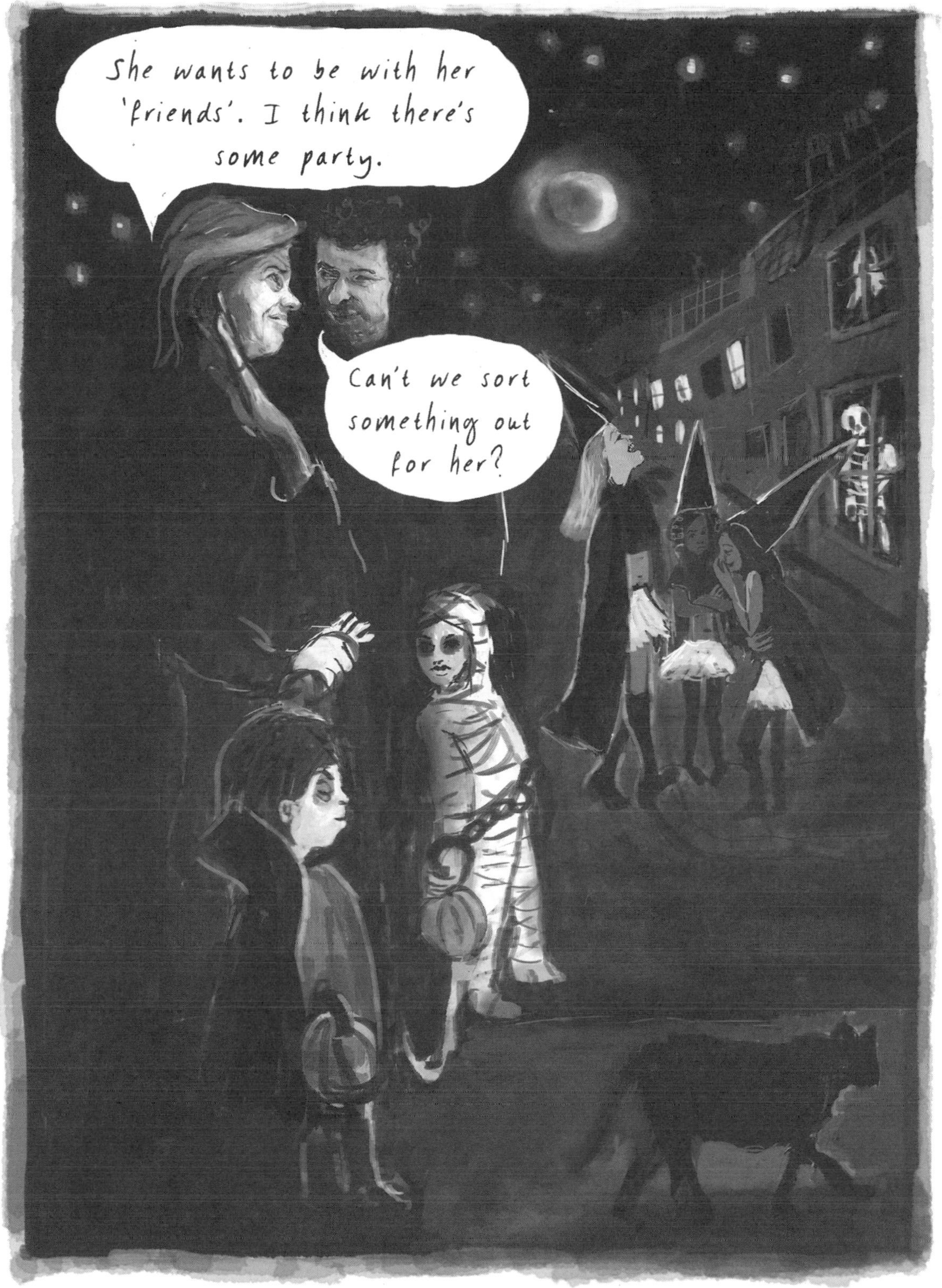
She wants to be with her 'friends'. I think there's some party.
Can't we sort something out for her?

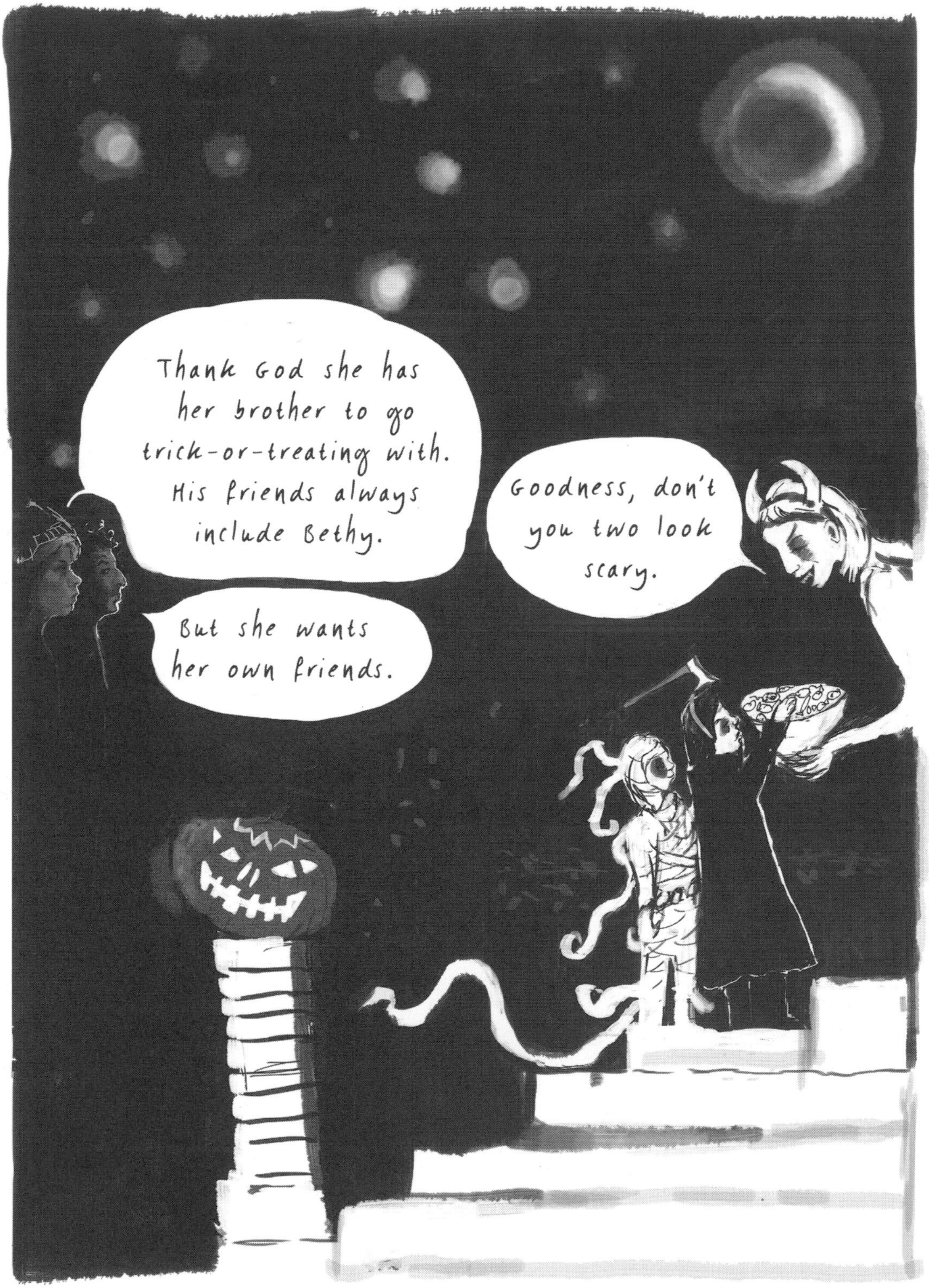
Thank God she has her brother to go trick-or-treating with. His friends always include Bethy.
But she wants her own friends.
Goodness, don't you two look scary.

Ring the doorbell, love.

Beth! Hi.
Mum! My class! My friends!
Oh, fuck!

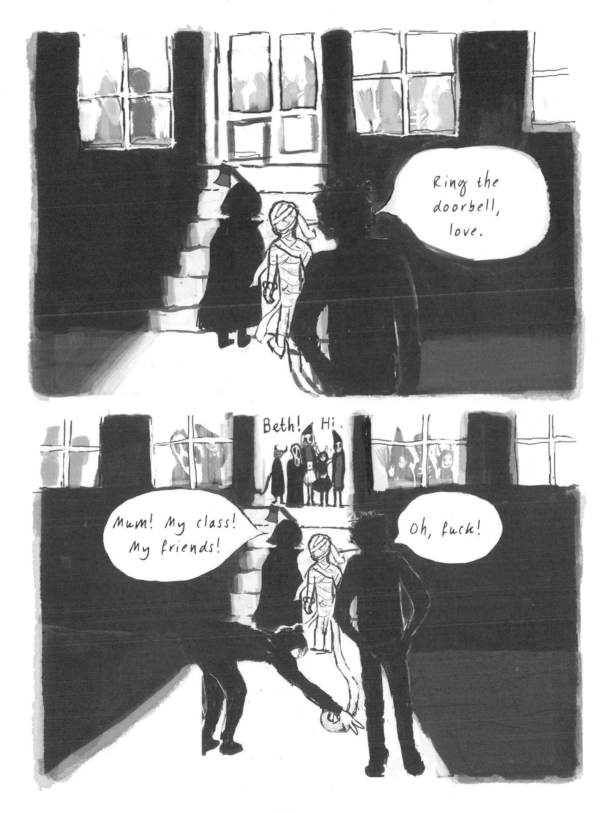

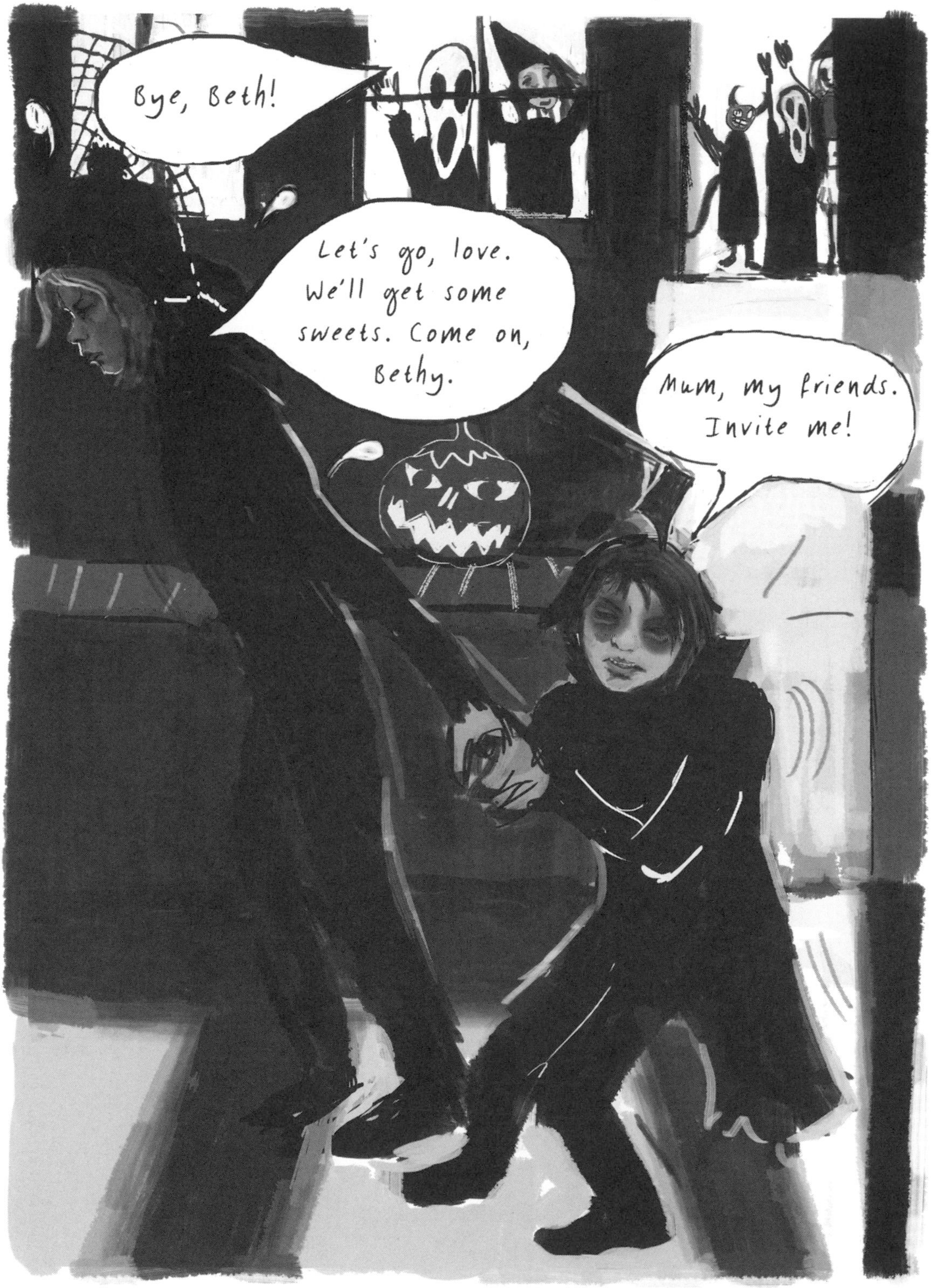
Bye, Beth!
Let's go, love. We'll get some sweets. Come on, Bethy.
Mum, my friends. Invite me!

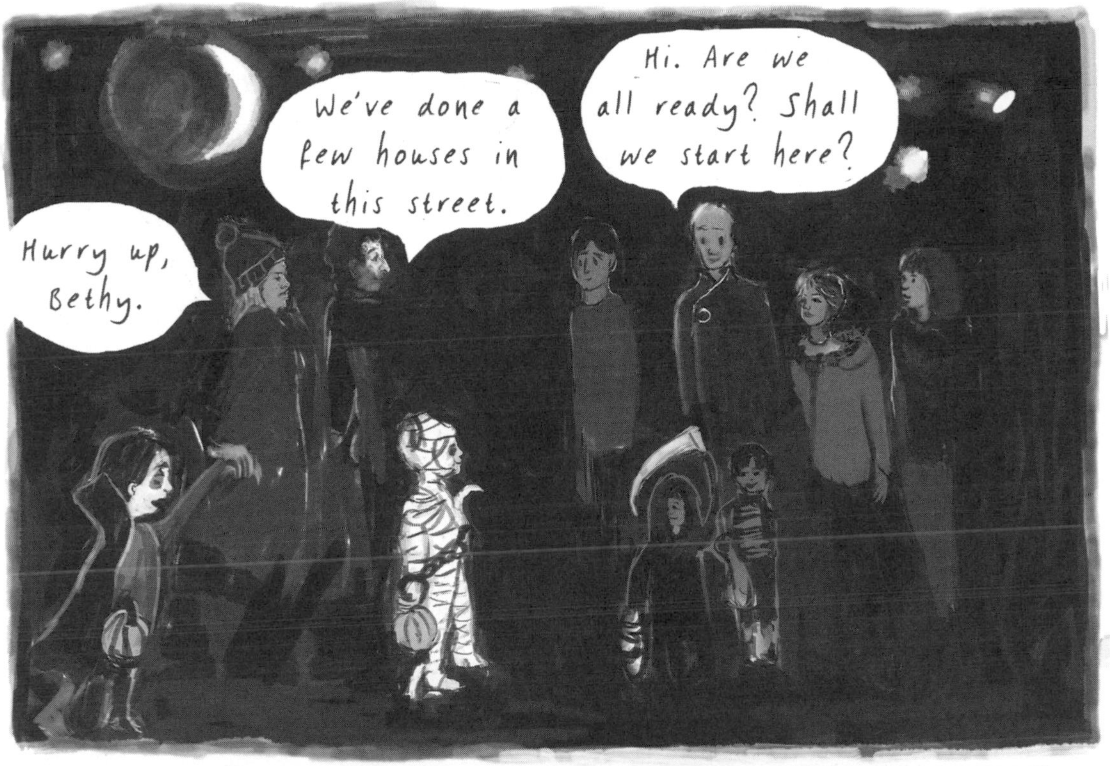
Hi. Are we all ready? Shall we start here?
We've done a few houses in this street.
Hurry up, Bethy.

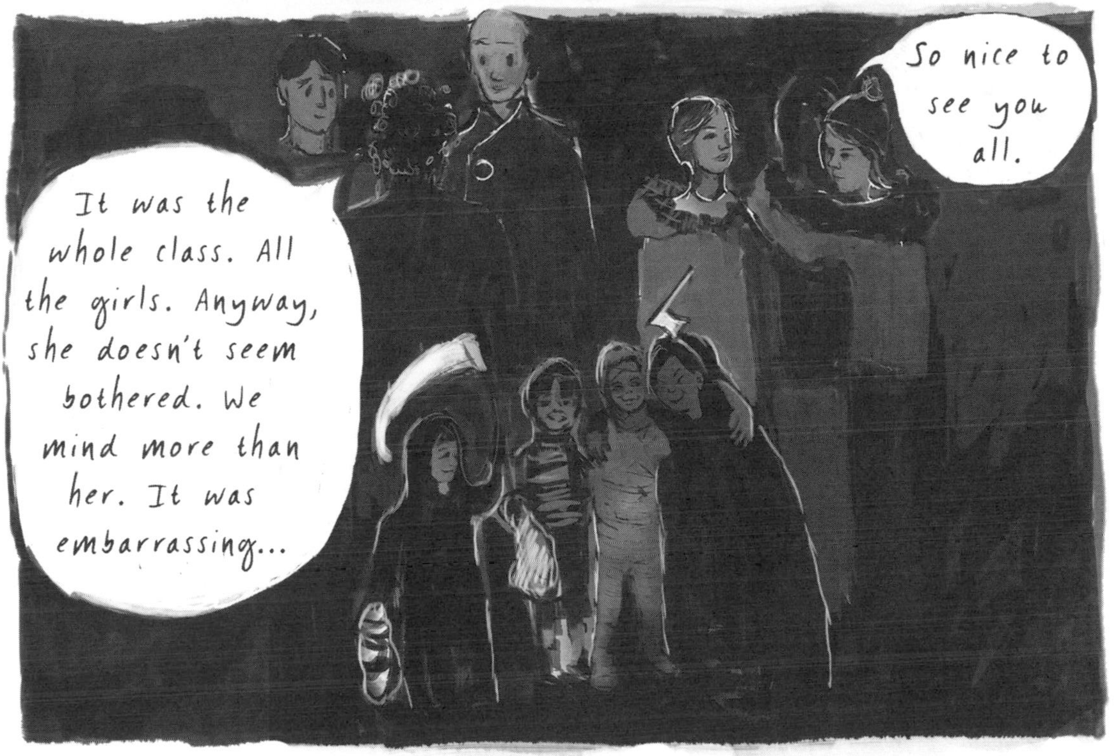
So nice to see you all.
It was the whole class. All the girls. Anyway, she doesn't seem bothered. We mind more than her. It was embarrassing...

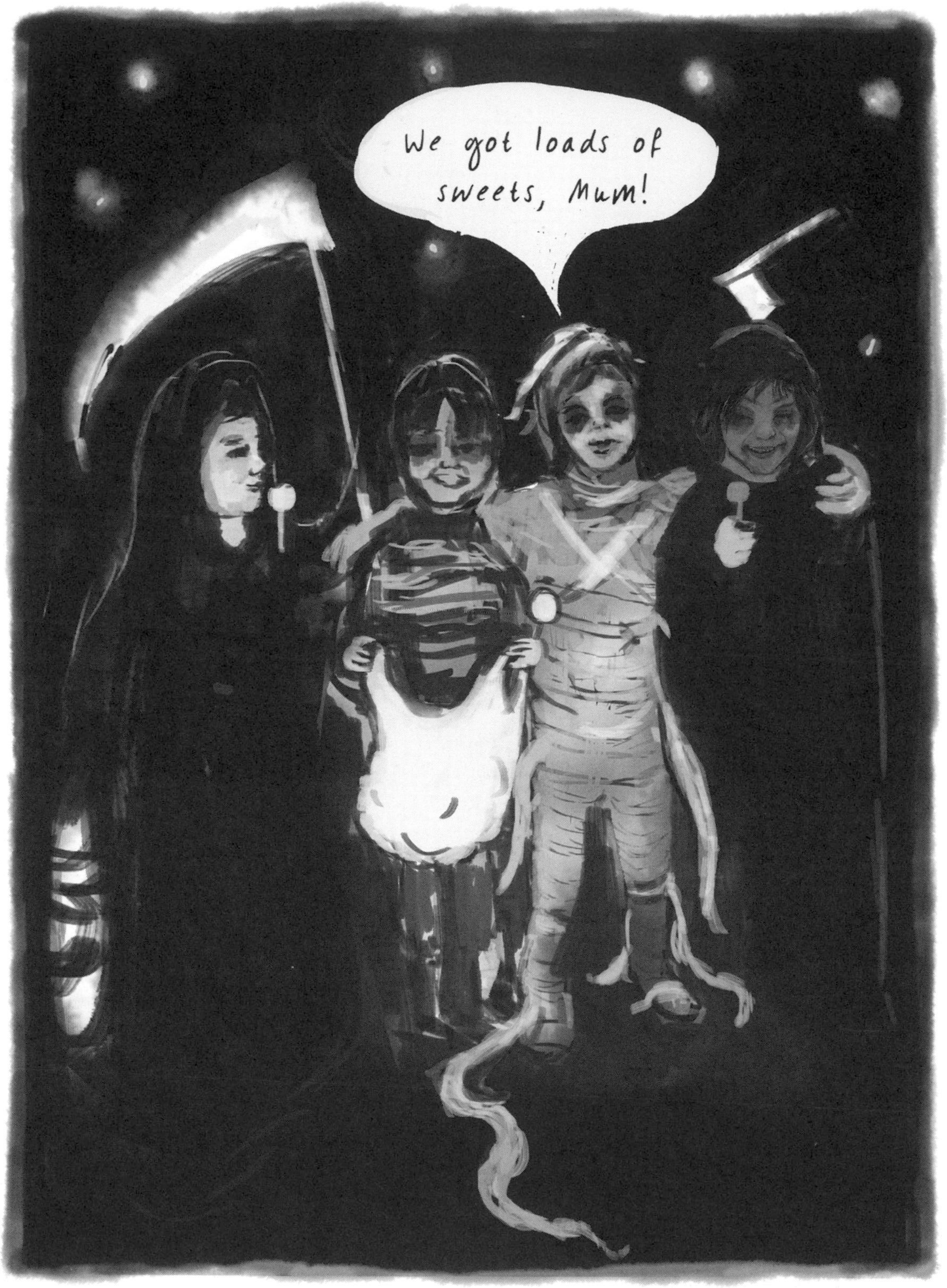
We got loads of sweets, Mum!

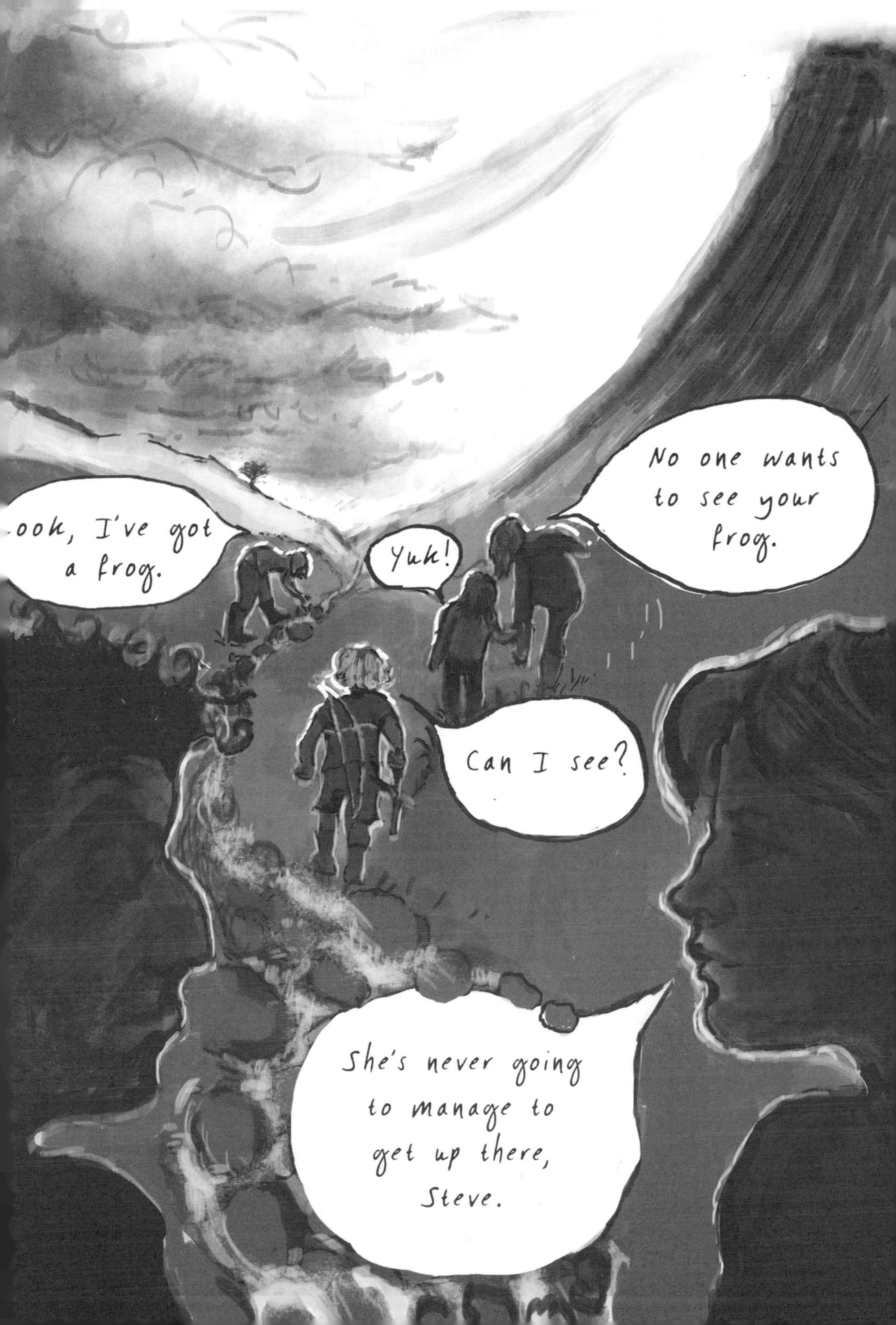
ook, I've got a frog.
Yuk!
No one wants to see your frog.
Can I see?
She's never going to manage to get up there, Steve.

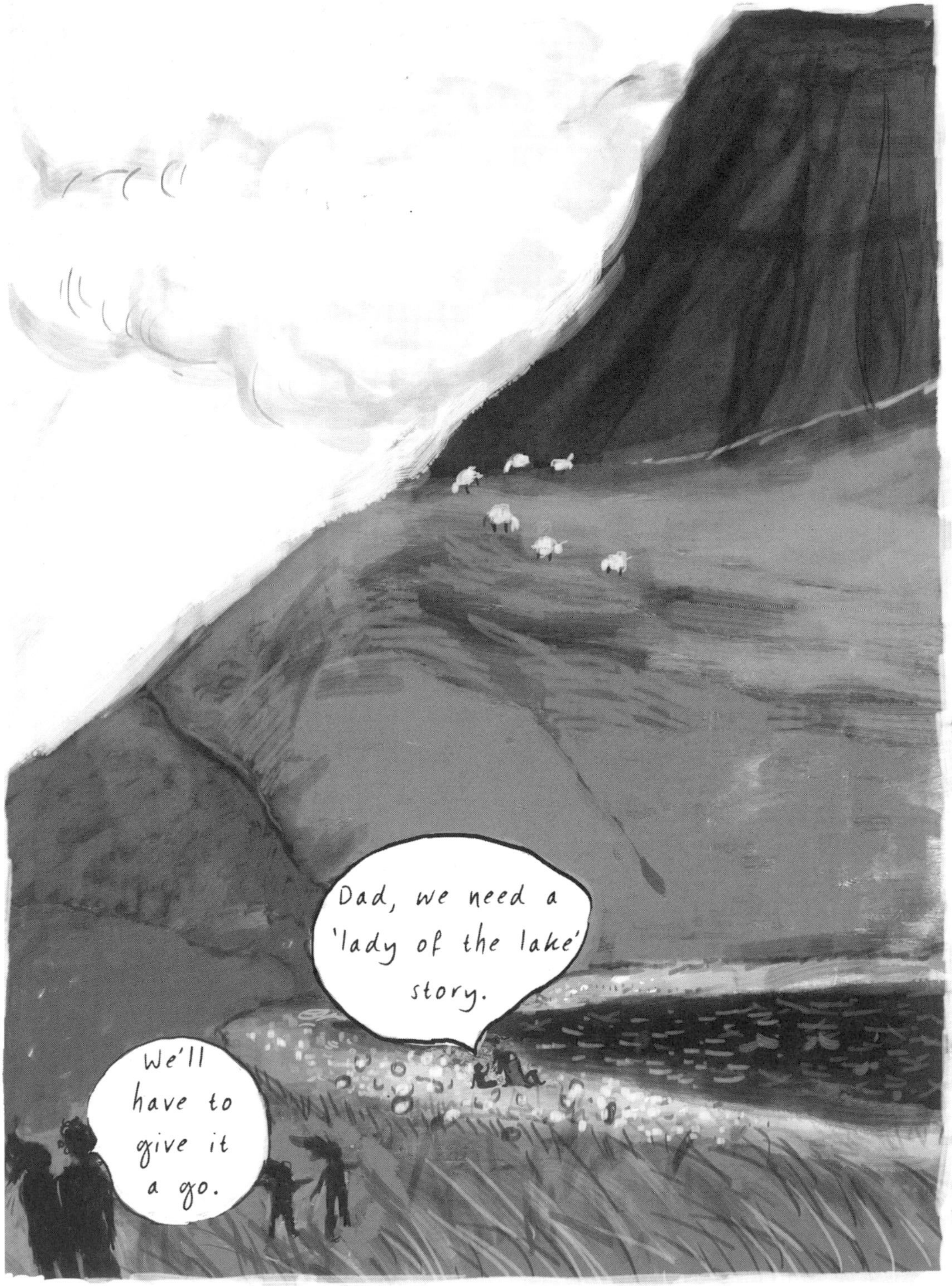
Dad, we need a 'lady of the lake' story.
We'll have to give it a go.

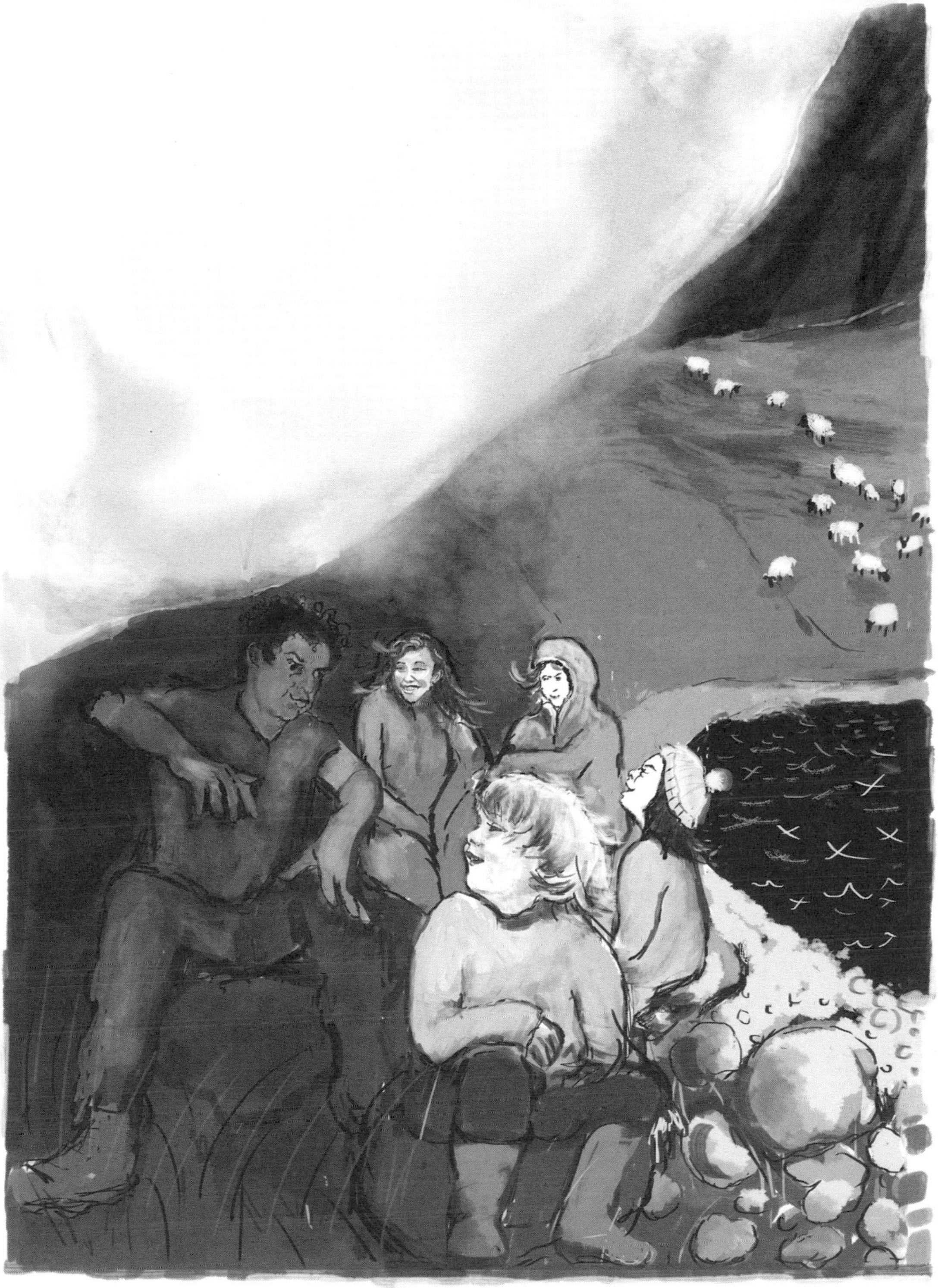

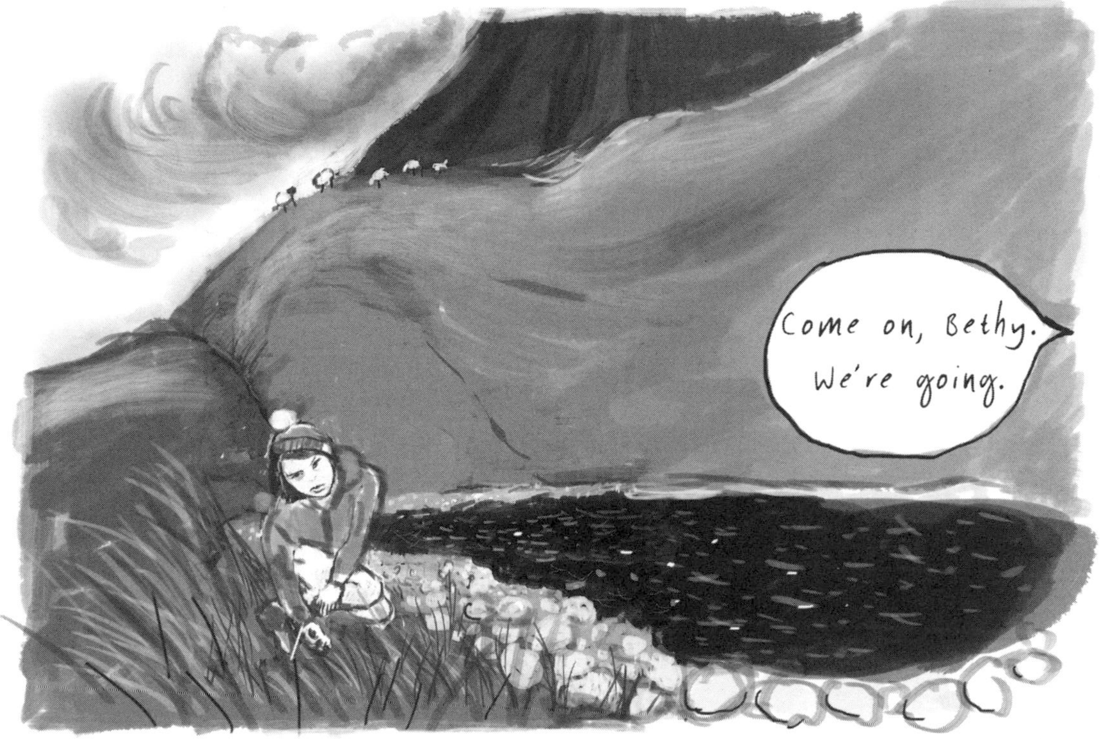
Come on, Bethy. We're going.

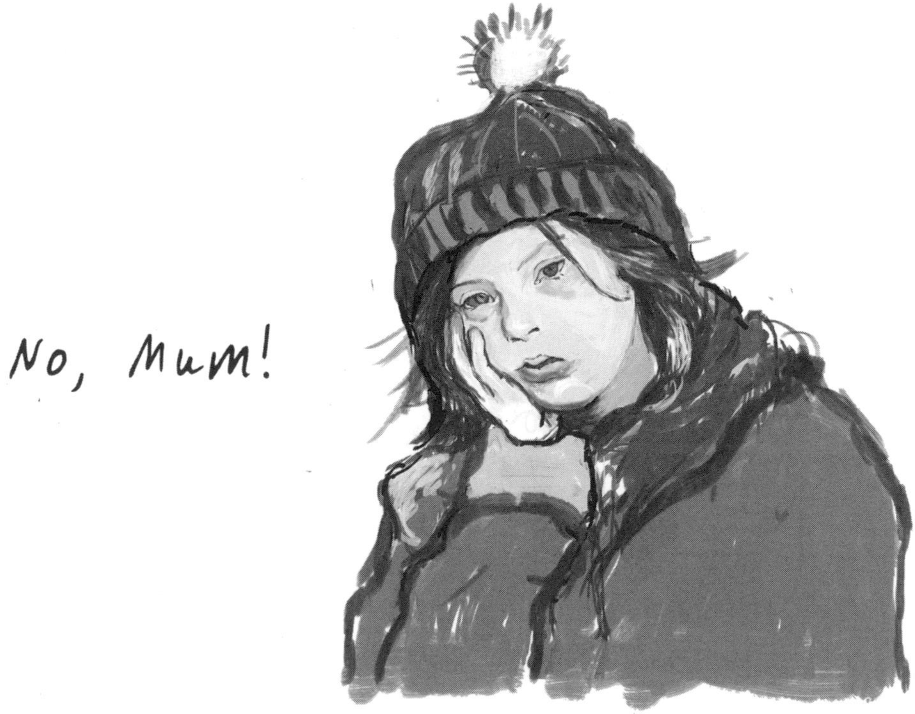
No, Mum!

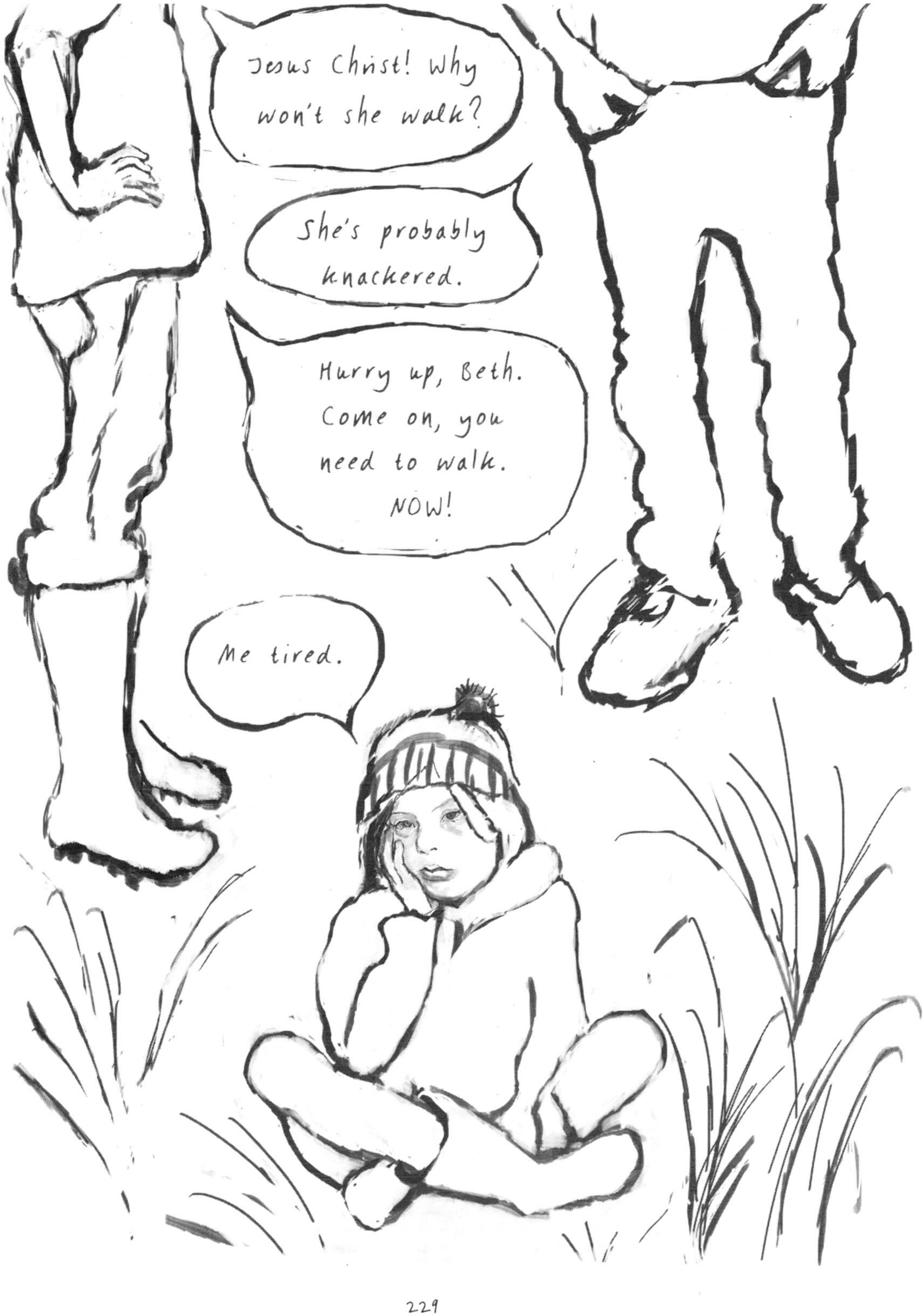
Jesus Christ! Why won't she walk?
She's probably knackered.
Hurry up, Beth. Come on, you need to walk. NOW!
Me tired.

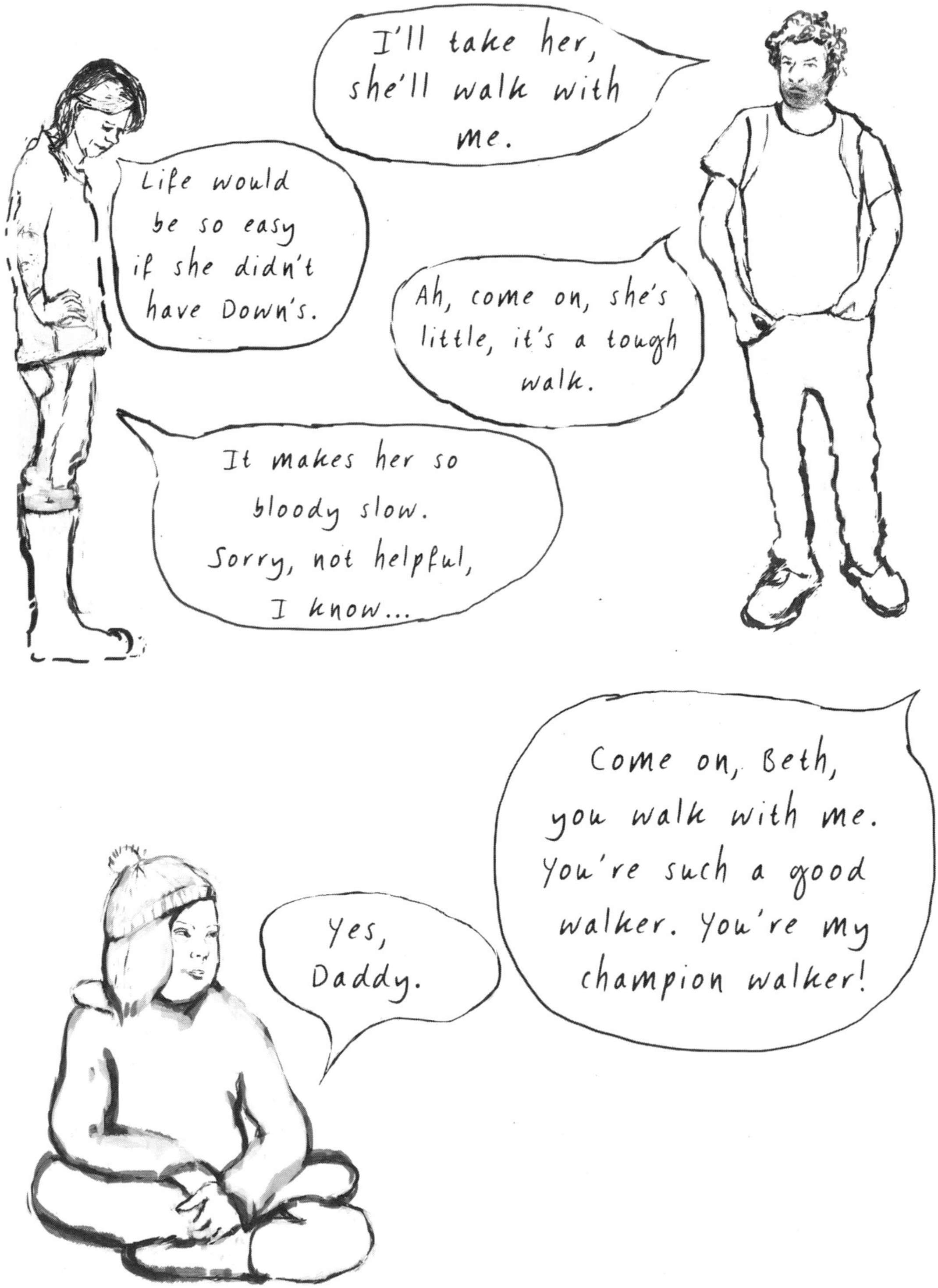
I'll take her, she'll walk with me.
Life would be so easy if she didn't have Down's.
Ah, come on, she's little, it's a tough walk.
It makes her so bloody slow. Sorry, not helpful, I know...
Come on, Beth, you walk with me. You're such a good walker. You're my champion walker!
Yes, Daddy.

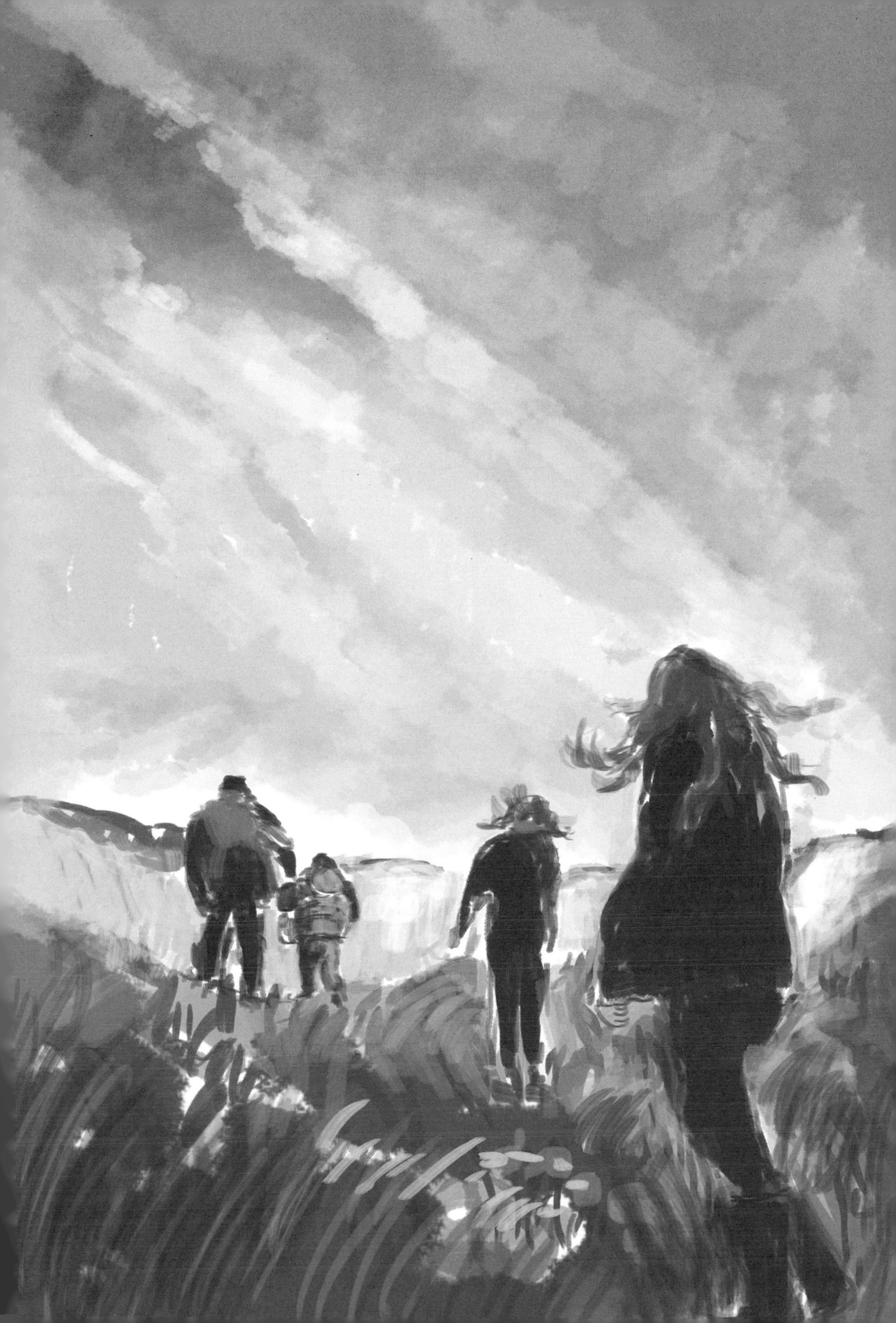

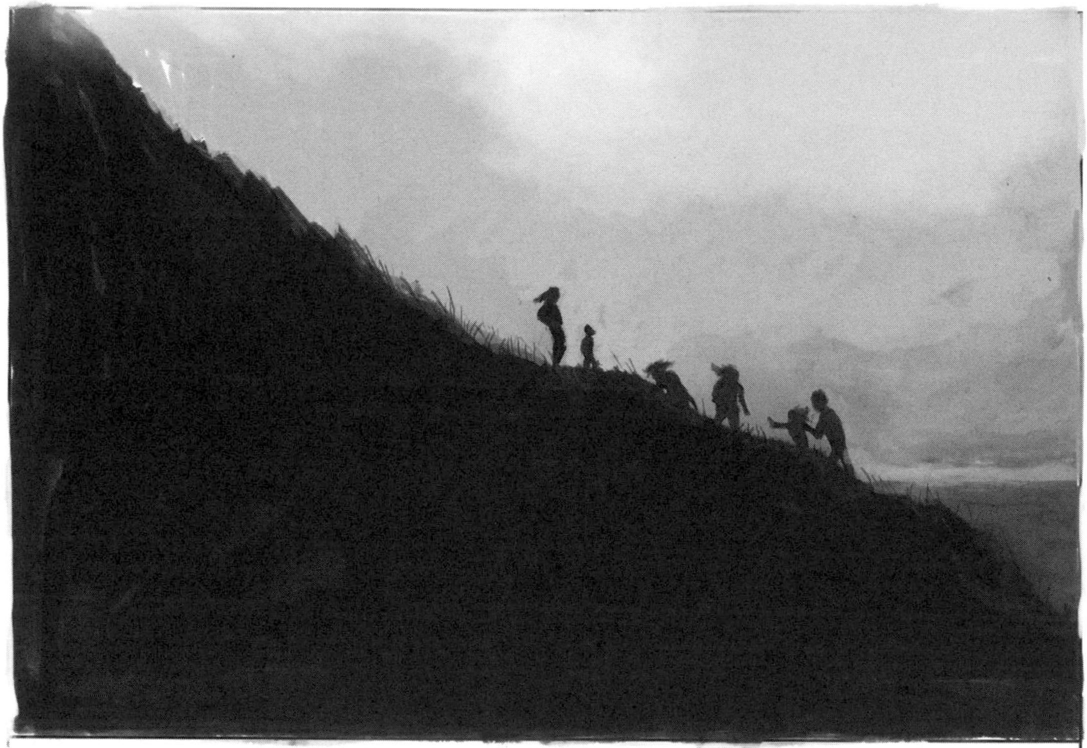

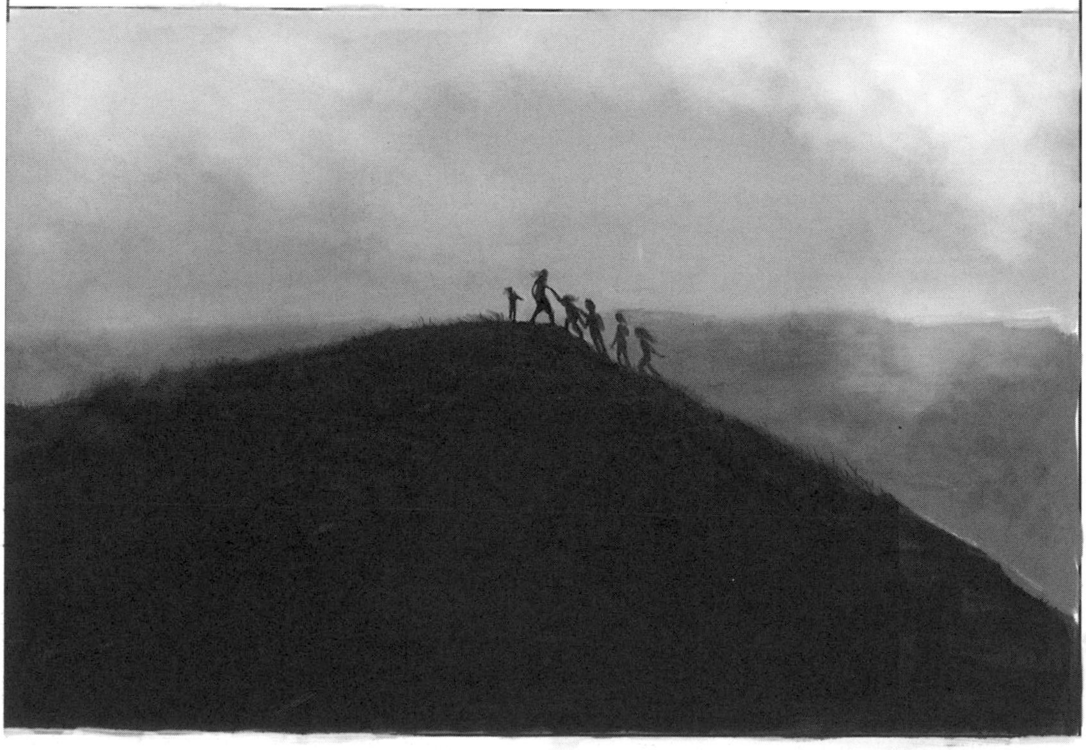

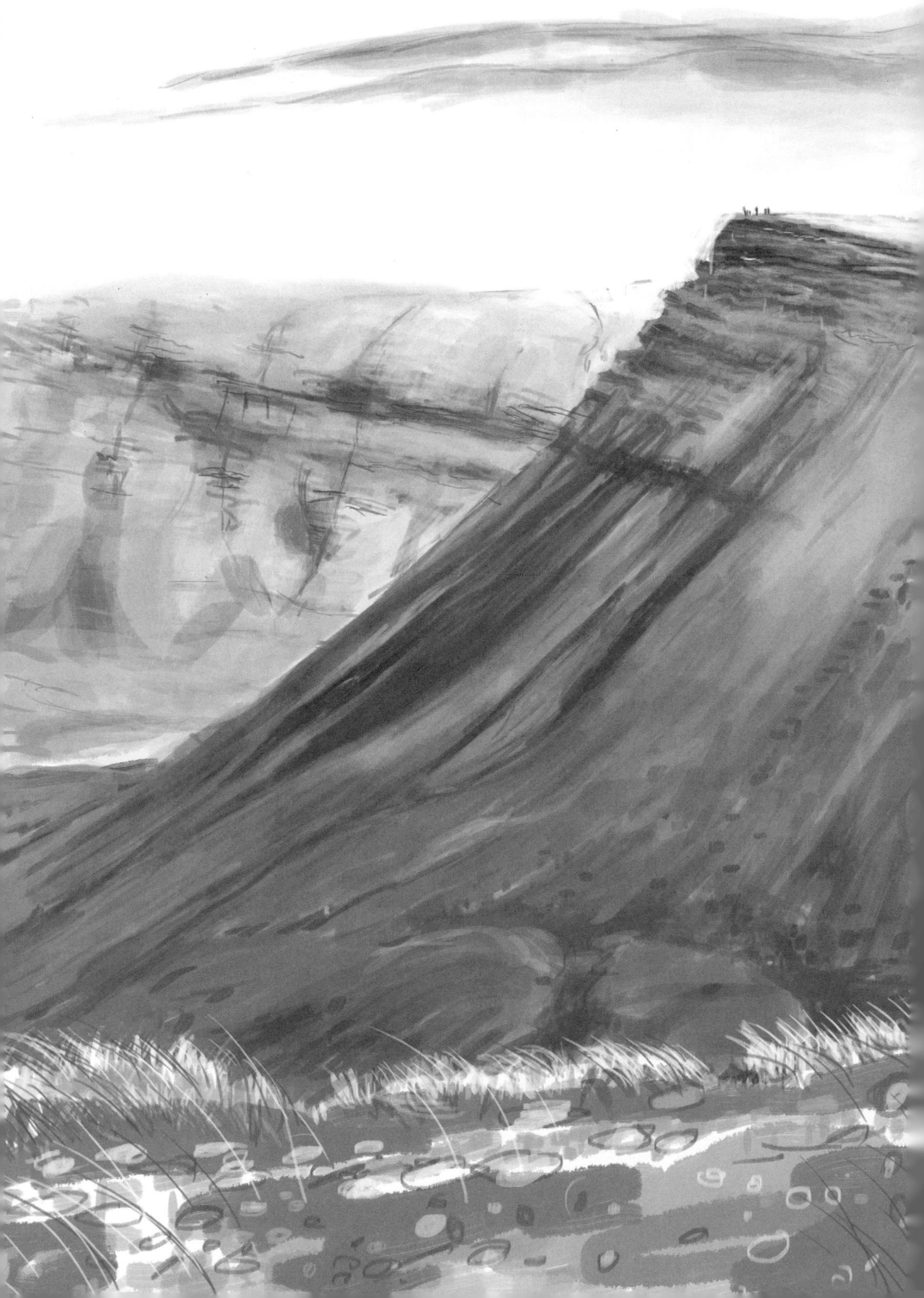

August 2012

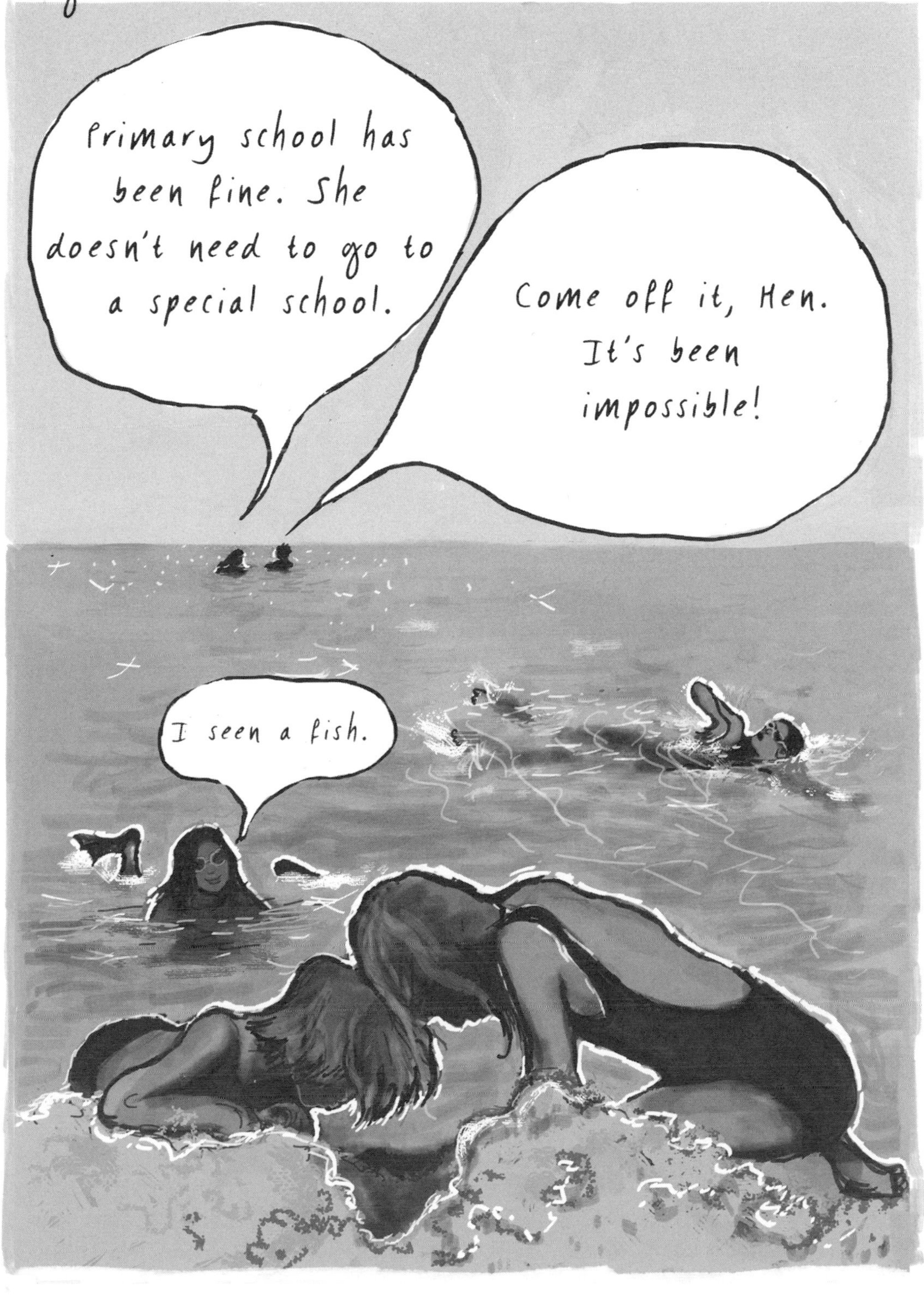
Primary school has been fine. She doesn't need to go to a special school.
Come off it, Hen. It's been impossible!
I seen a fish.

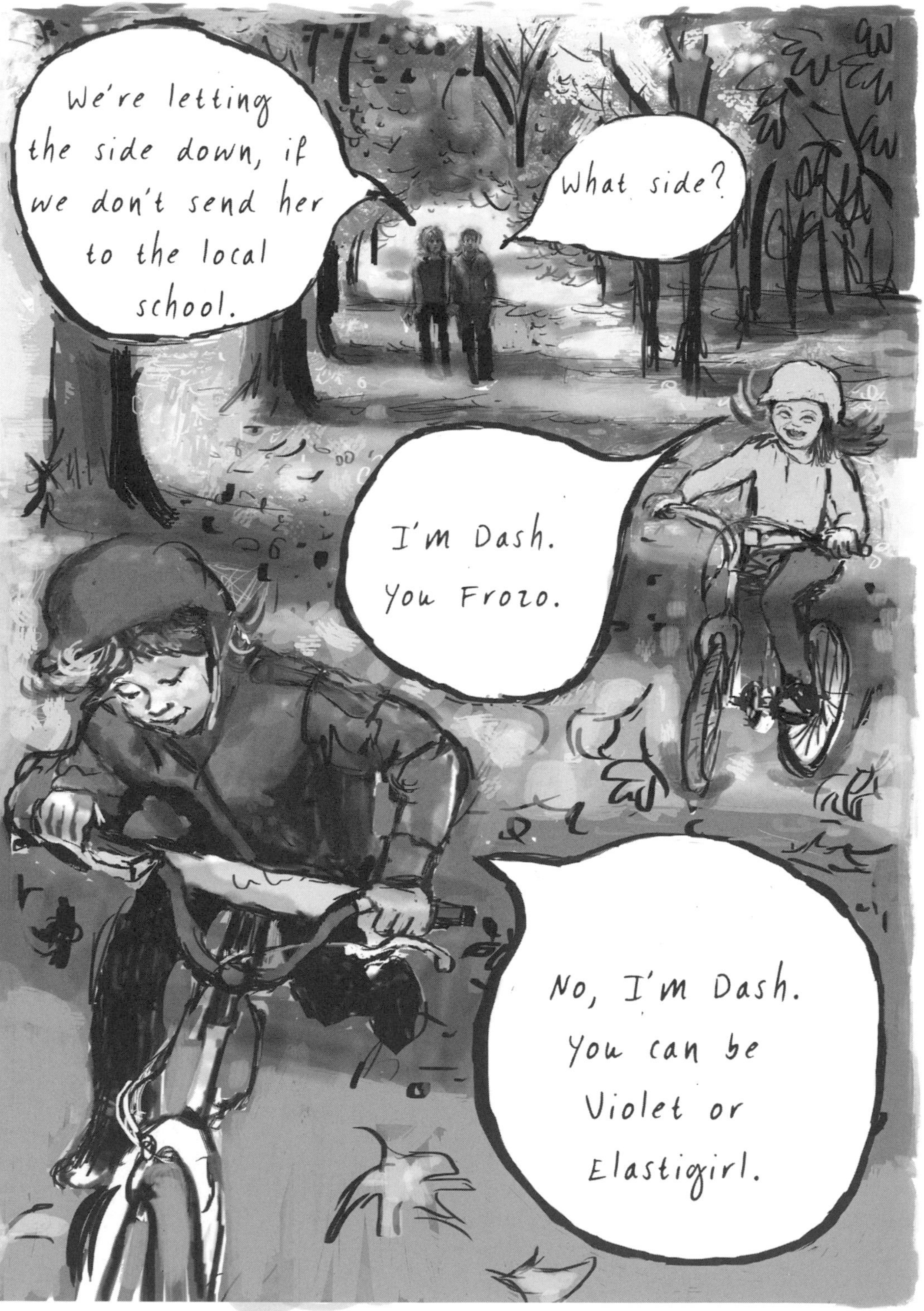
We're letting the side down, if we don't send her to the local school.
What side?
I'm Dash. You Frozo.
No, I'm Dash. You can be Violet or Elastigirl.

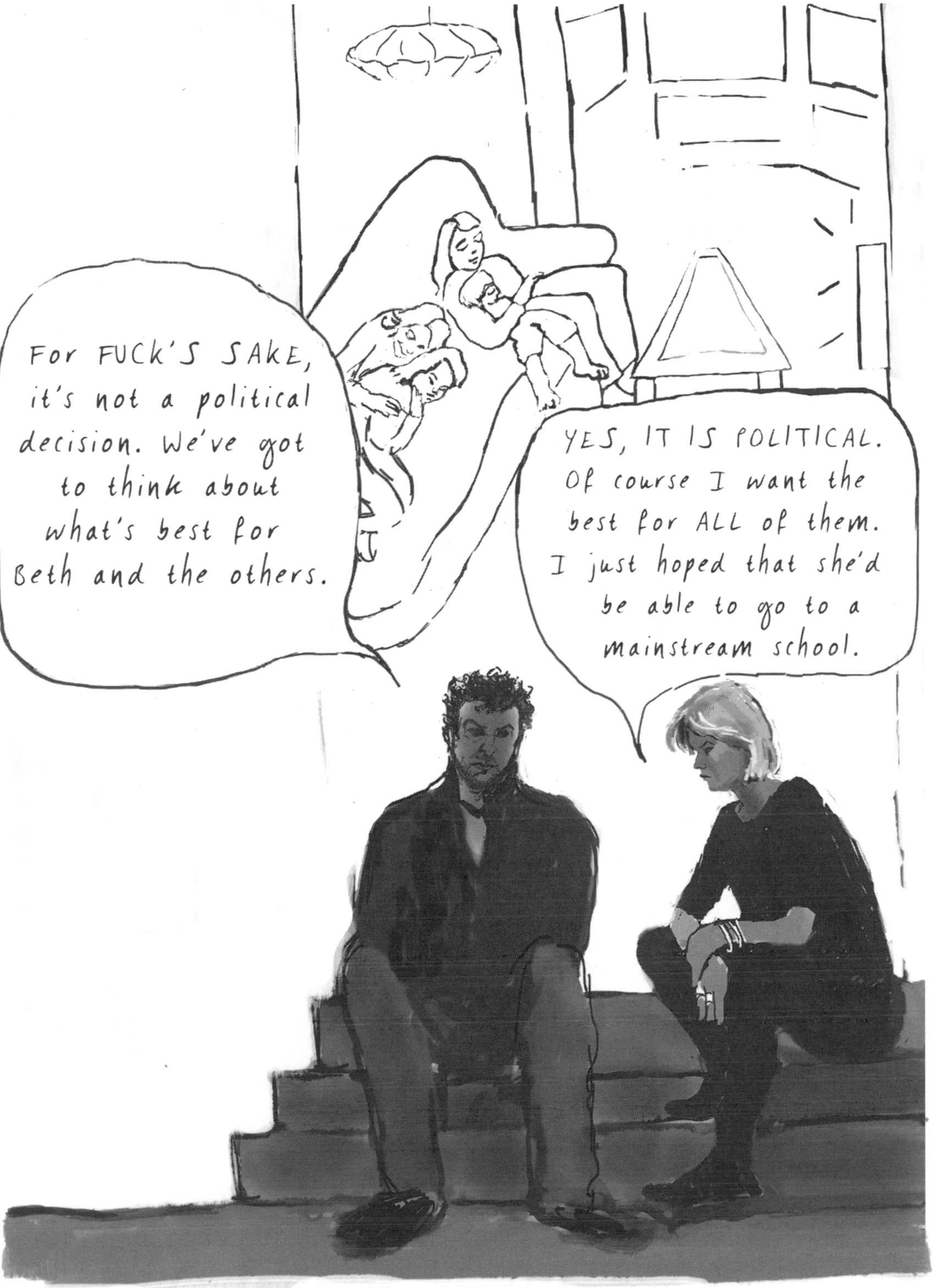
For FUCK'S SAKE, it's not a political decision. We've got to think about what's best for Beth and the others.
YES, IT IS POLITICAL. Of course I want the best for ALL of them. I just hoped that she'd be able to go to a mainstream school.

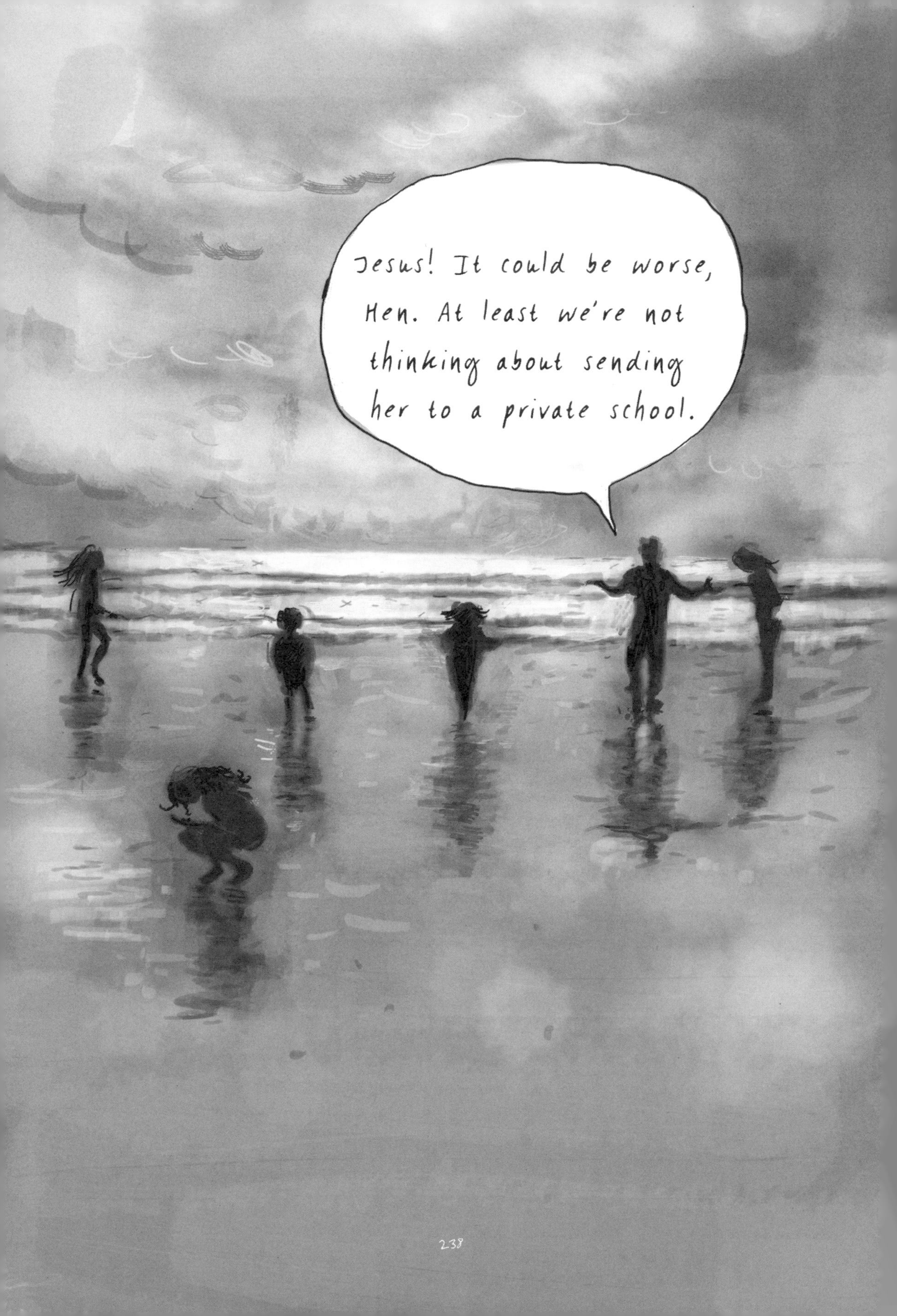
Jesus! It could be worse, Hen. At least we're not thinking about sending her to a private school.

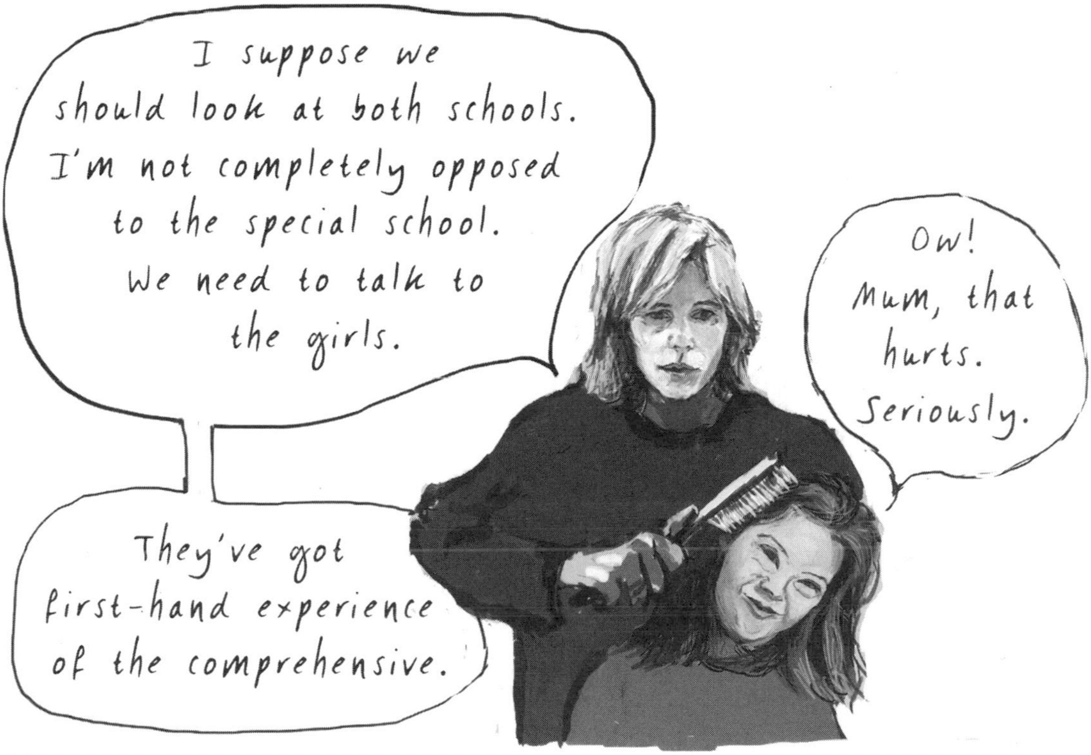
I suppose we should look at both schools. I'm not completely opposed to the special school. We need to talk to the girls.
They've got first-hand experience of the comprehensive.
Ow! Mum, that hurts. Seriously.

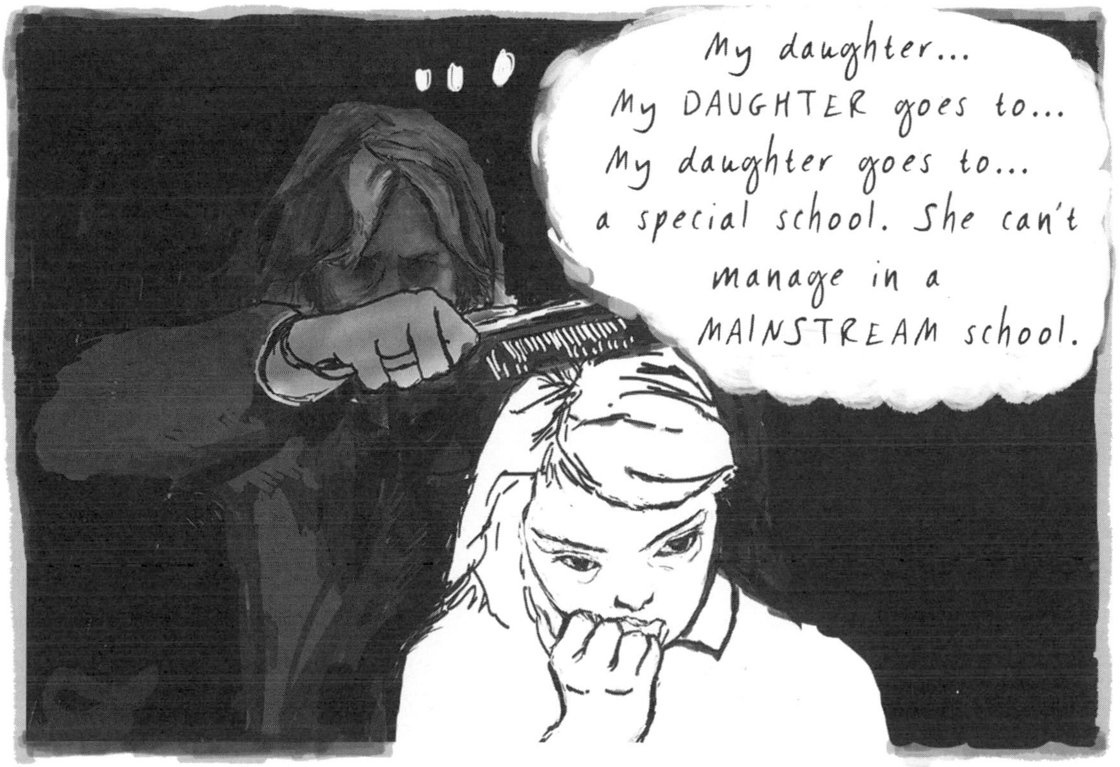
...
My daughter... My DAUGHTER goes to... My daughter goes to... a special school. She can't manage in a MAINSTREAM school.

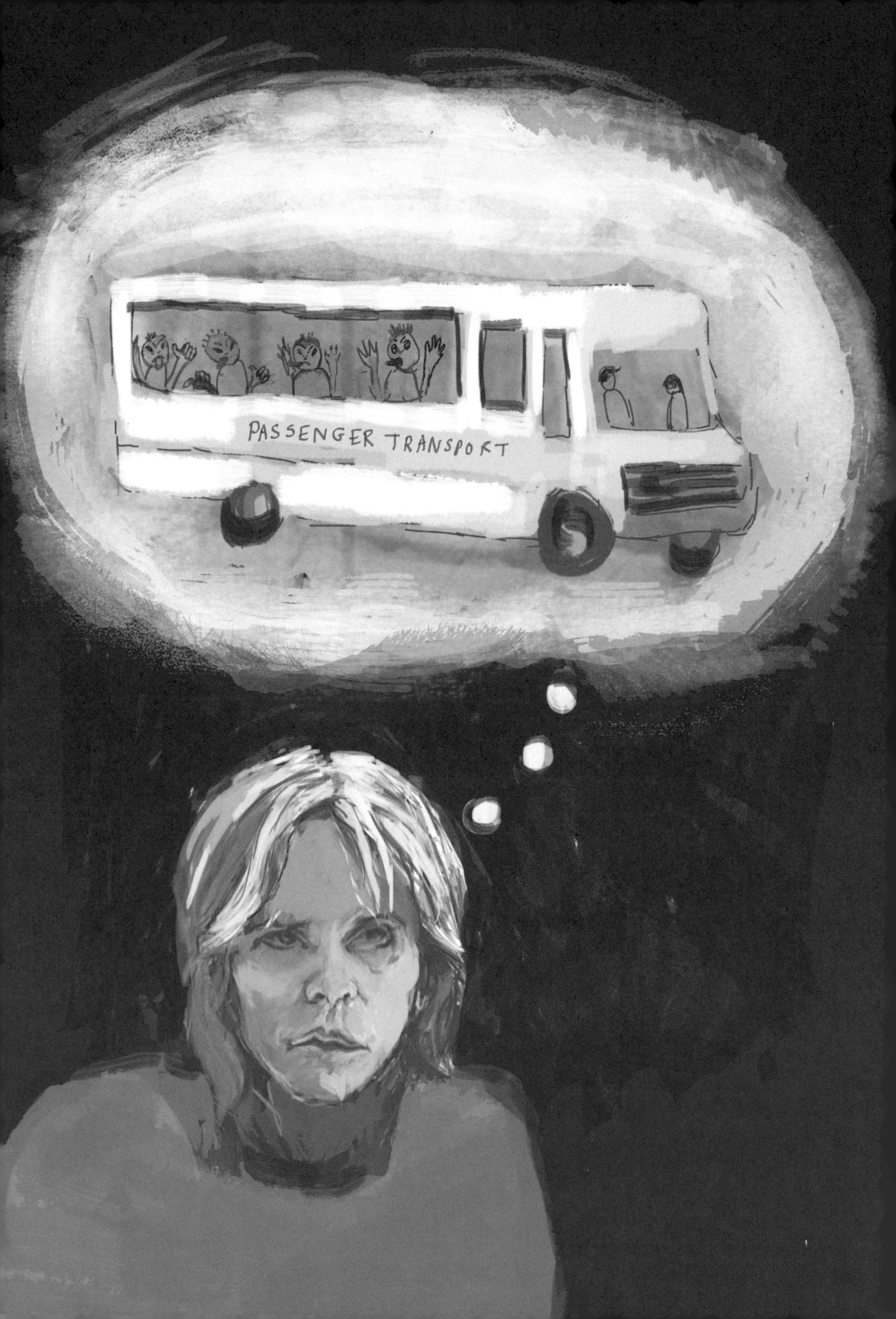
PASSENGER TRANSPORT

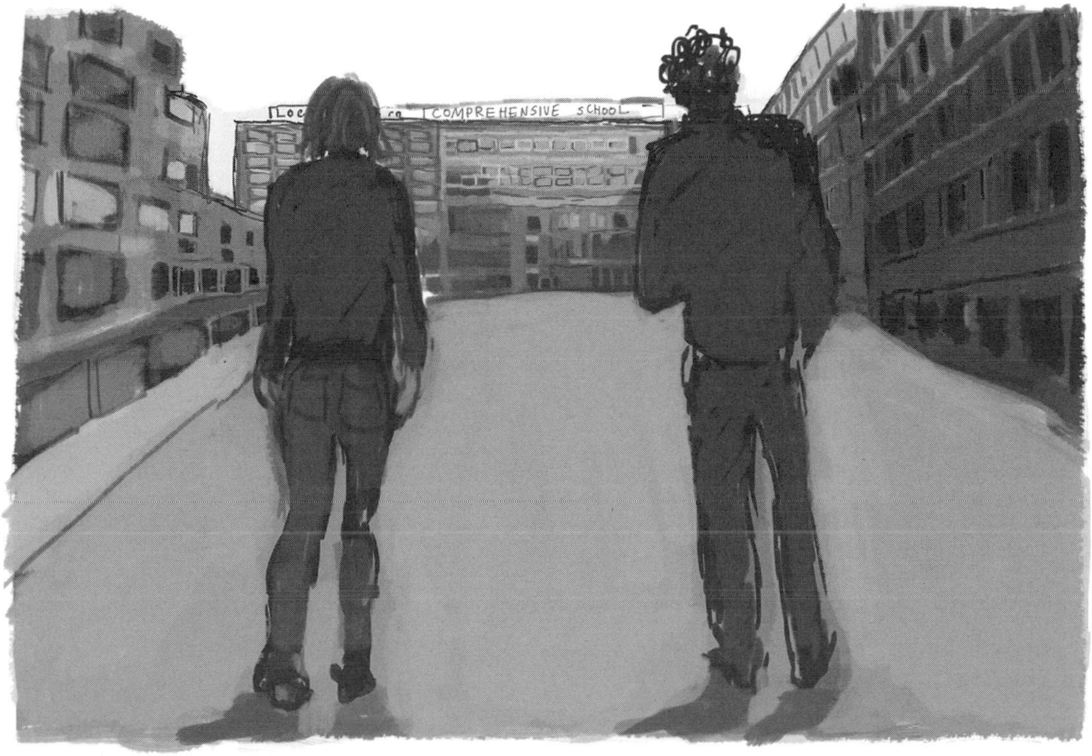
COMPREHENSIVE SCHOOL

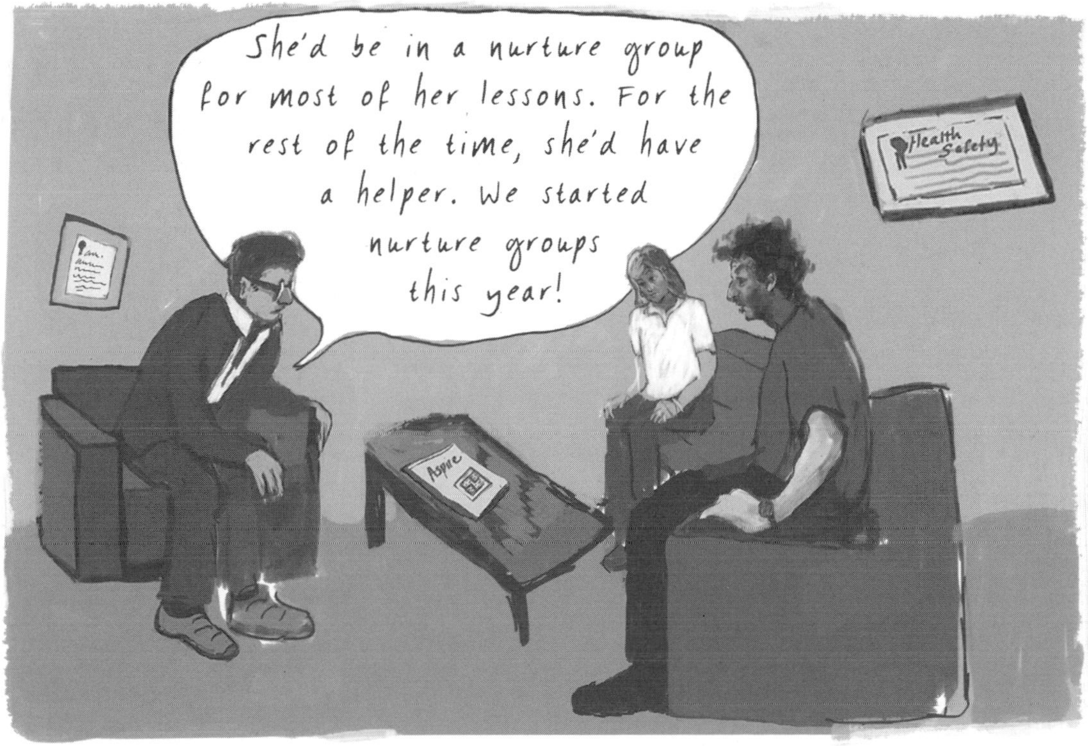
She'd be in a nurture group for most of her lessons. For the rest of the time, she'd have a helper. We started nurture groups this year!
Health Safety

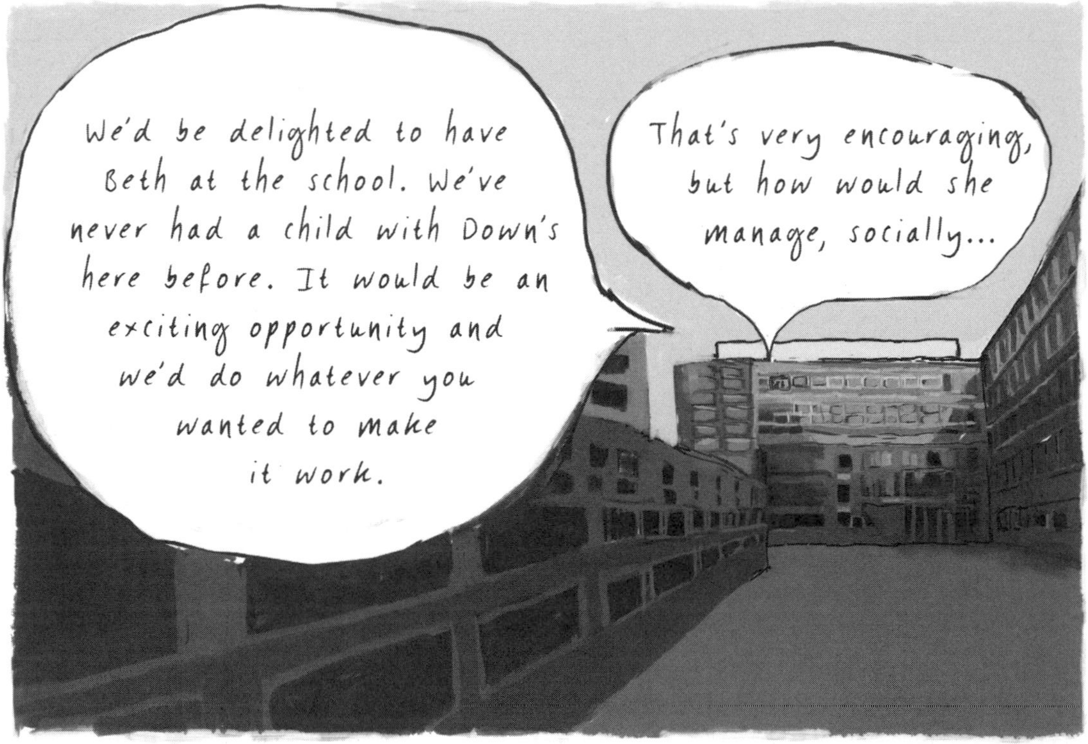
We'd be delighted to have Beth at the school. We've never had a child with Down's here before. It would be an exciting opportunity and we'd do whatever you wanted to make it work.
That's very encouraging, but how would she manage, socially...

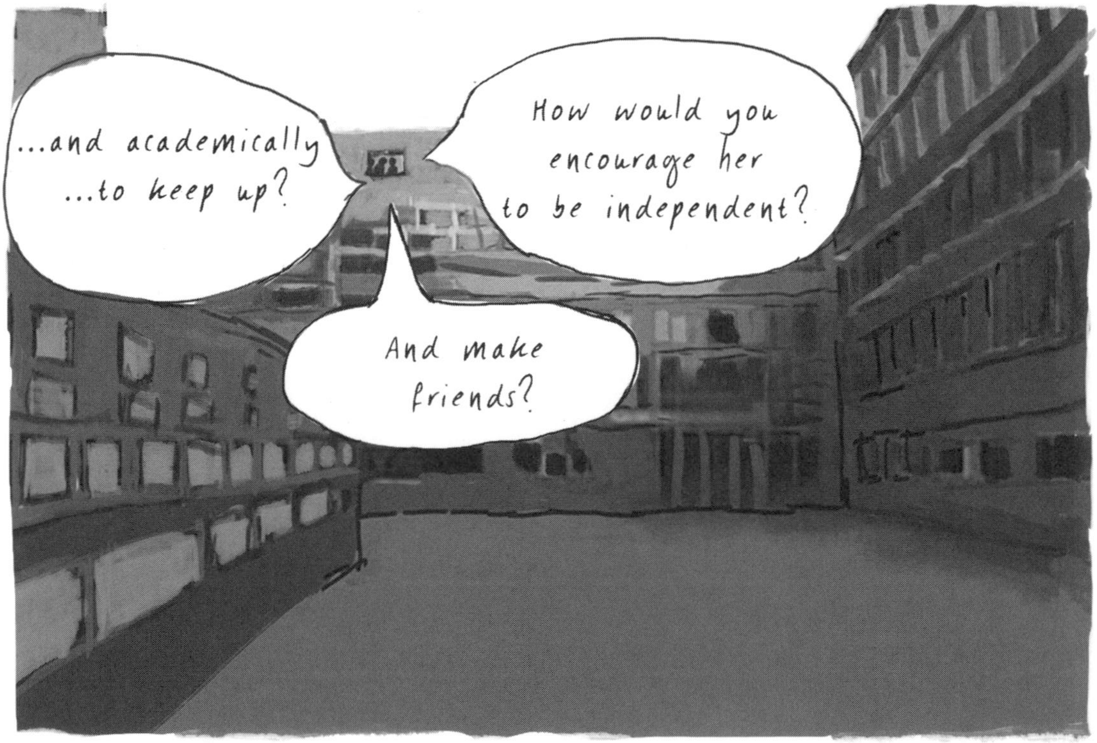
...and academically ...to keep up?
How would you encourage her to be independent?
And make friends?

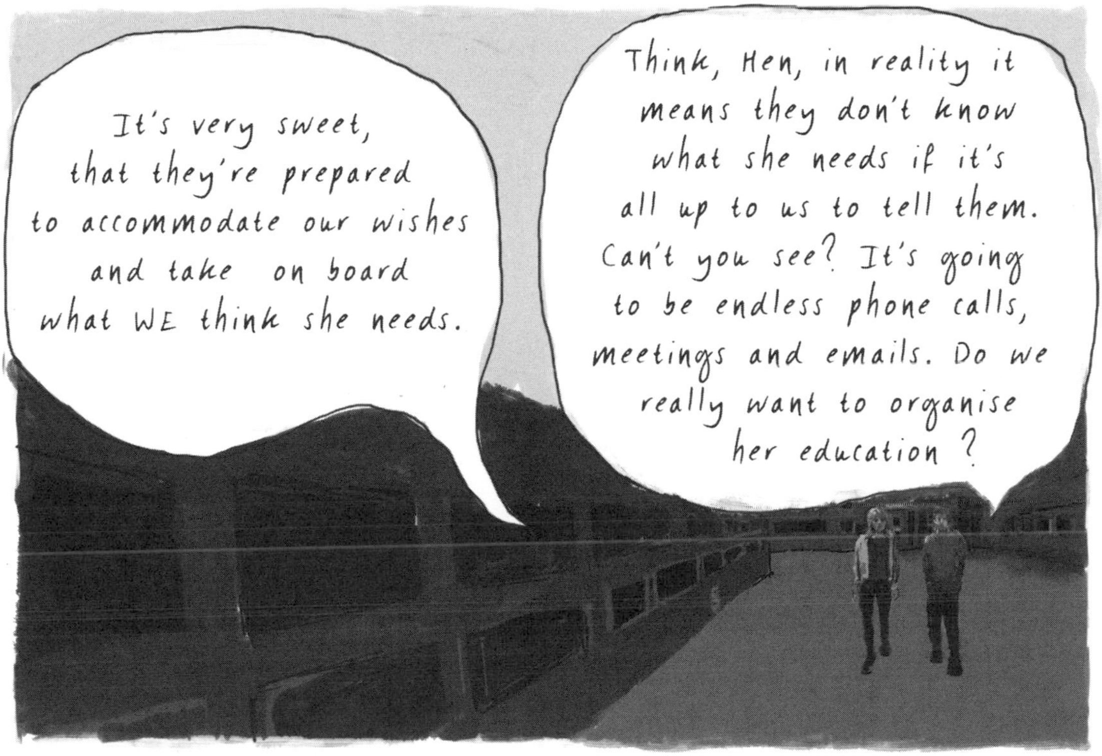

It's very sweet, that they're prepared to accommodate our wishes and take on board what WE think she needs.
Think, Hen, in reality it means they don't know what she needs if it's all up to us to tell them. Can't you see? It's going to be endless phone calls, meetings and emails. Do we really want to organise her education?

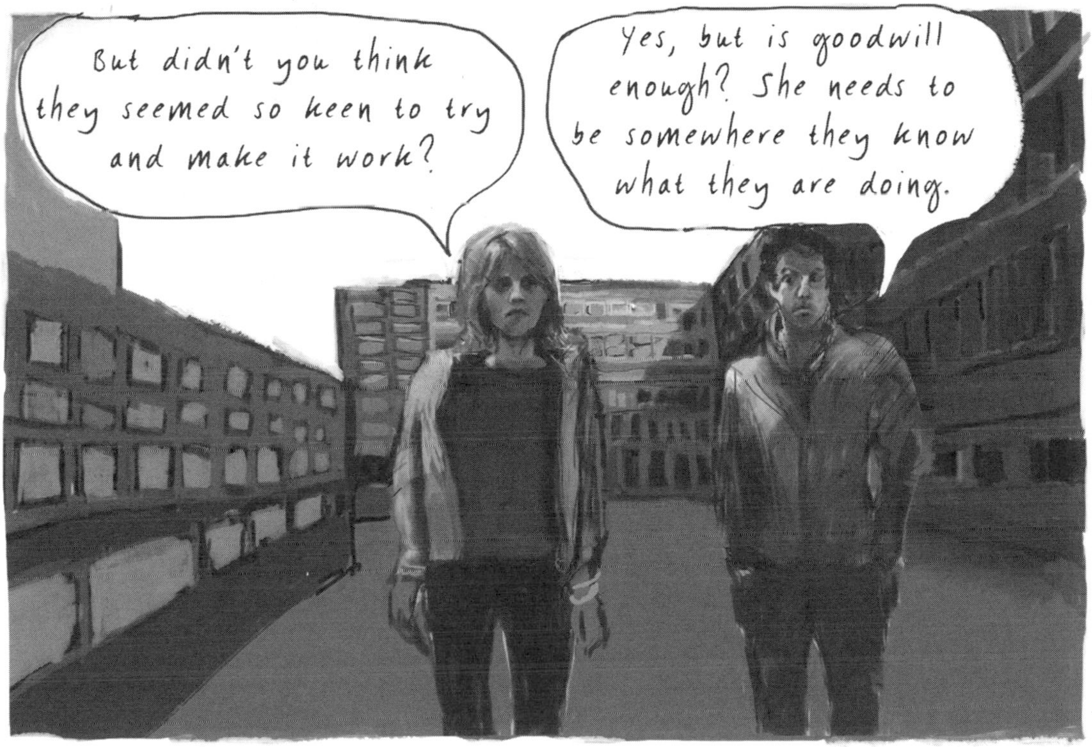

But didn't you think they seemed so keen to try and make it work?
Yes, but is goodwill enough? She needs to be somewhere they know what they are doing.

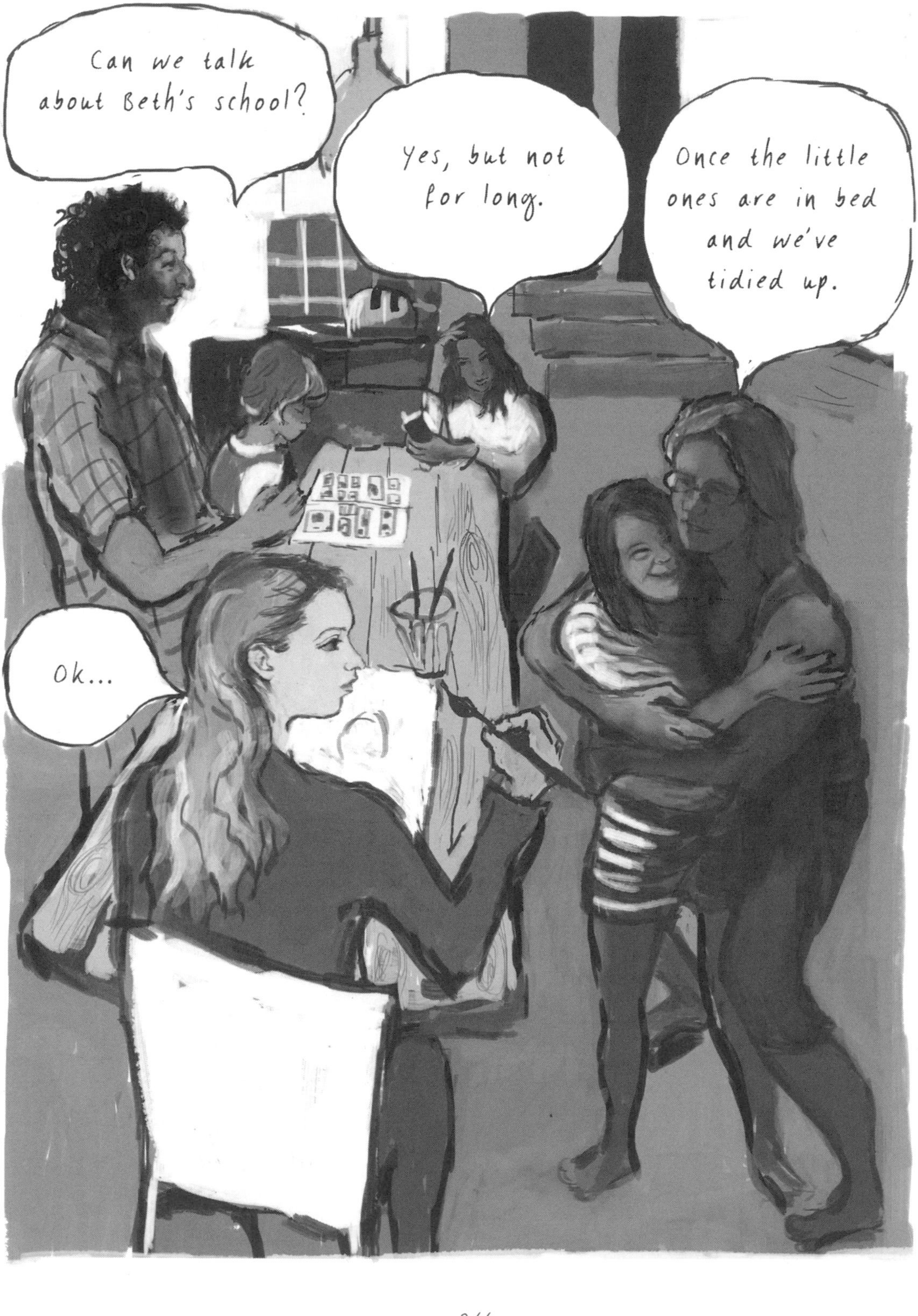
Can we talk about Beth's school?
Yes, but not for long.
Once the little ones are in bed and we've tidied up.
Ok...

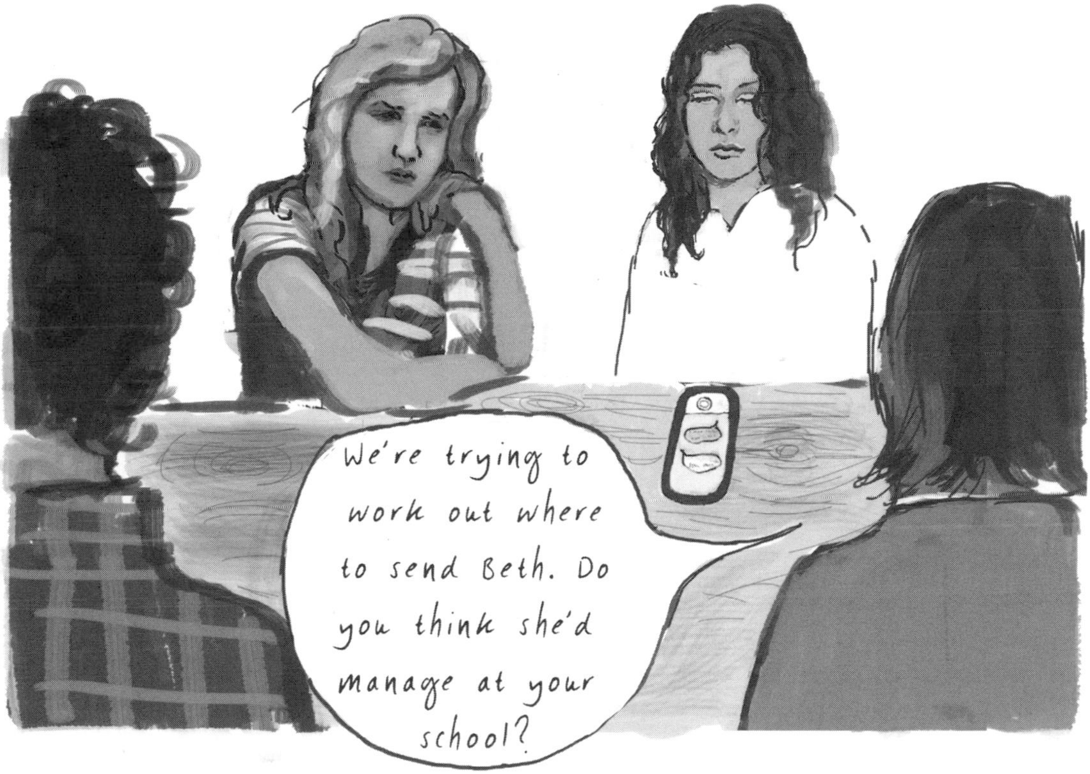
We're trying to work out where to send Beth. Do you think she'd manage at your school?

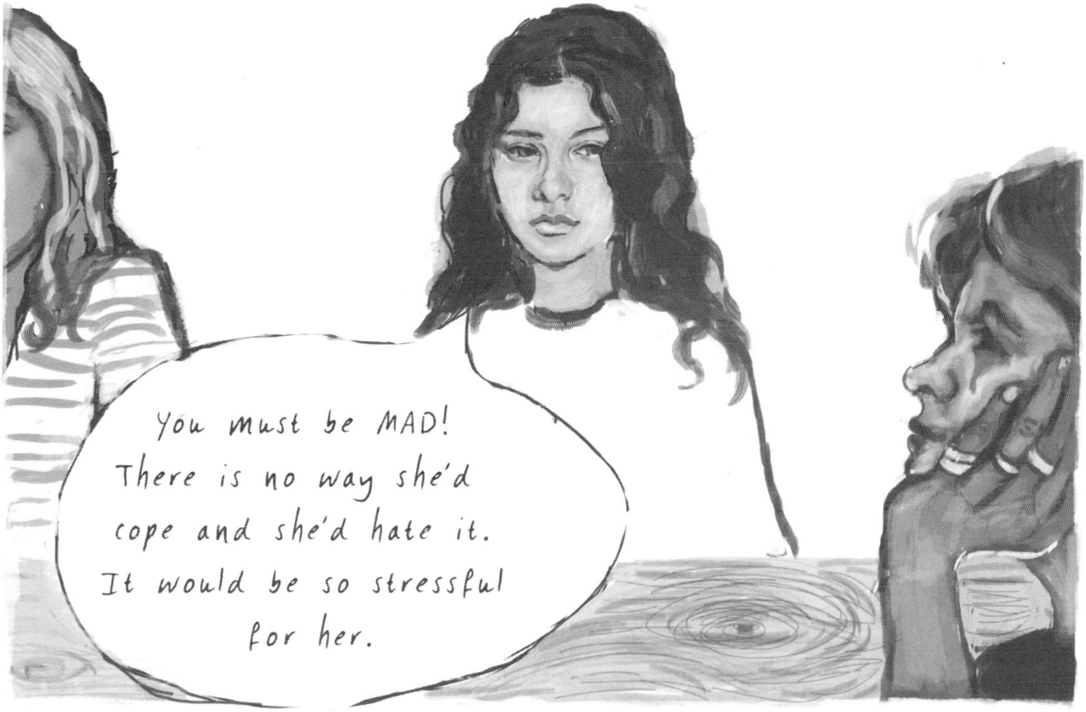
You must be MAD! There is no way she'd cope and she'd hate it. It would be so stressful for her.

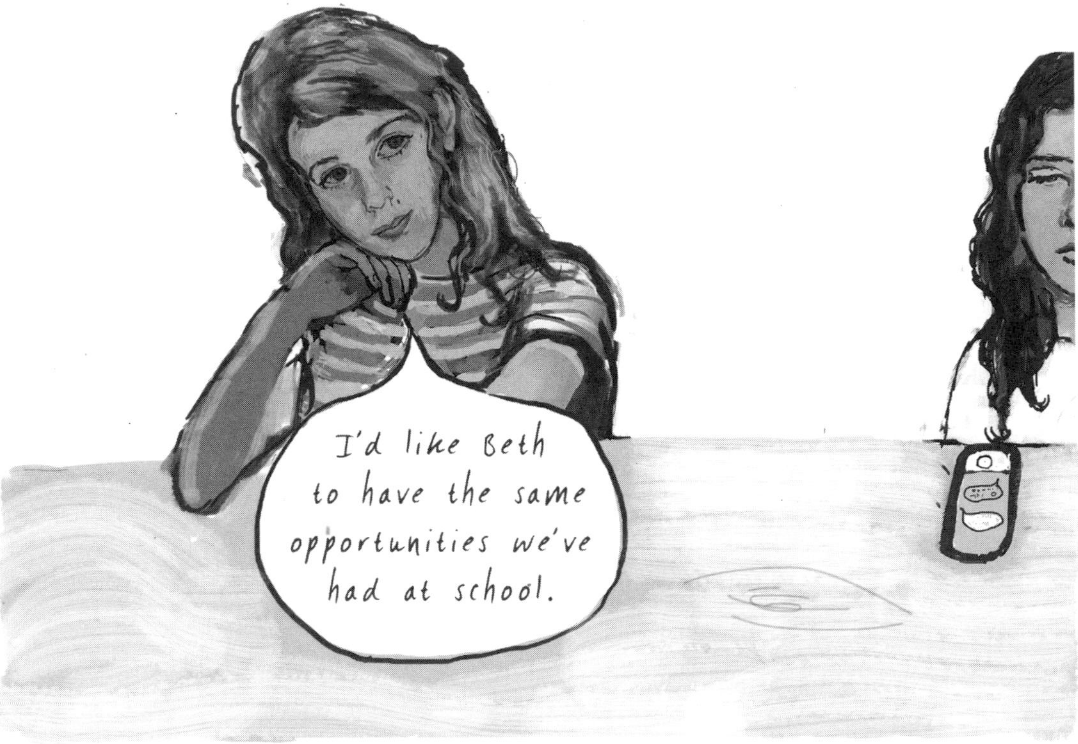
I'd like Beth to have the same opportunities we've had at school.

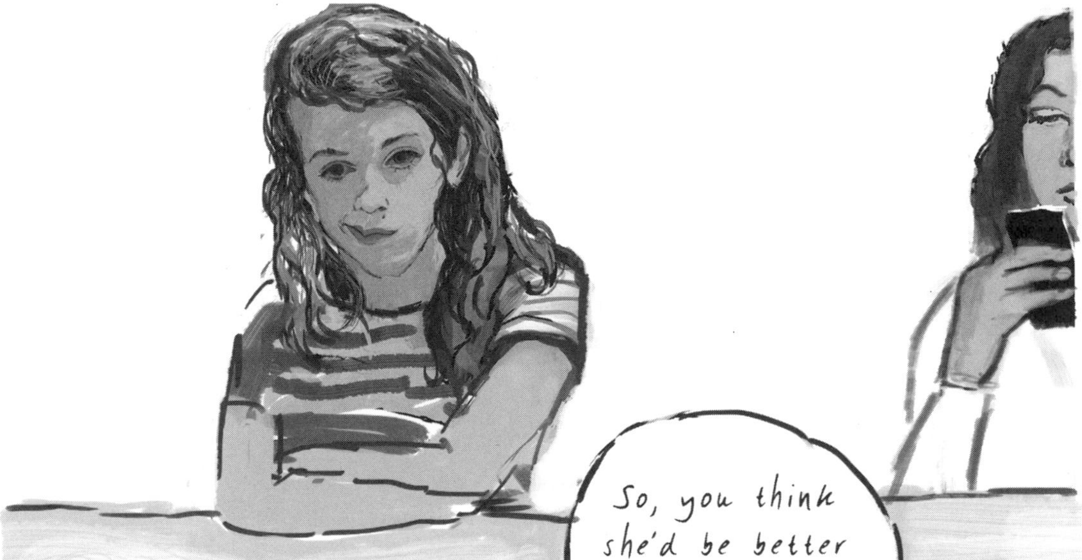
So, you think she'd be better off at your school, then?

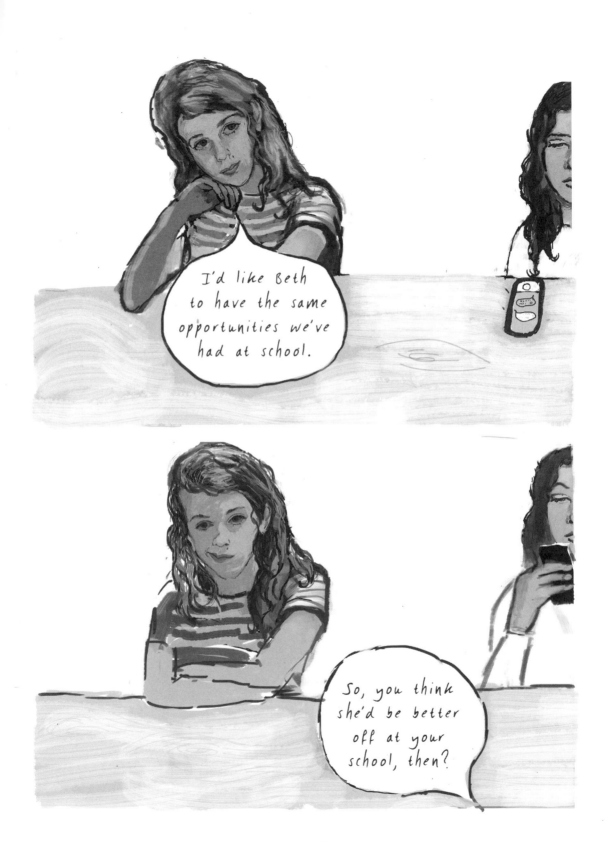

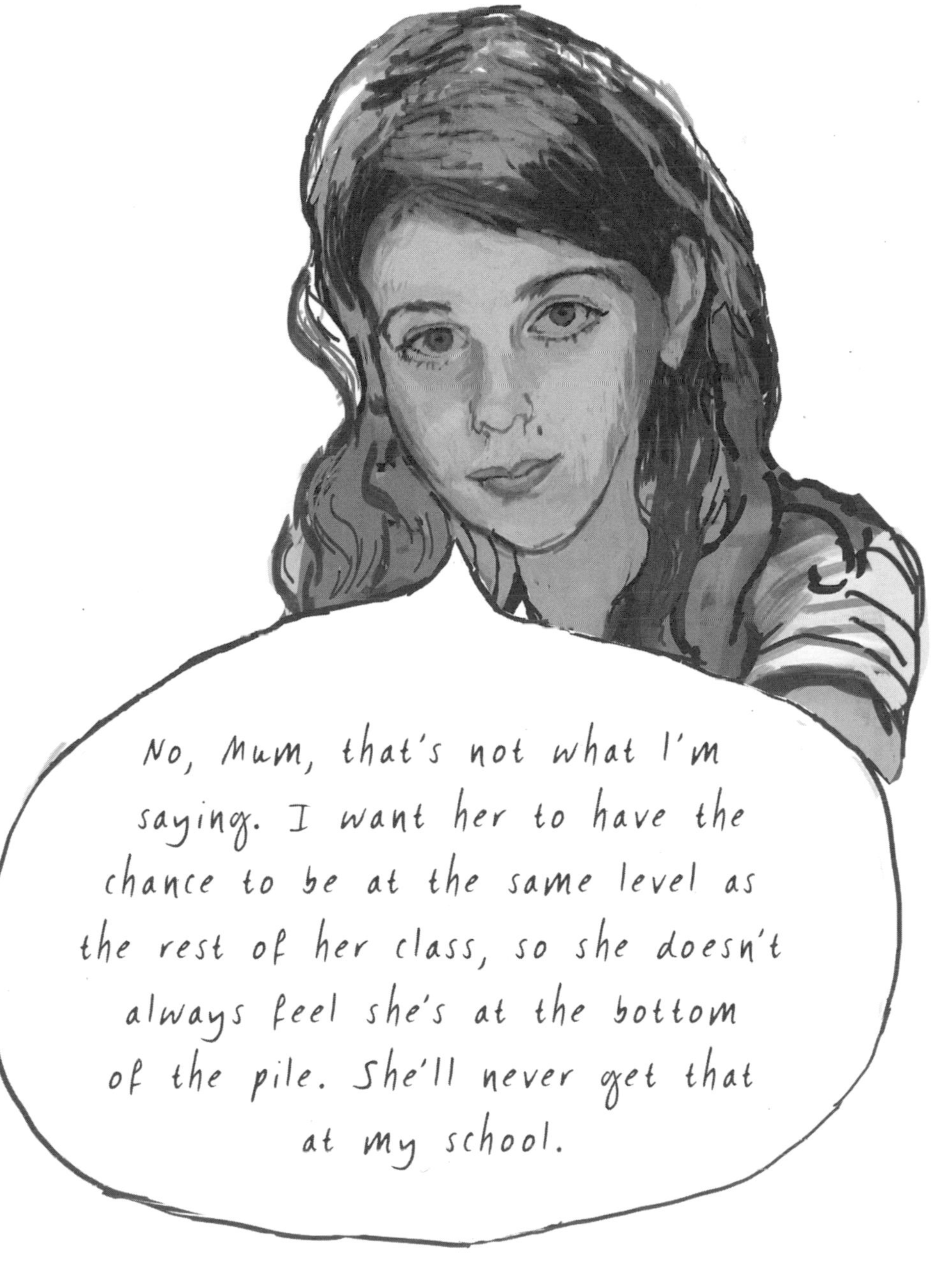
No, Mum, that's not what I'm saying. I want her to have the chance to be at the same level as the rest of her class, so she doesn't always feel she's at the bottom of the pile. She'll never get that at my school.

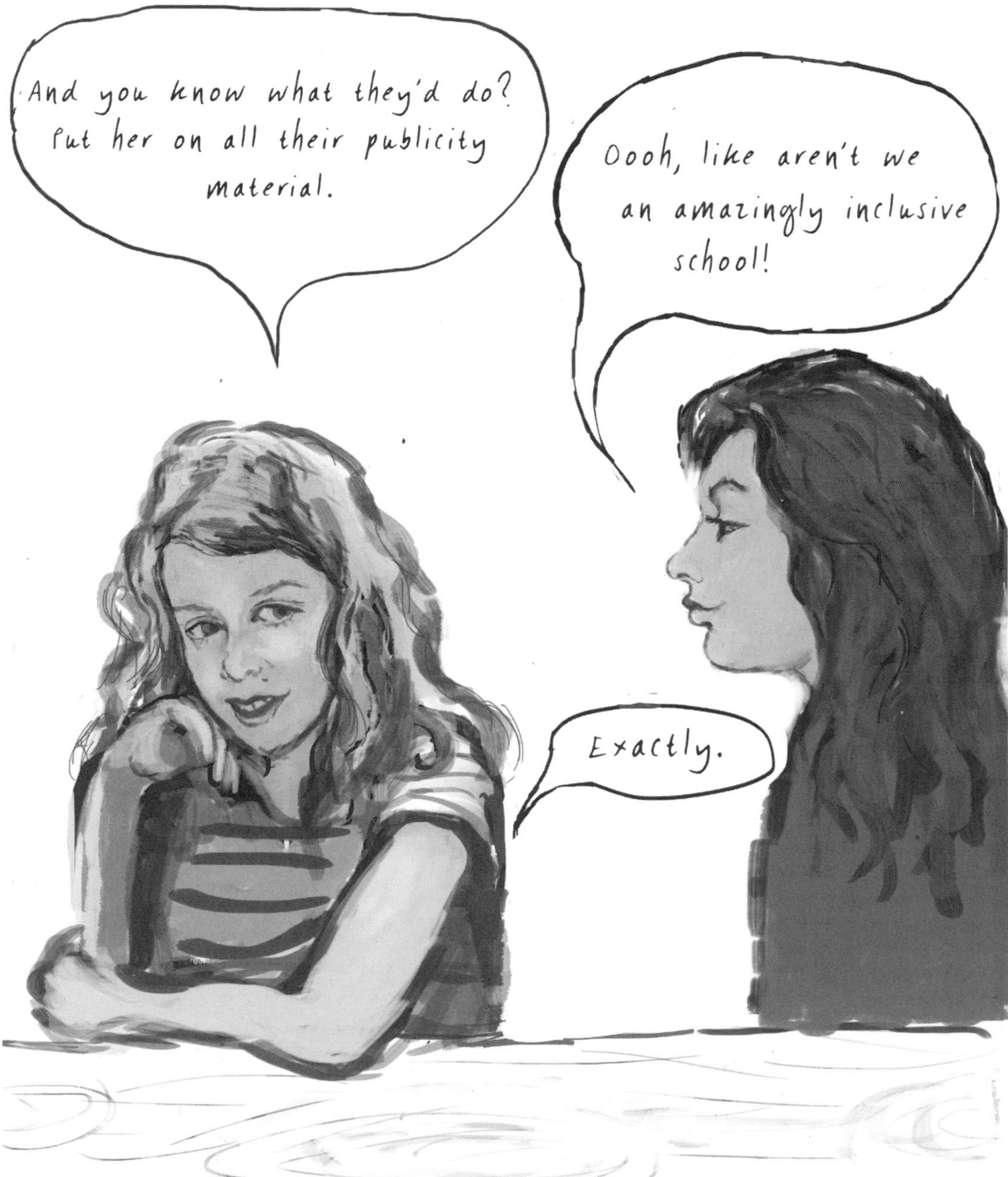
And you know what they'd do? Put her on all their publicity material.
Oooh, like aren't we an amazingly inclusive school!
Exactly.

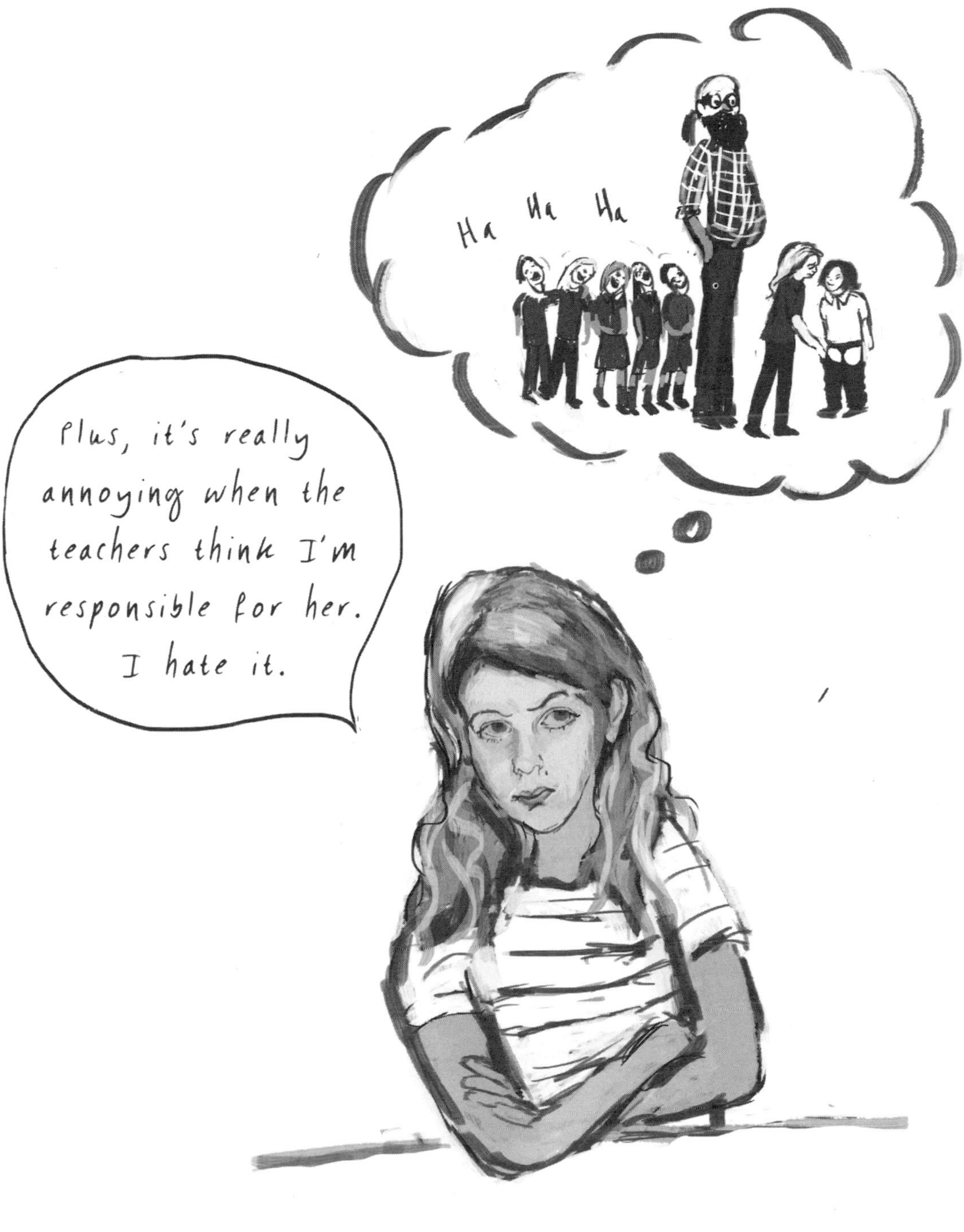
Ha Ha Ha
Plus, it's really annoying when the teachers think I'm responsible for her. I hate it.

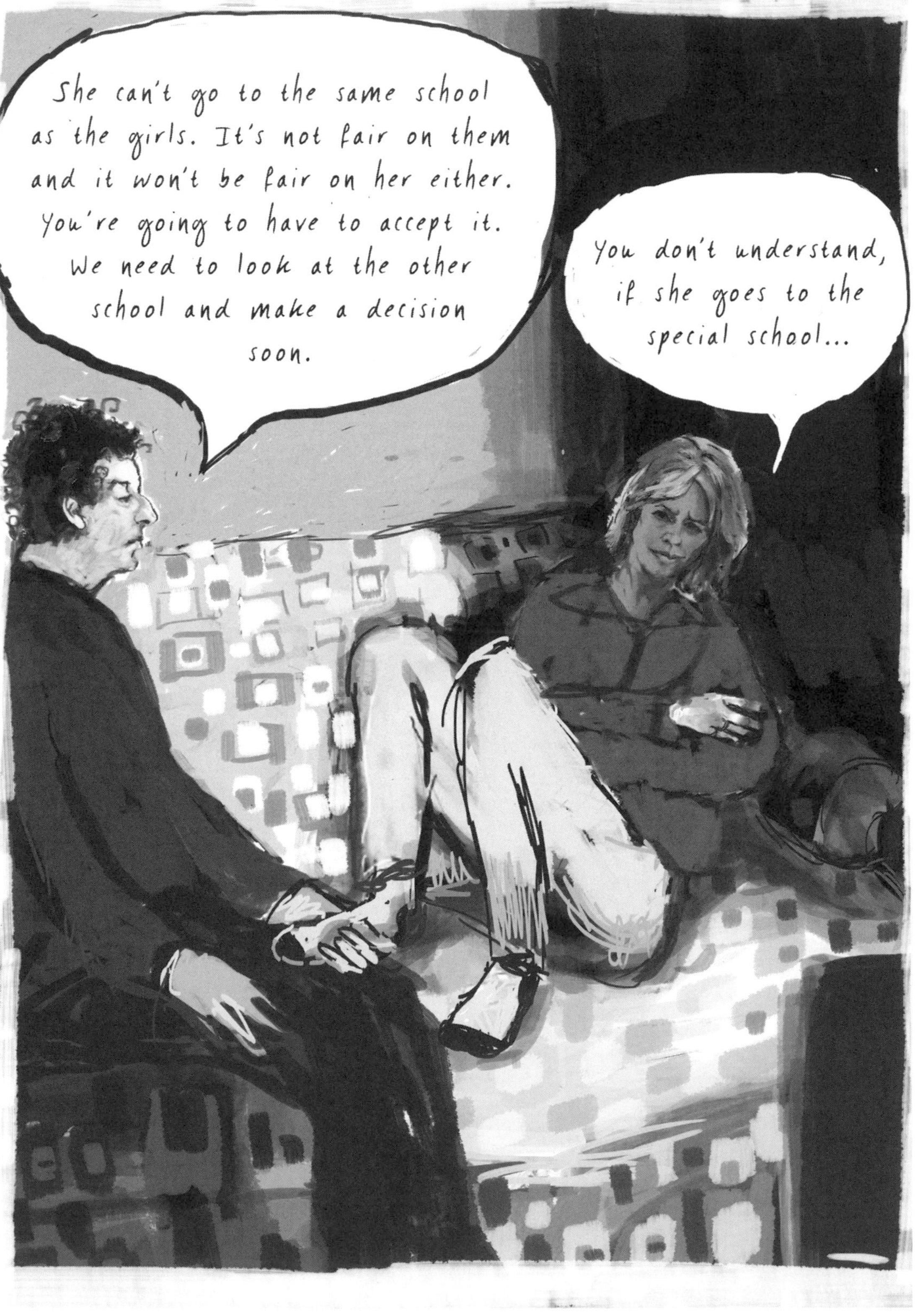
She can't go to the same school as the girls. It's not fair on them and it won't be fair on her either. You're going to have to accept it. We need to look at the other school and make a decision soon.
You don't understand, if she goes to the special school...

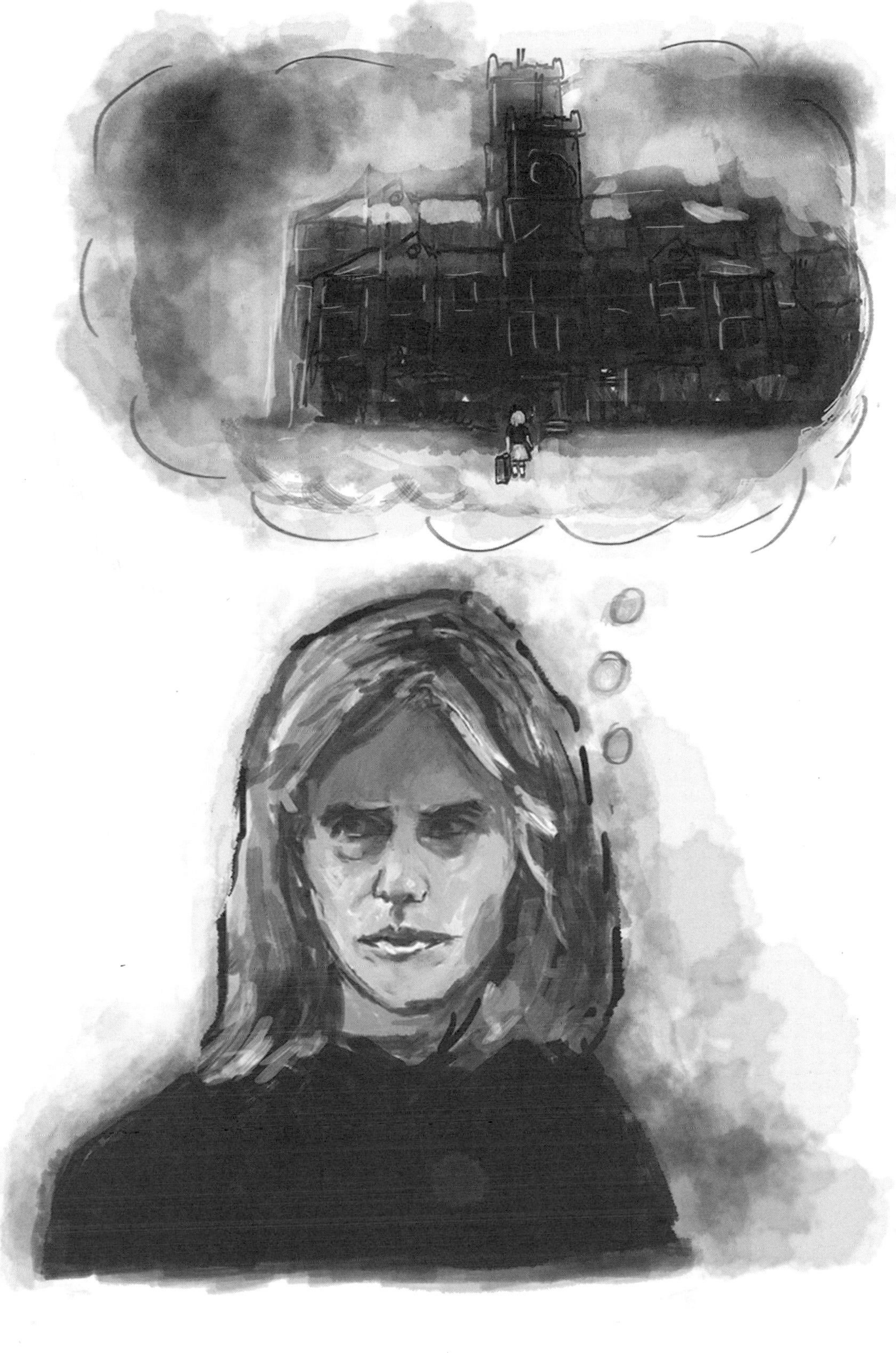

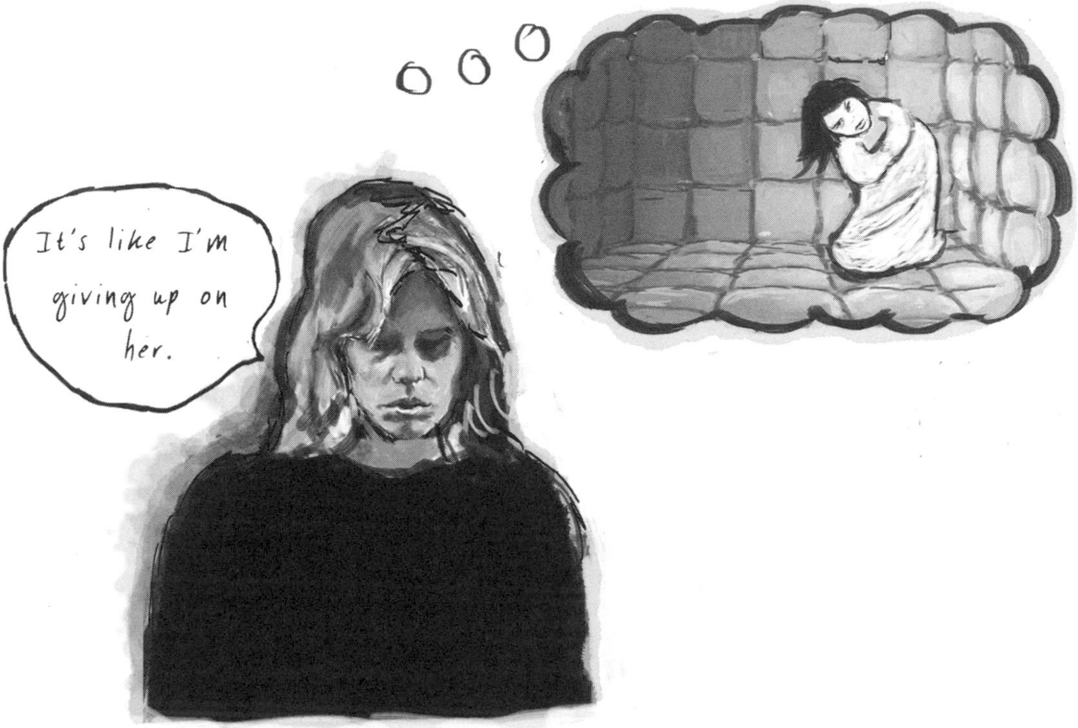
It's like I'm giving up on her.

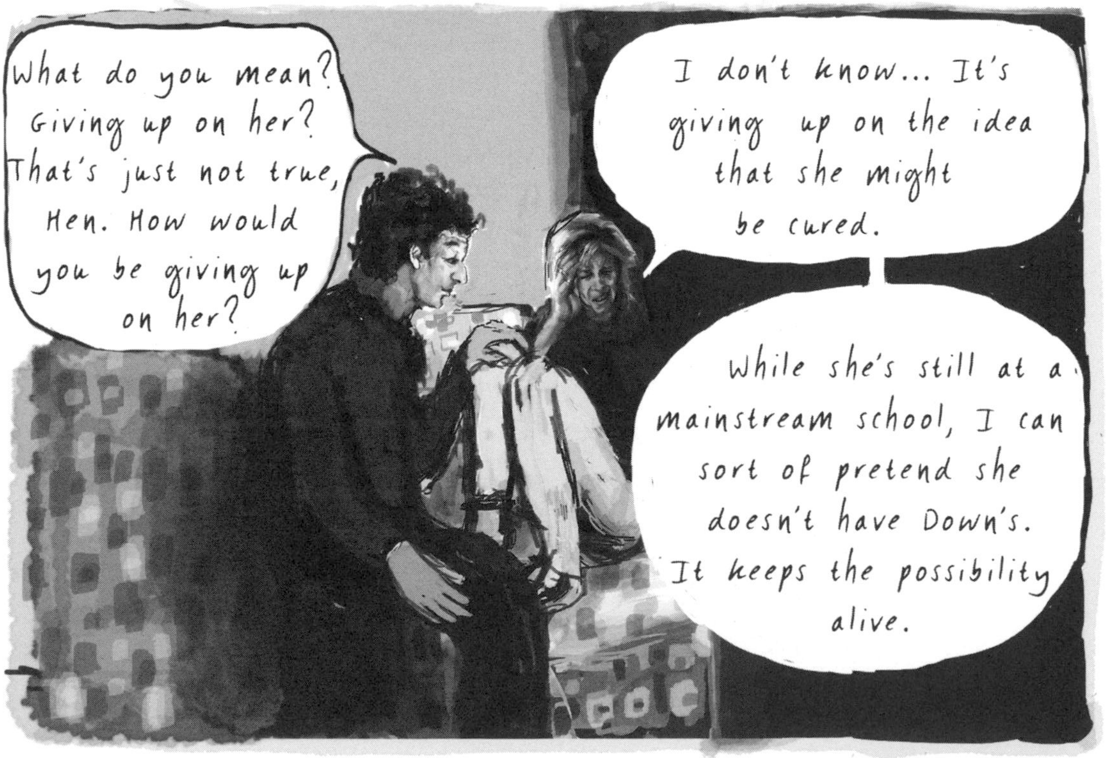
What do you mean? Giving up on her? That's just not true, Hen. How would you be giving up on her?
I don't know... It's giving up on the idea that she might be cured.
While she's still at a mainstream school, I can sort of pretend she doesn't have Down's. It keeps the possibility alive.

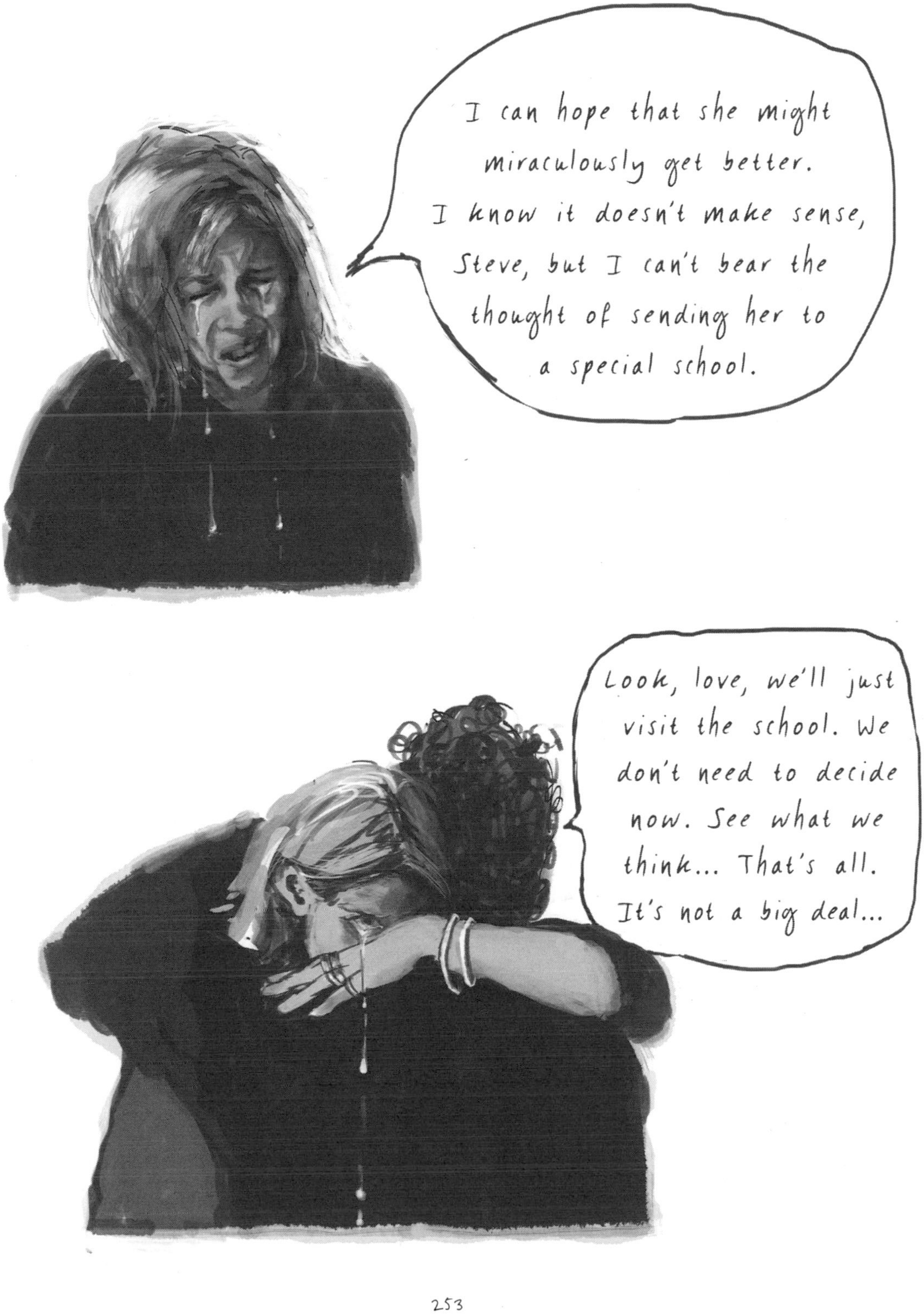
I can hope that she might miraculously get better. I know it doesn't make sense, Steve, but I can't bear the thought of sending her to a special school.
Look, love, we'll just visit the school. We don't need to decide now. See what we think... That's all. It's not a big deal...

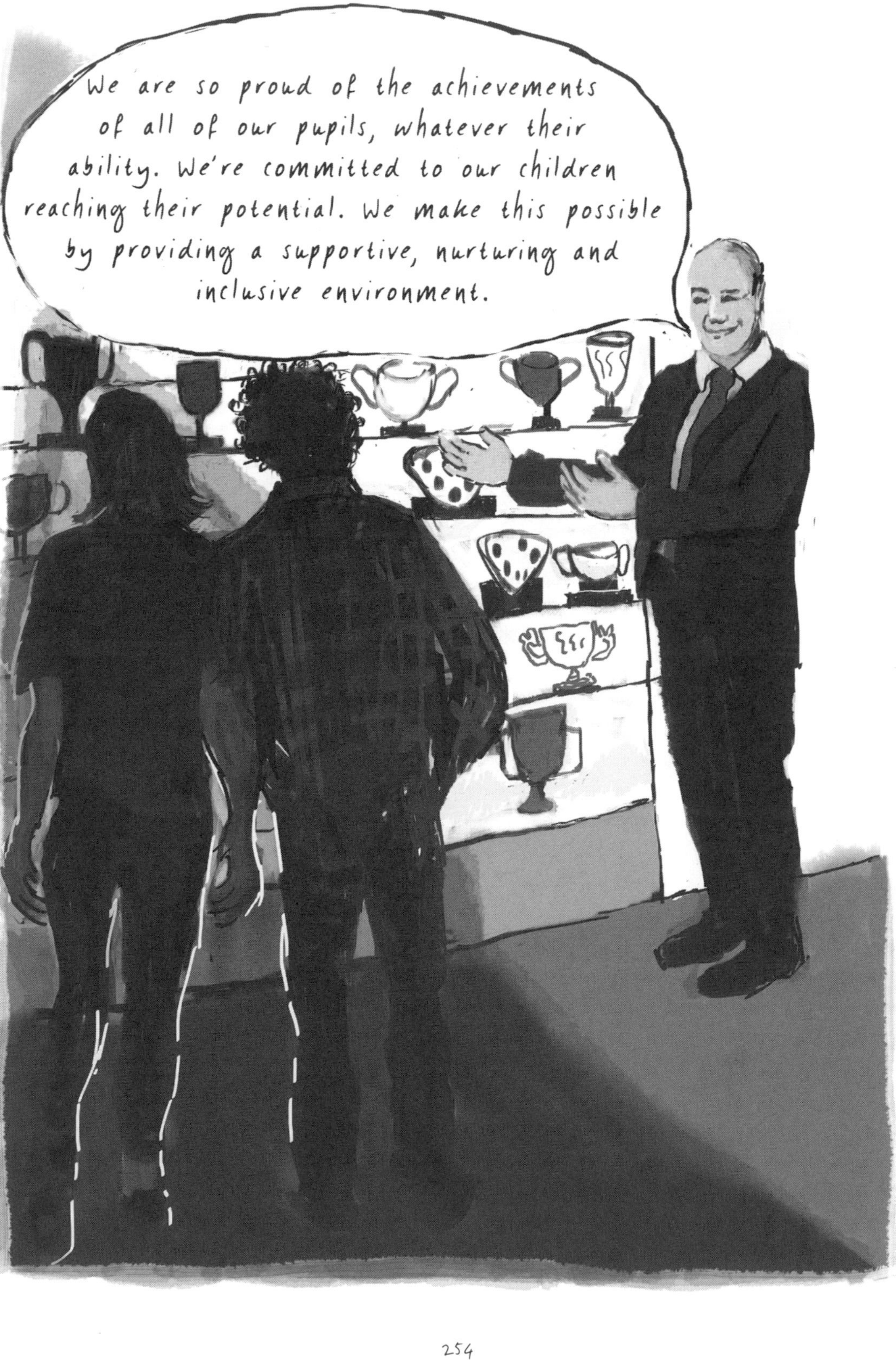
We are so proud of the achievements of all of our pupils, whatever their ability. We're committed to our children reaching their potential. We make this possible by providing a supportive, nurturing and inclusive environment.

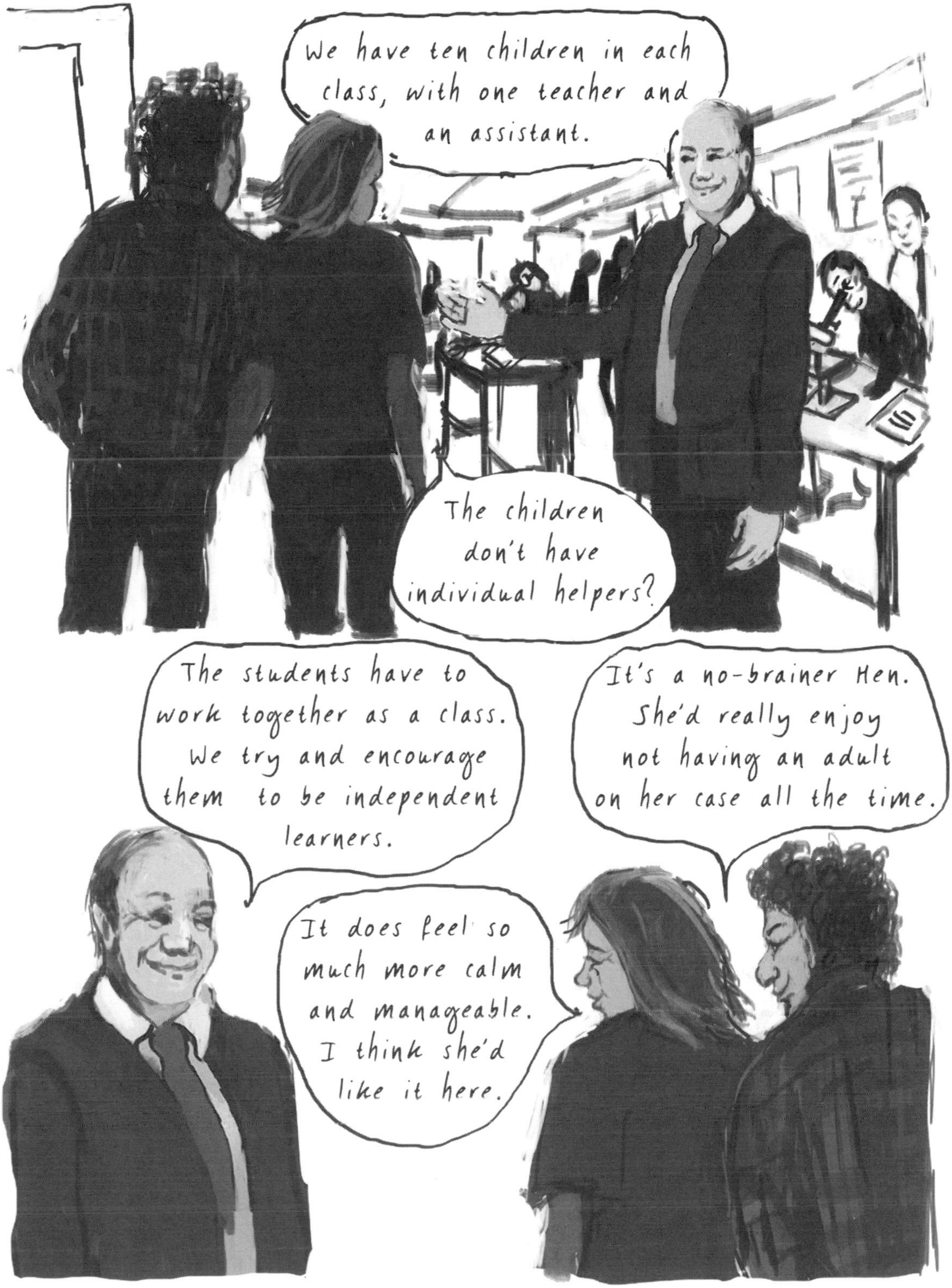
We have ten children in each class, with one teacher and an assistant.
The children don't have individual helpers?
The students have to work together as a class. We try and encourage them to be independent learners.
It's a no-brainer Hen. She'd really enjoy not having an adult on her case all the time.
It does feel so much more calm and manageable. I think she'd like it here.

Part Five

1D

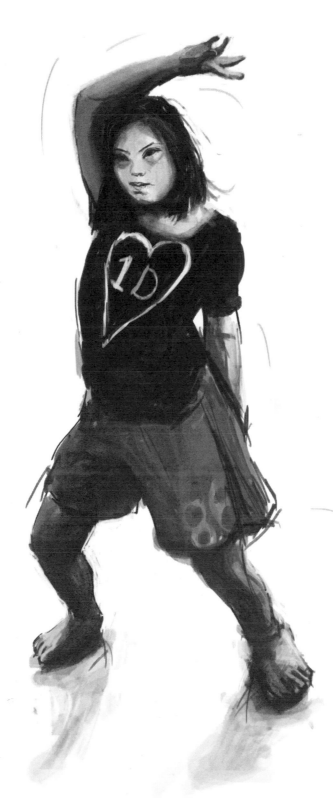

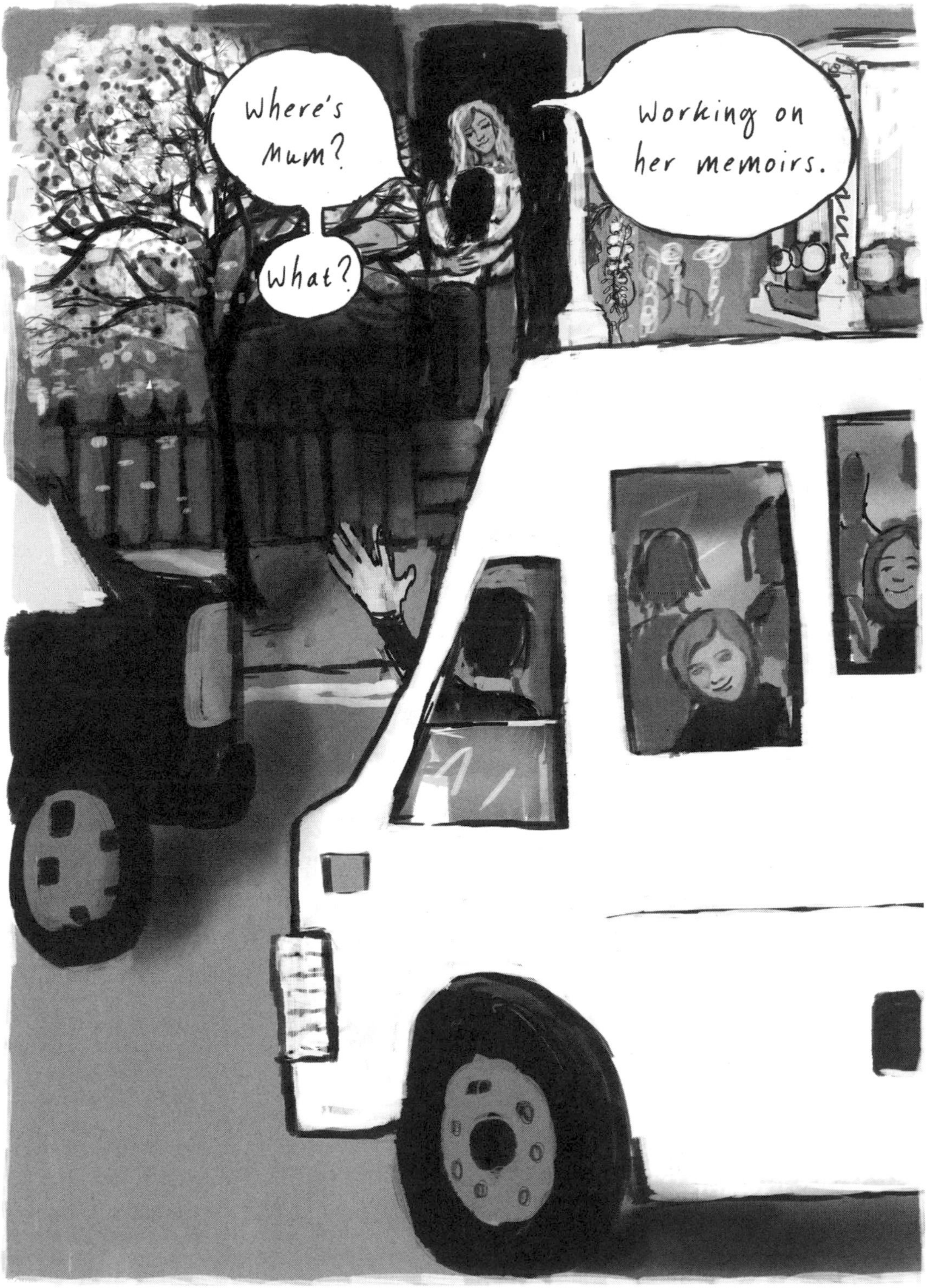
Where's Mum?
What?
Working on her memoirs.

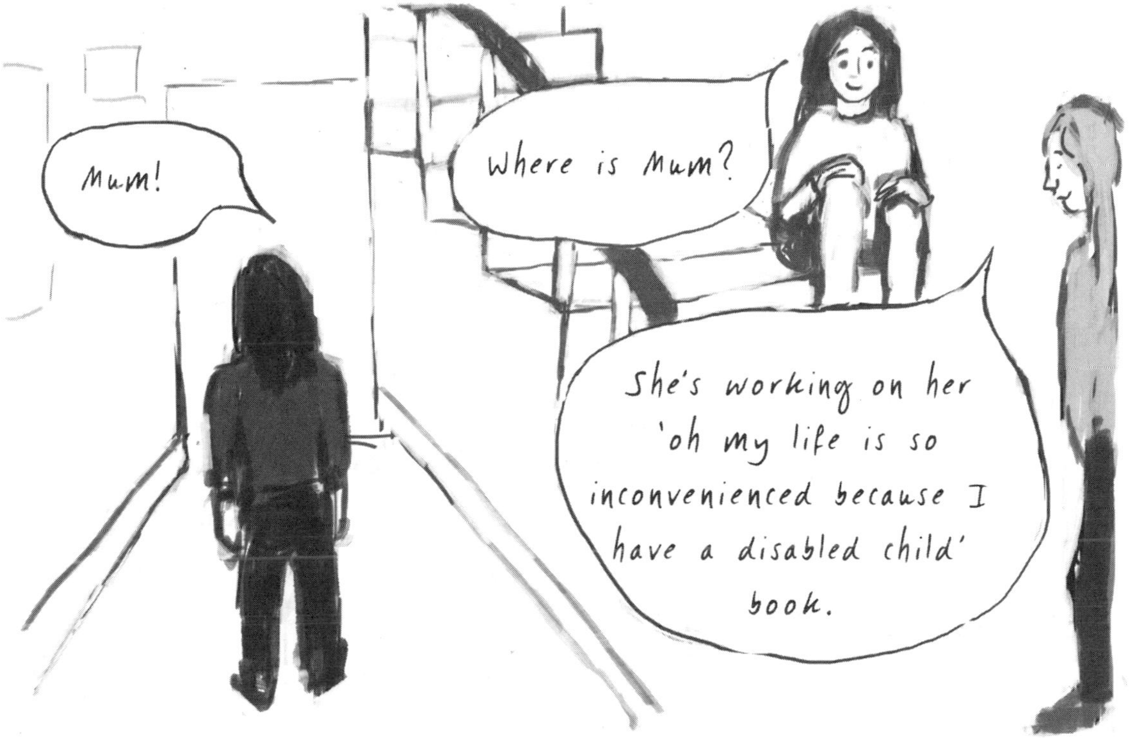
Mum!
Where is Mum?
She's working on her 'oh my life is so inconvenienced because I have a disabled child' book.

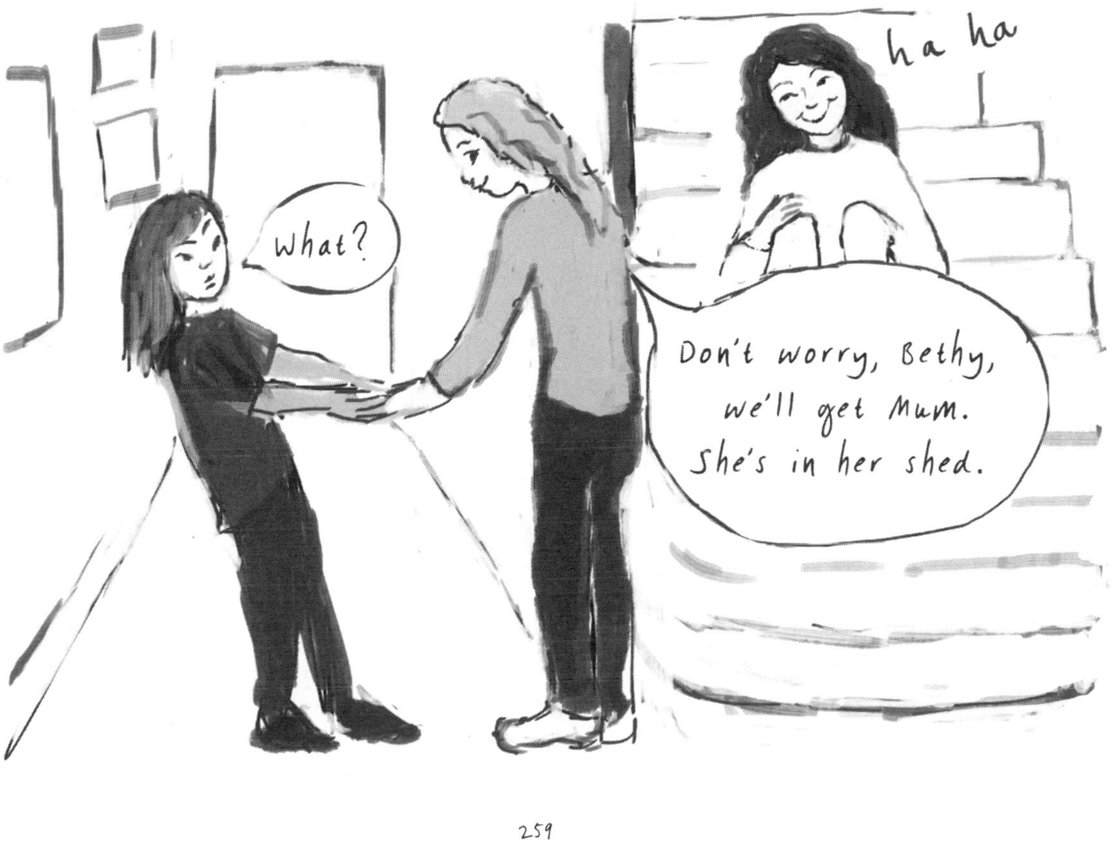
ha ha
What?
Don't worry, Bethy, we'll get Mum. She's in her shed.

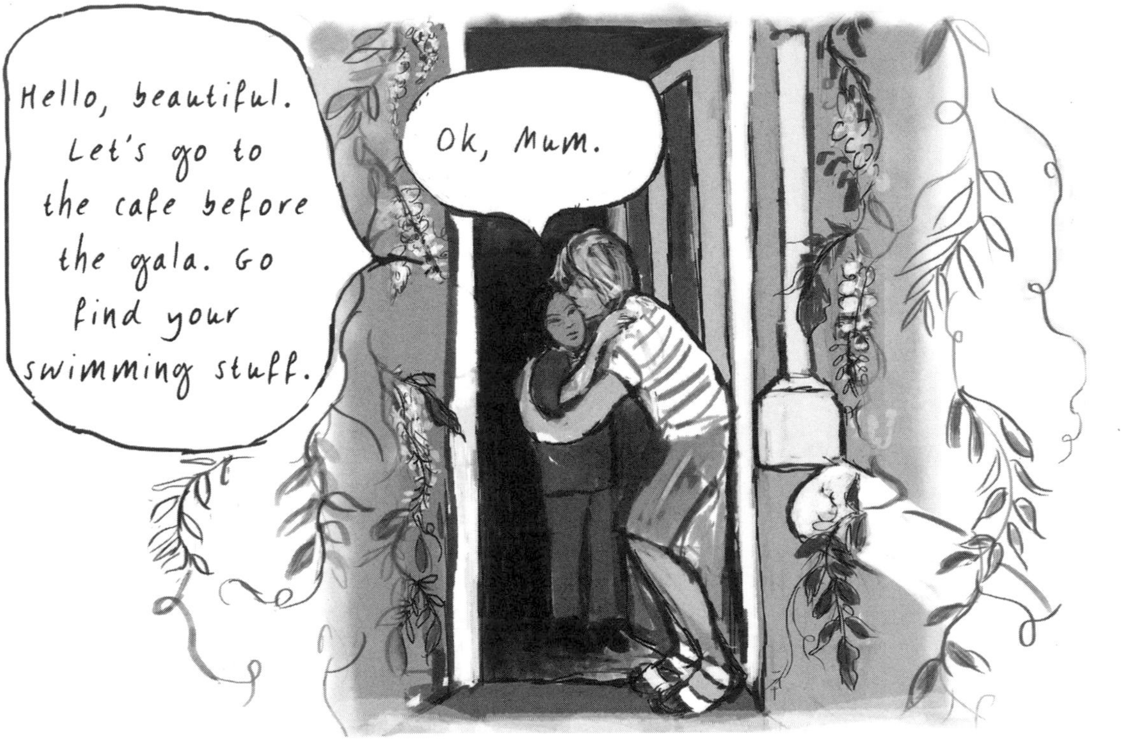
Hello, beautiful. Let's go to the cafe before the gala. Go find your swimming stuff.
Ok, Mum.

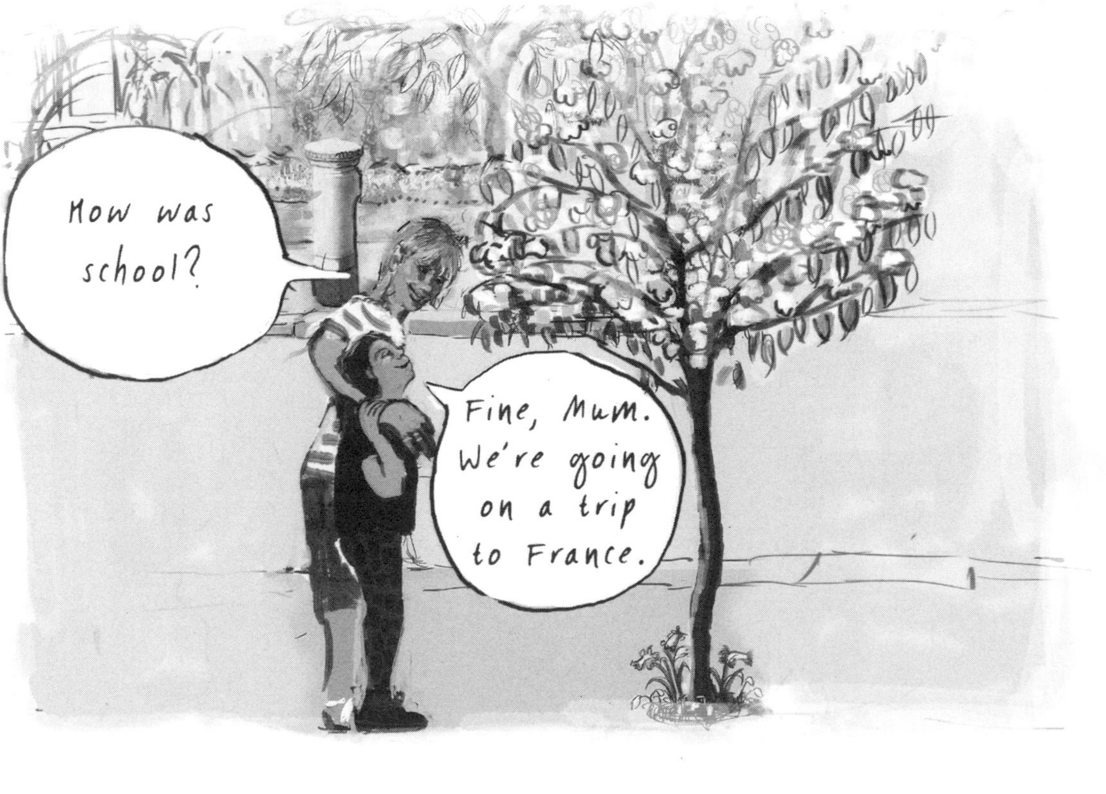
How was school?
Fine, Mum. We're going on a trip to France.

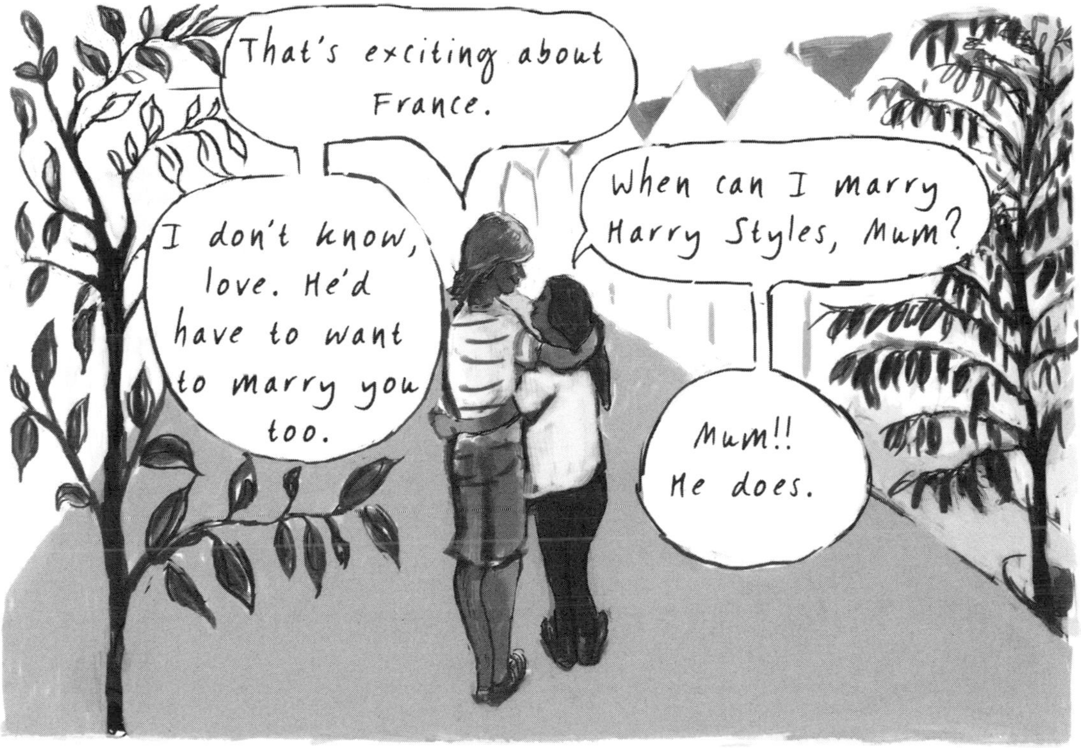
That's exciting about France.
I don't know, love. He'd have to want to marry you too.
When can I marry Harry Styles, Mum?
Mum!! He does.

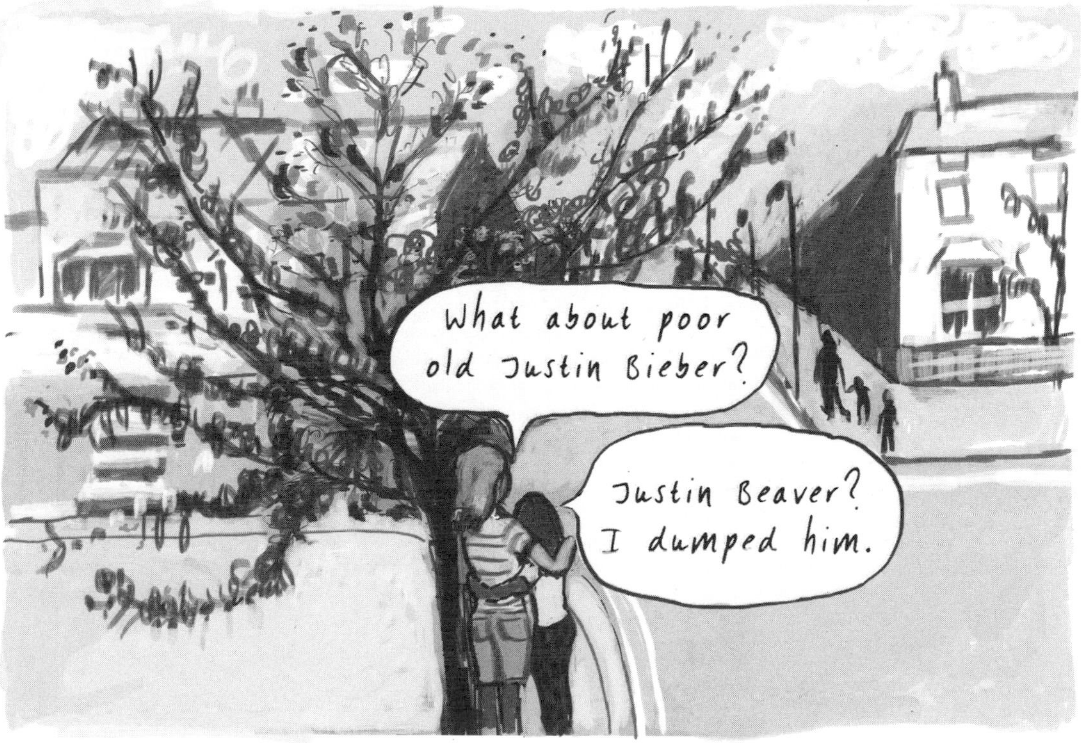
What about poor old Justin Bieber?
Justin Beaver? I dumped him.

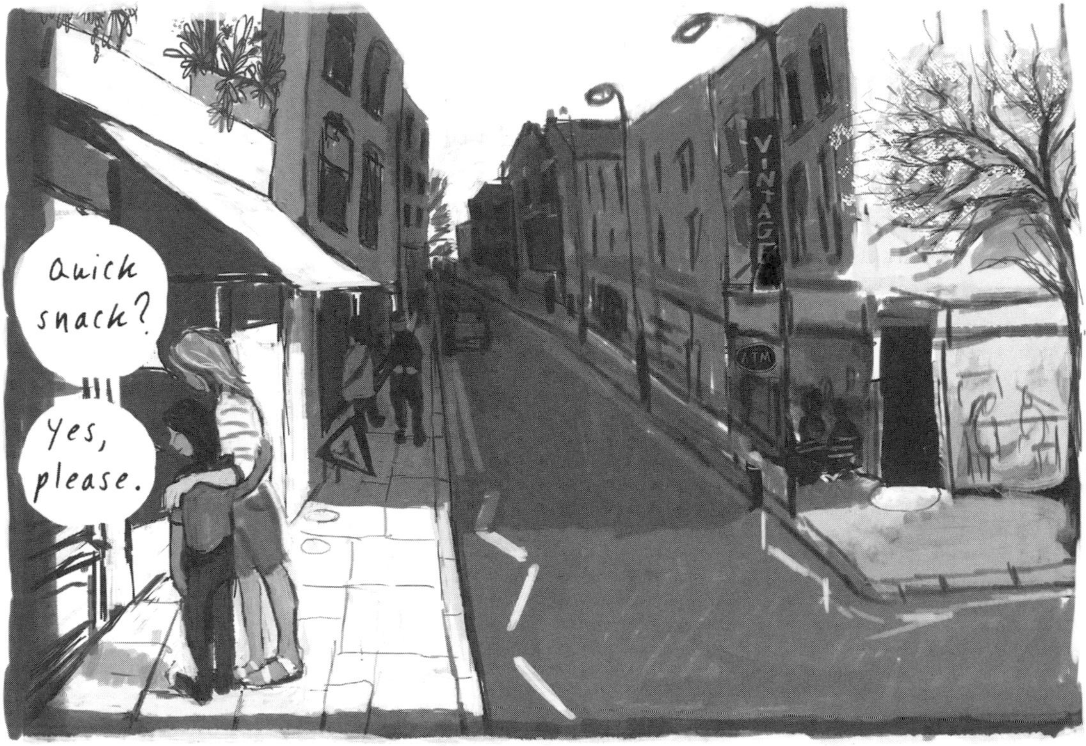
Quick snack?
Yes, please.
VINTAGE
ATM

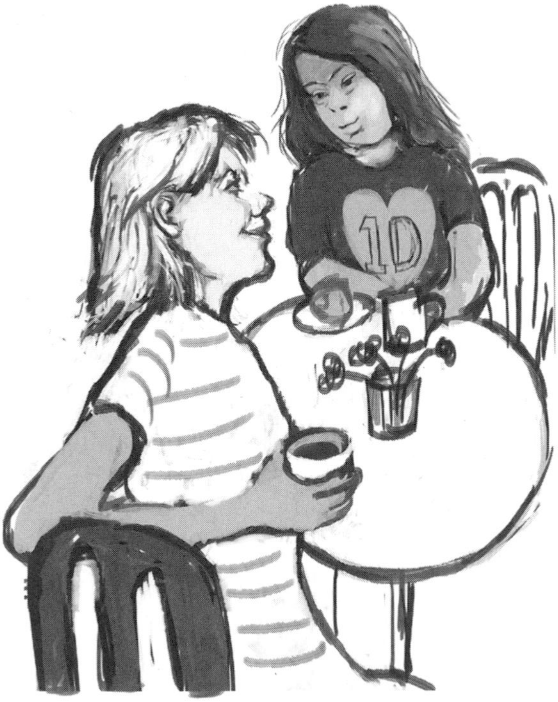
1D

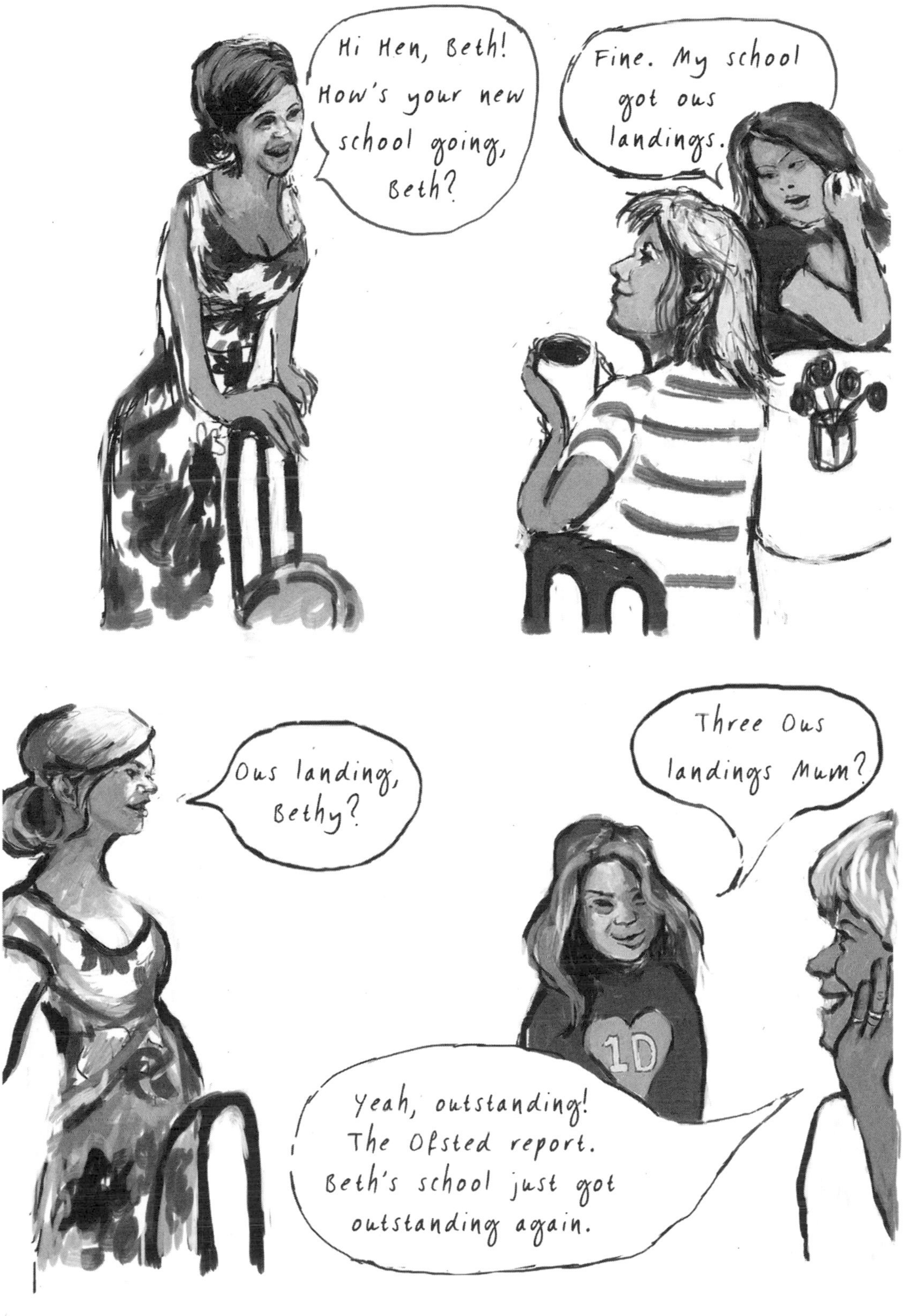
Hi Hen, Beth! How's your new school going, Beth?
Fine. My school got ous landings.
Ous landing, Bethy?
Three Ous landings Mum?
Yeah, outstanding! The Ofsted report. Beth's school just got outstanding again.

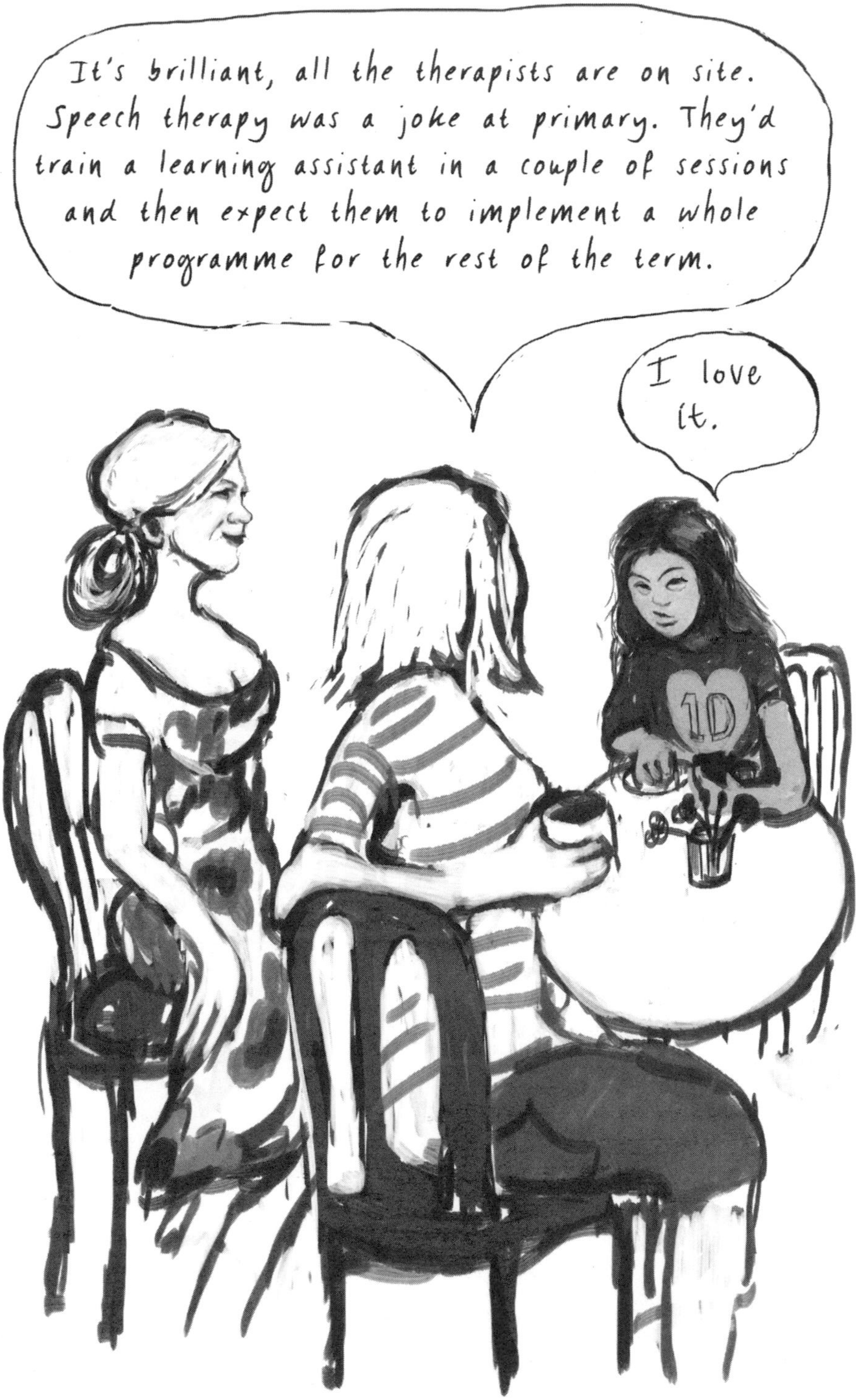
It's brilliant, all the therapists are on site. Speech therapy was a joke at primary. They'd train a learning assistant in a couple of sessions and then expect them to implement a whole programme for the rest of the term.
I love it.
1D

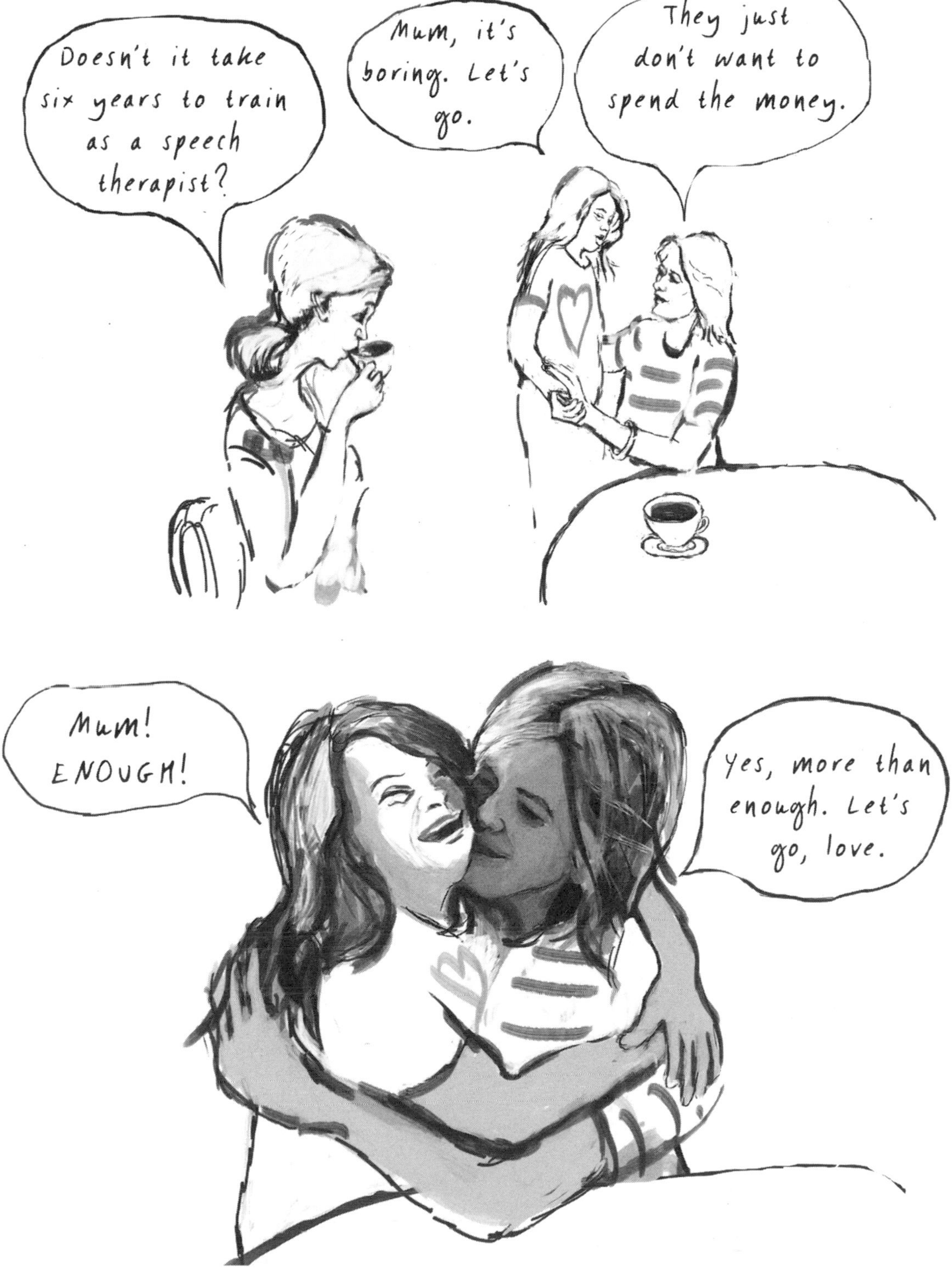
Doesn't it take six years to train as a speech therapist?
Mum, it's boring. Let's go.
They just don't want to spend the money.
Mum! ENOUGH!
Yes, more than enough. Let's go, love.

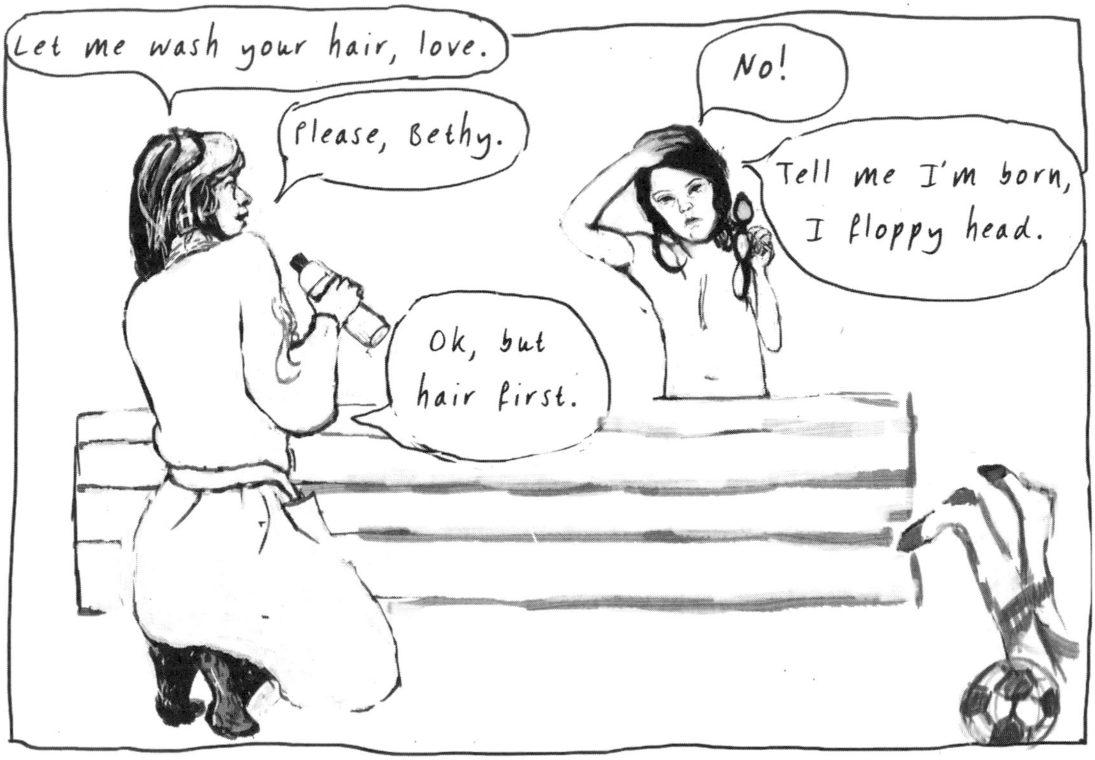
Let me wash your hair, love.
Please, Bethy.
No!
Tell me I'm born, I floppy head.
Ok, but hair first.

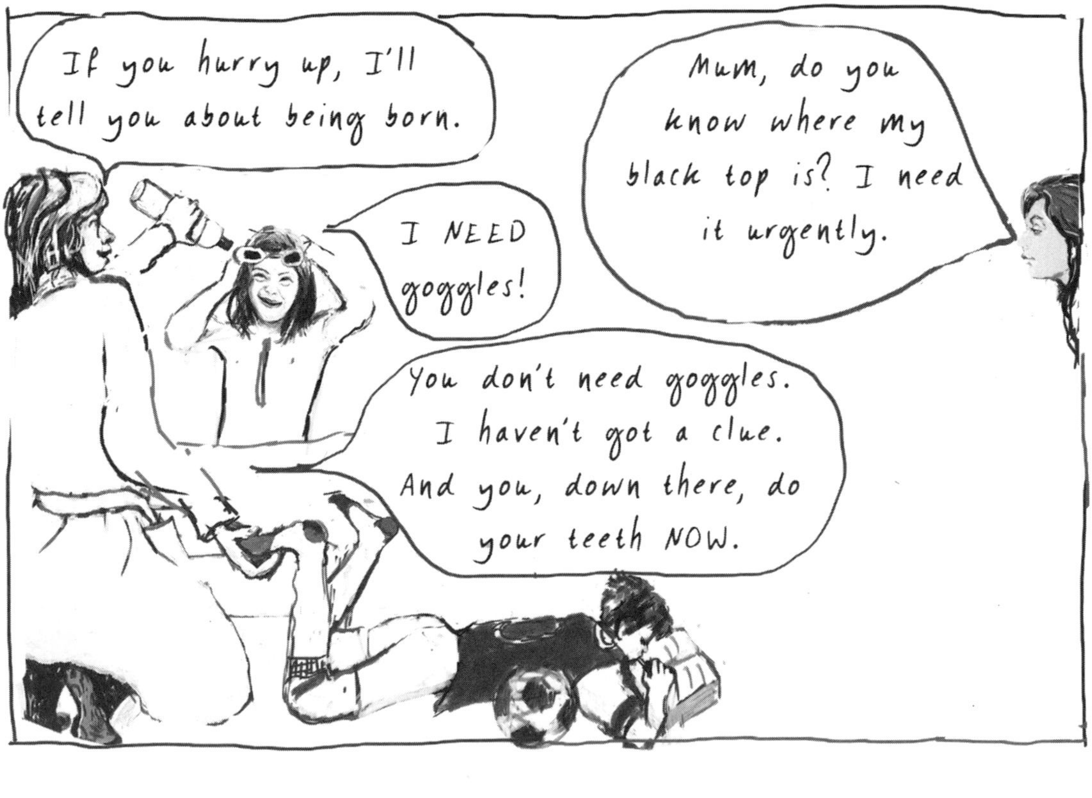
If you hurry up, I'll tell you about being born.
I NEED goggles!
Mum, do you know where my black top is? I need it urgently.
You don't need goggles. I haven't got a clue. And you, down there, do your teeth NOW.

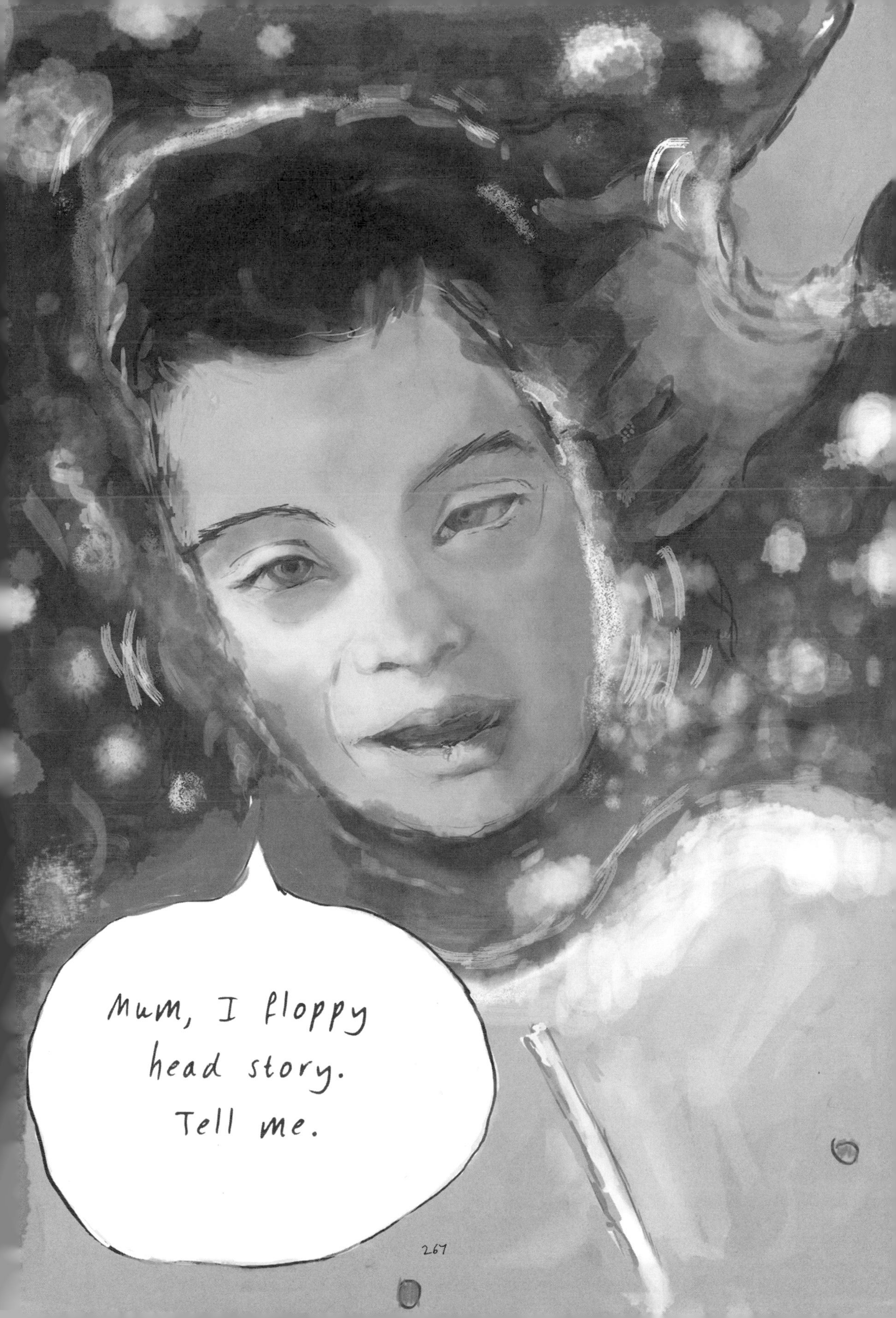
Mum, I floppy head story. Tell me.

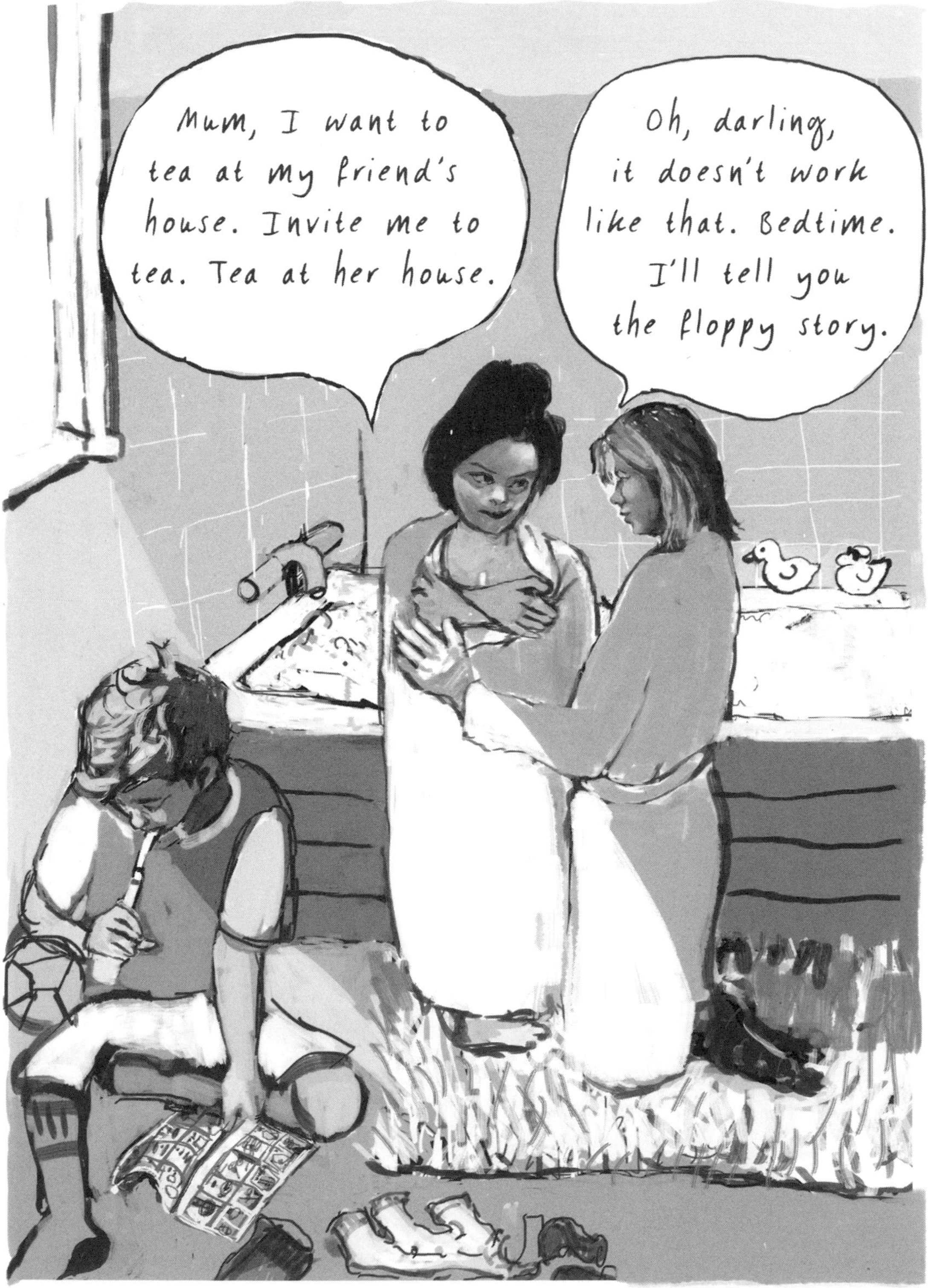
Mum, I want to tea at my friend's house. Invite me to tea. Tea at her house.
Oh, darling, it doesn't work like that. Bedtime. I'll tell you the floppy story.

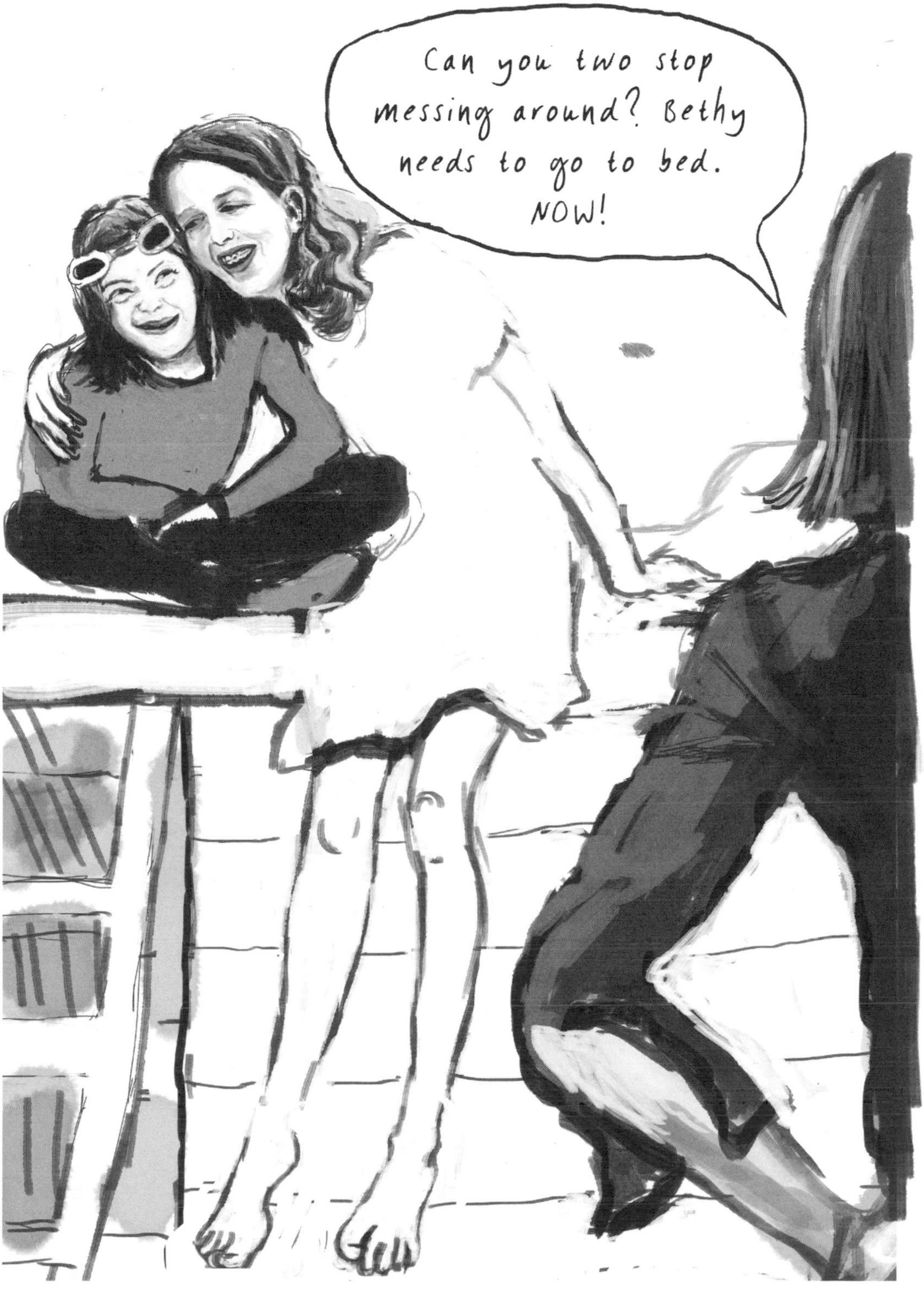
Can you two stop messing around? Bethy needs to go to bed. NOW!

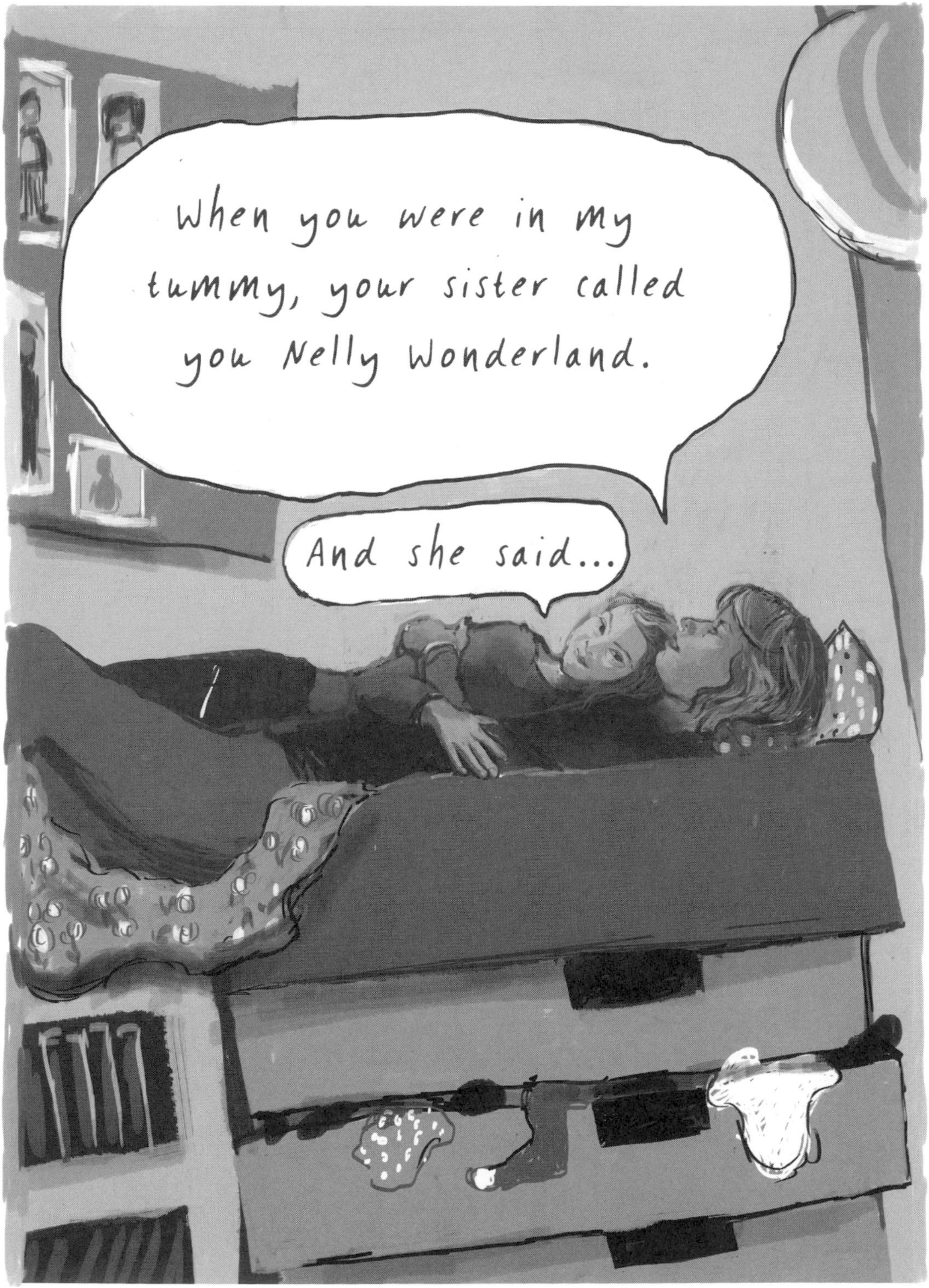
When you were in my tummy, your sister called you Nelly Wonderland.
And she said...

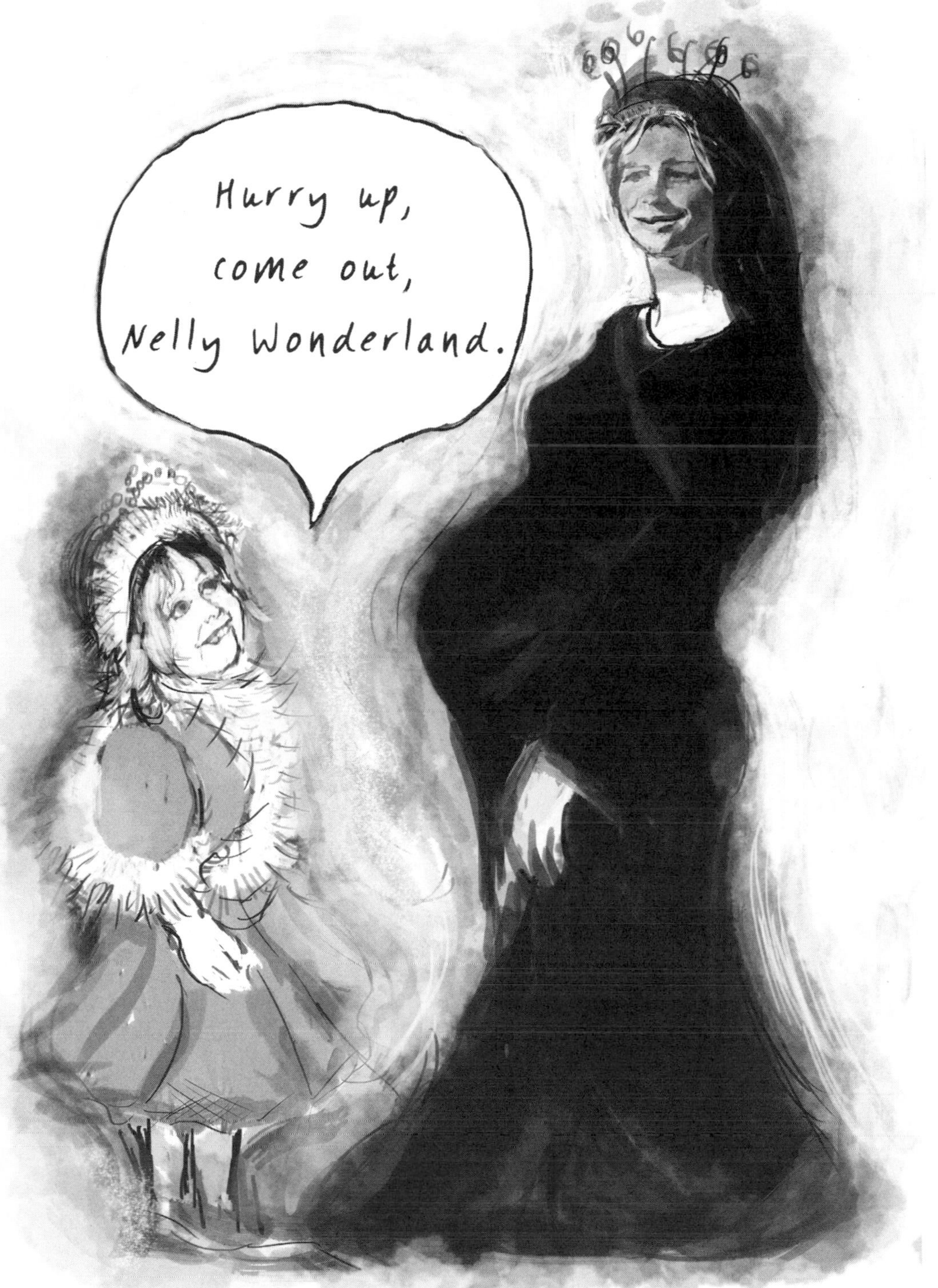
Hurry up, come out, Nelly Wonderland.

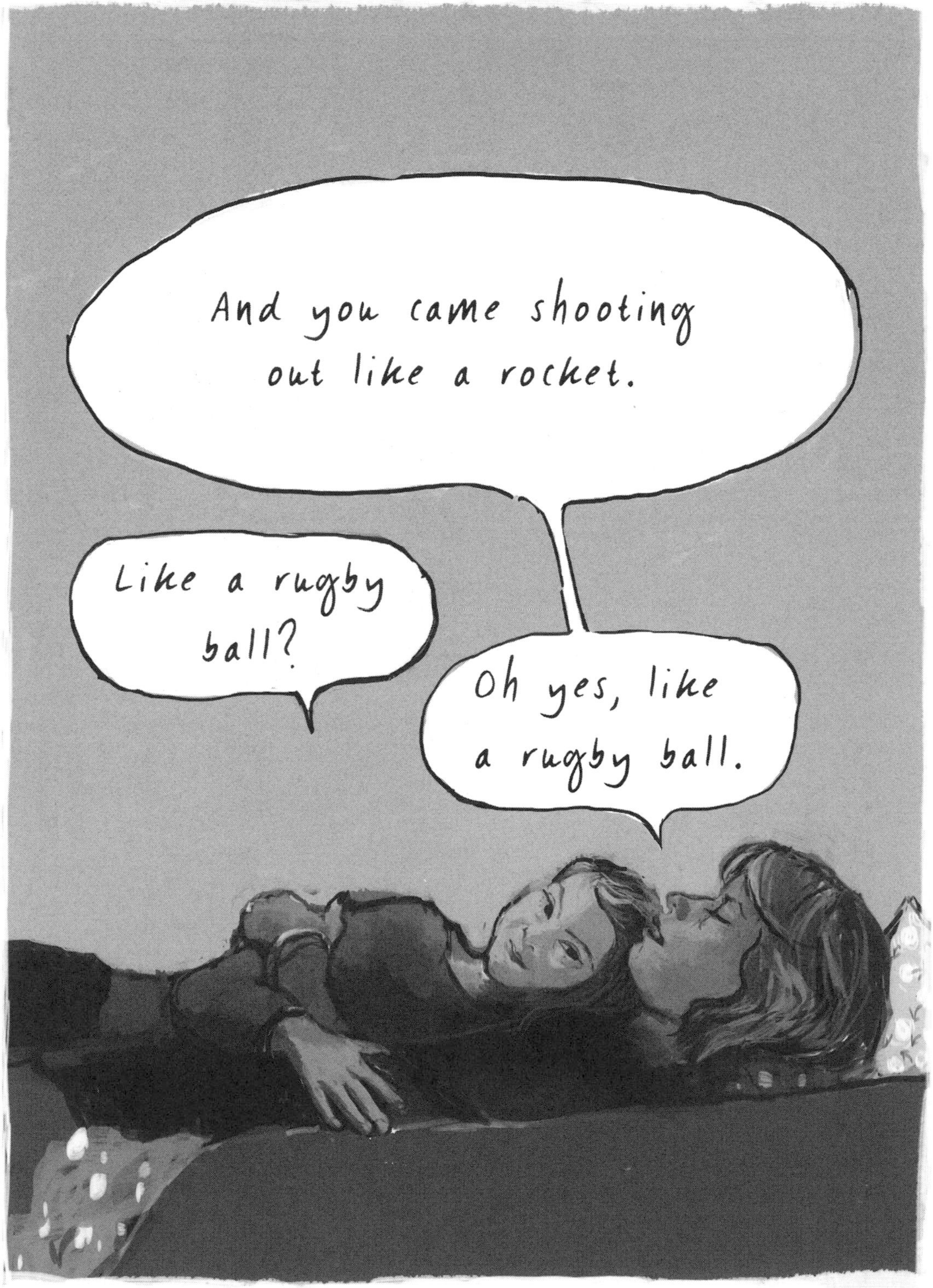
And you came shooting out like a rocket.
Like a rugby ball?
Oh yes, like a rugby ball.

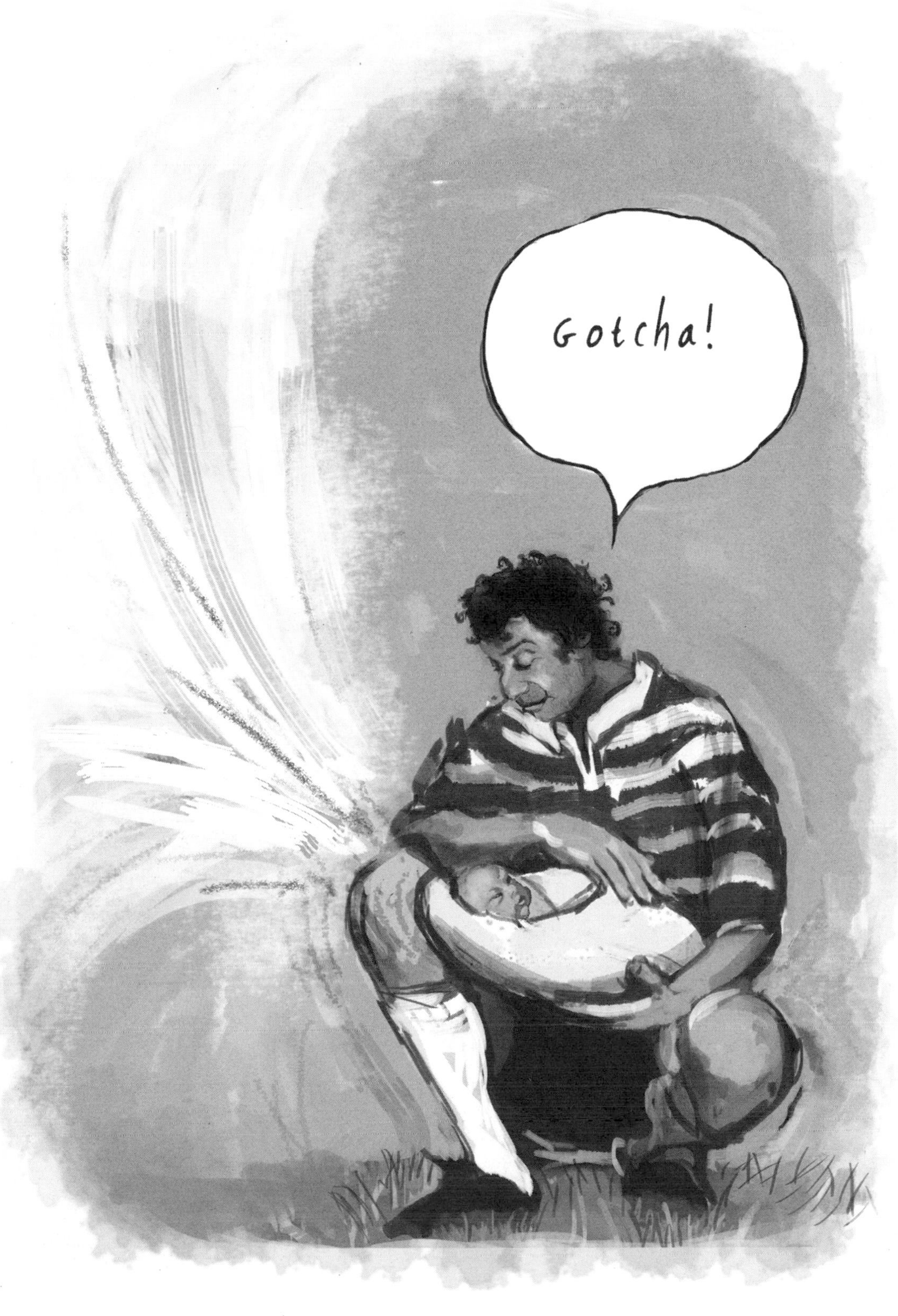
Gotcha!

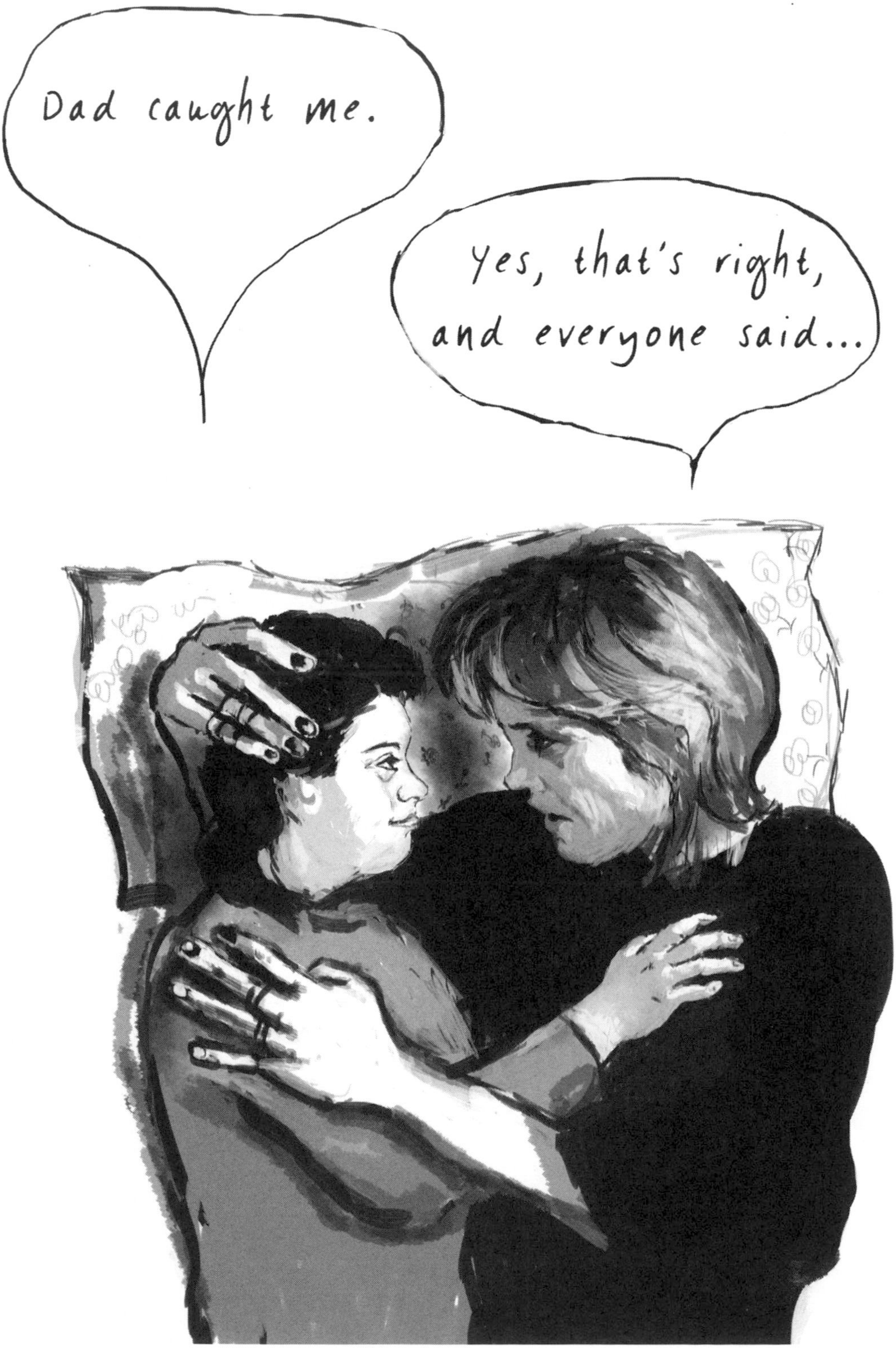
Dad caught me.
Yes, that's right, and everyone said...

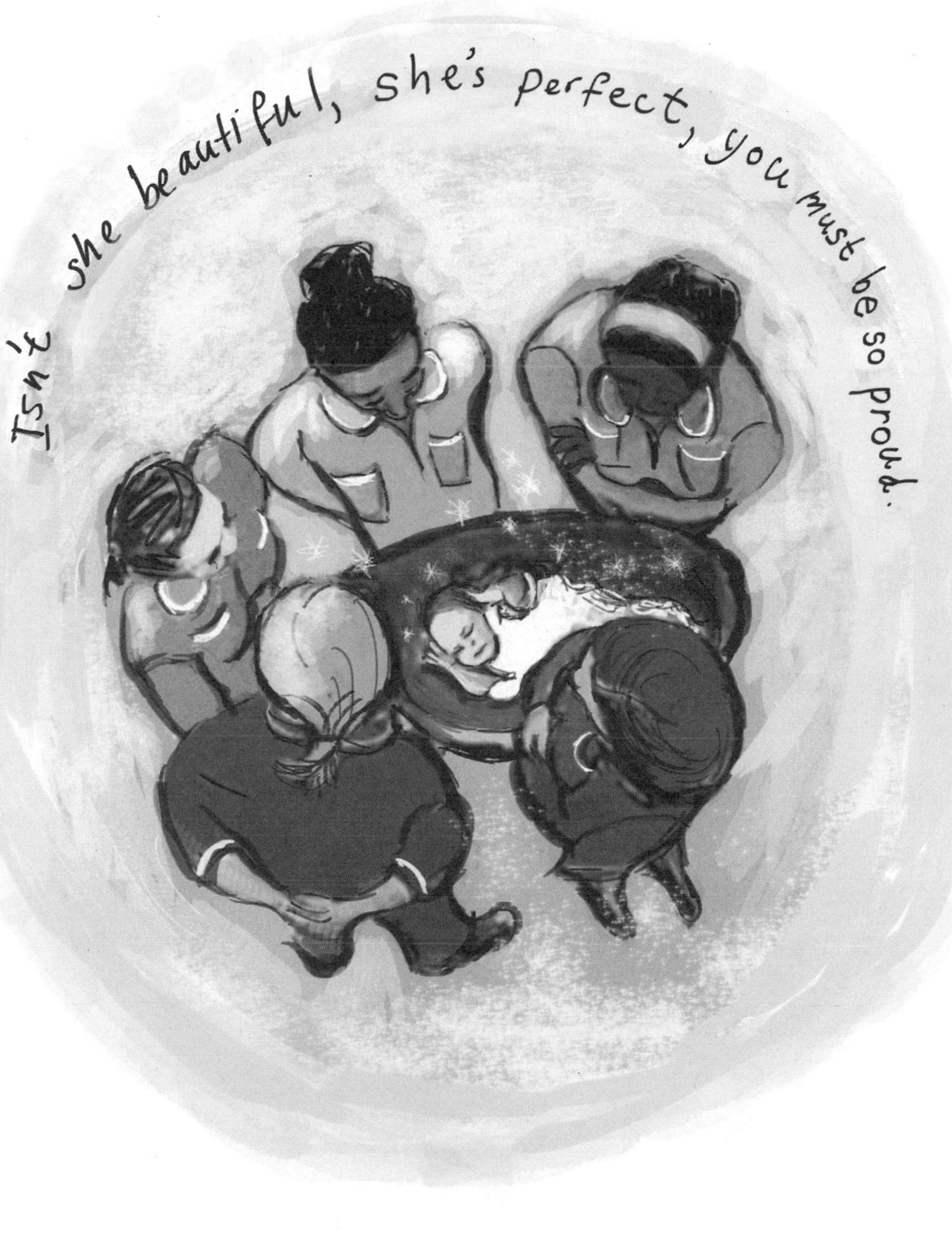
Isn't she beautiful, she's perfect, you must be so proud.

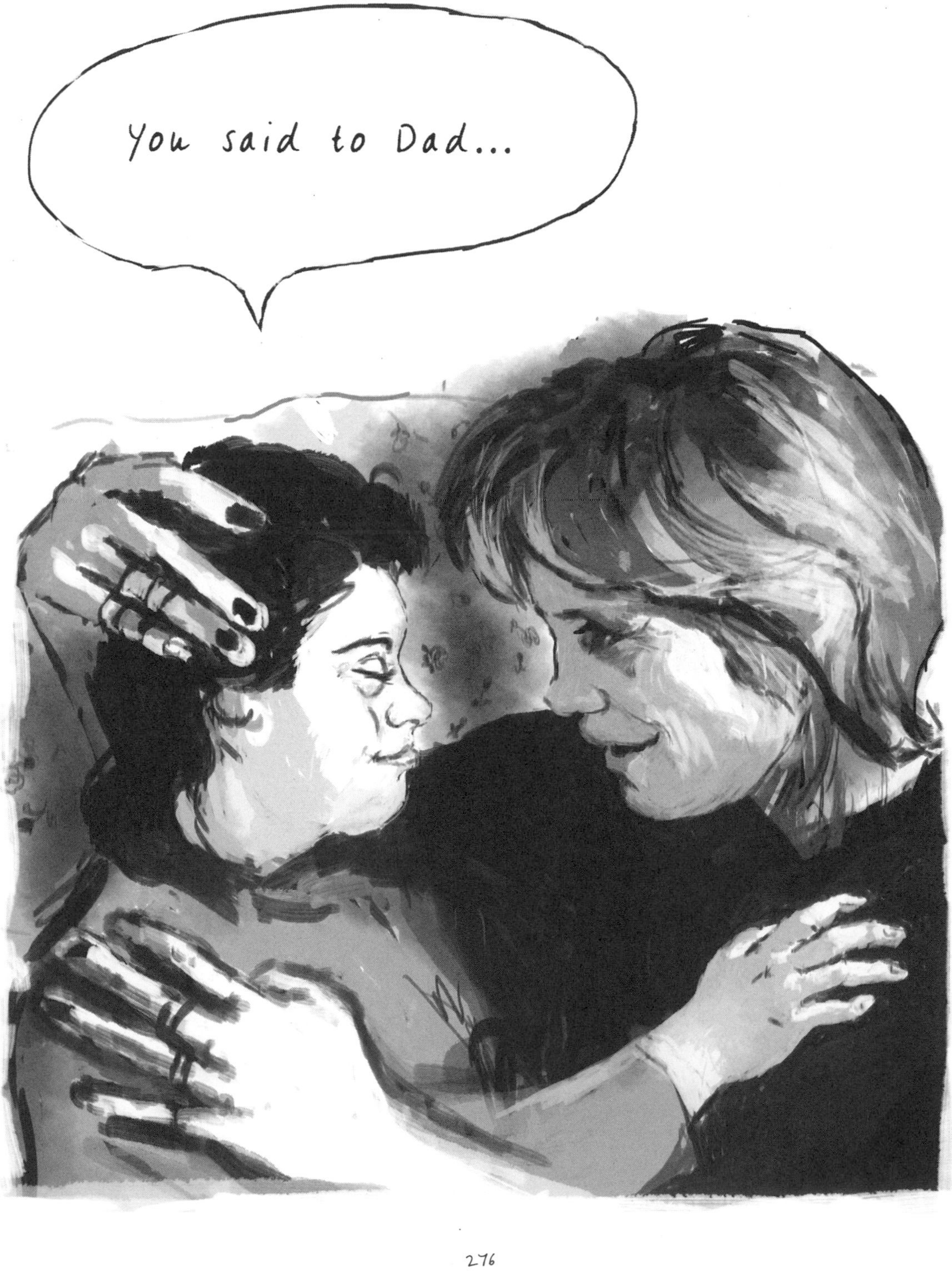
You said to Dad...

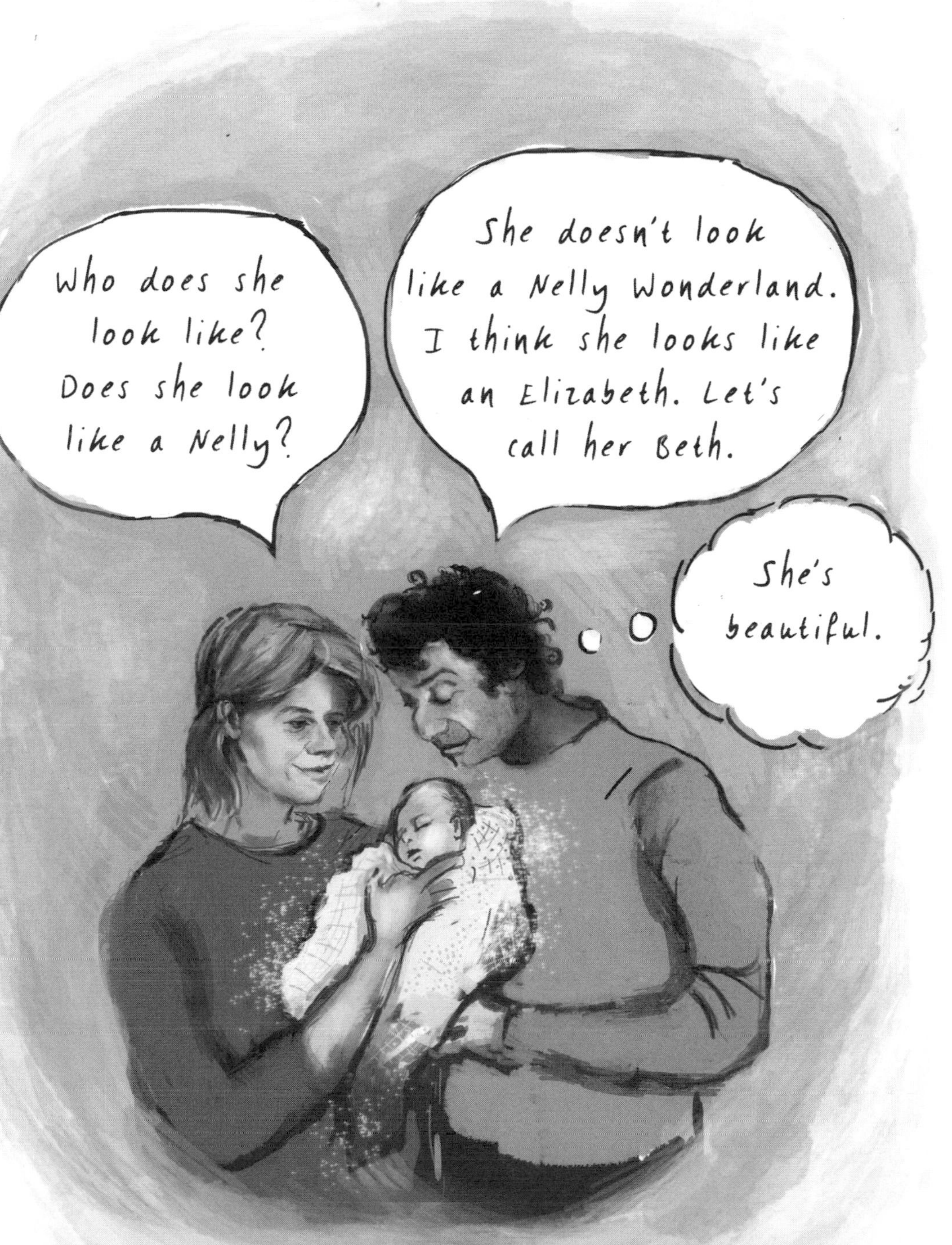
Who does she look like? Does she look like a Nelly?
She doesn't look like a Nelly Wonderland. I think she looks like an Elizabeth. Let's call her Beth.
She's beautiful.

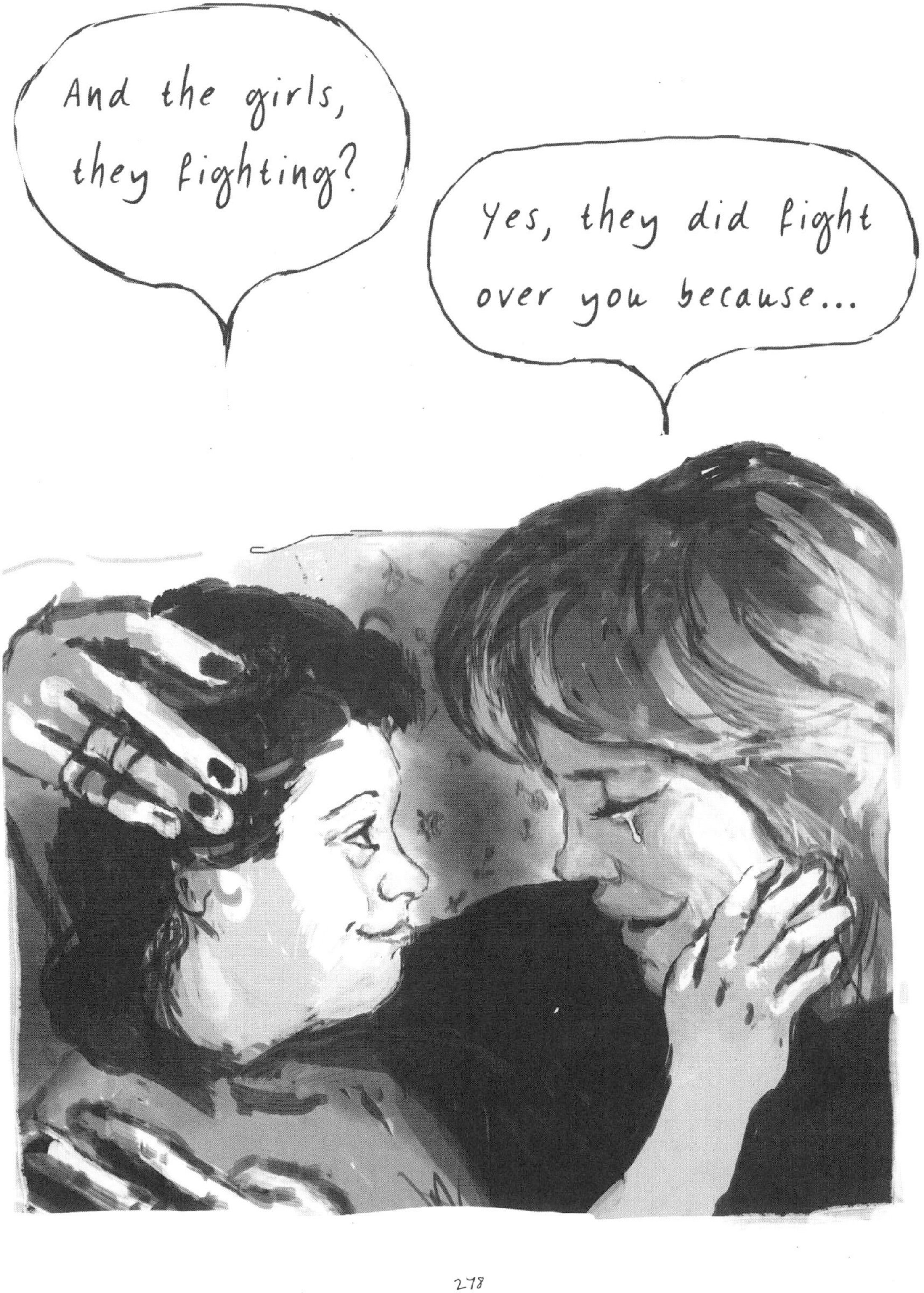
And the girls, they fighting?
Yes, they did fight over you because...

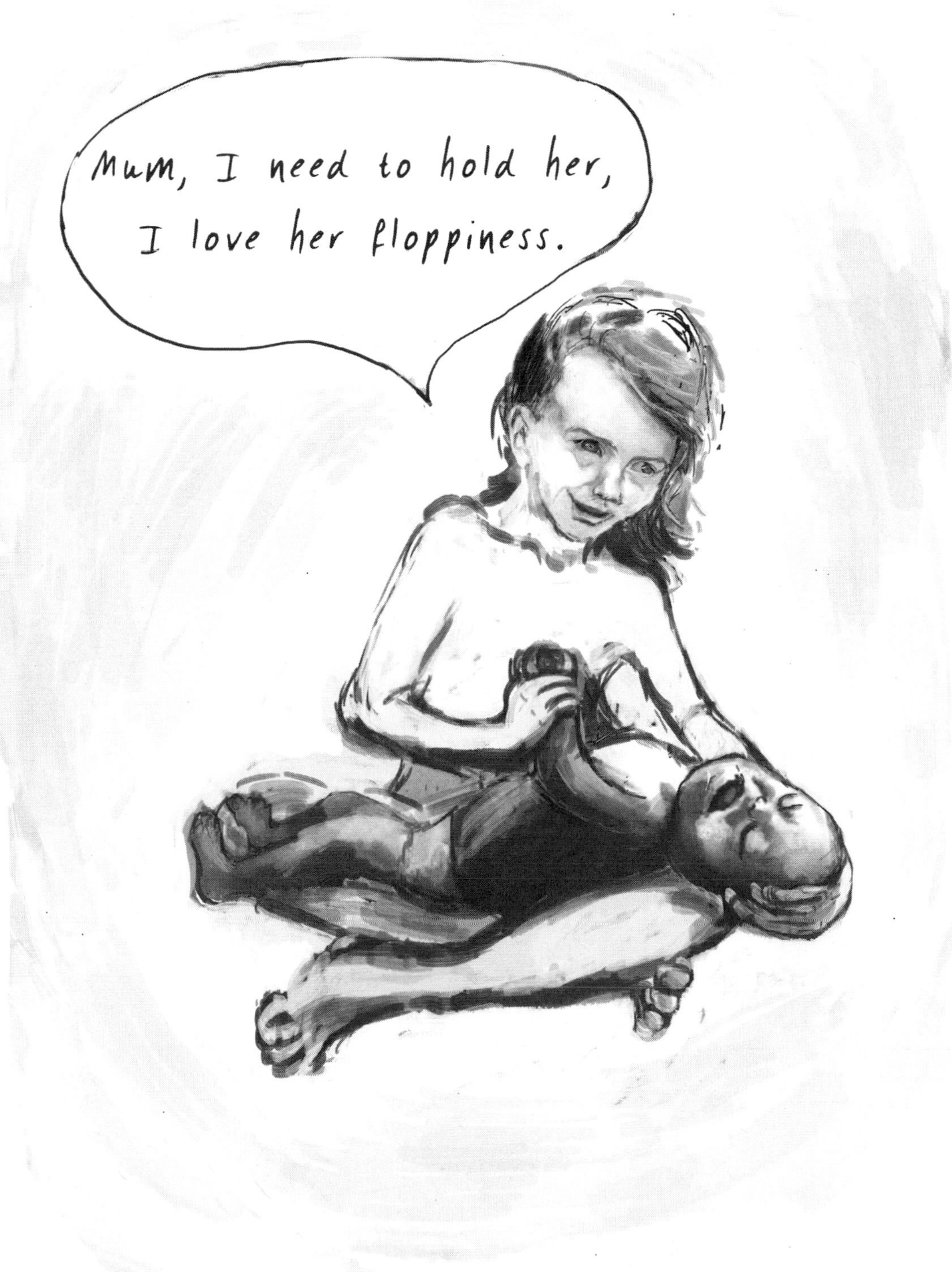
Mum, I need to hold her,
I love her floppiness.

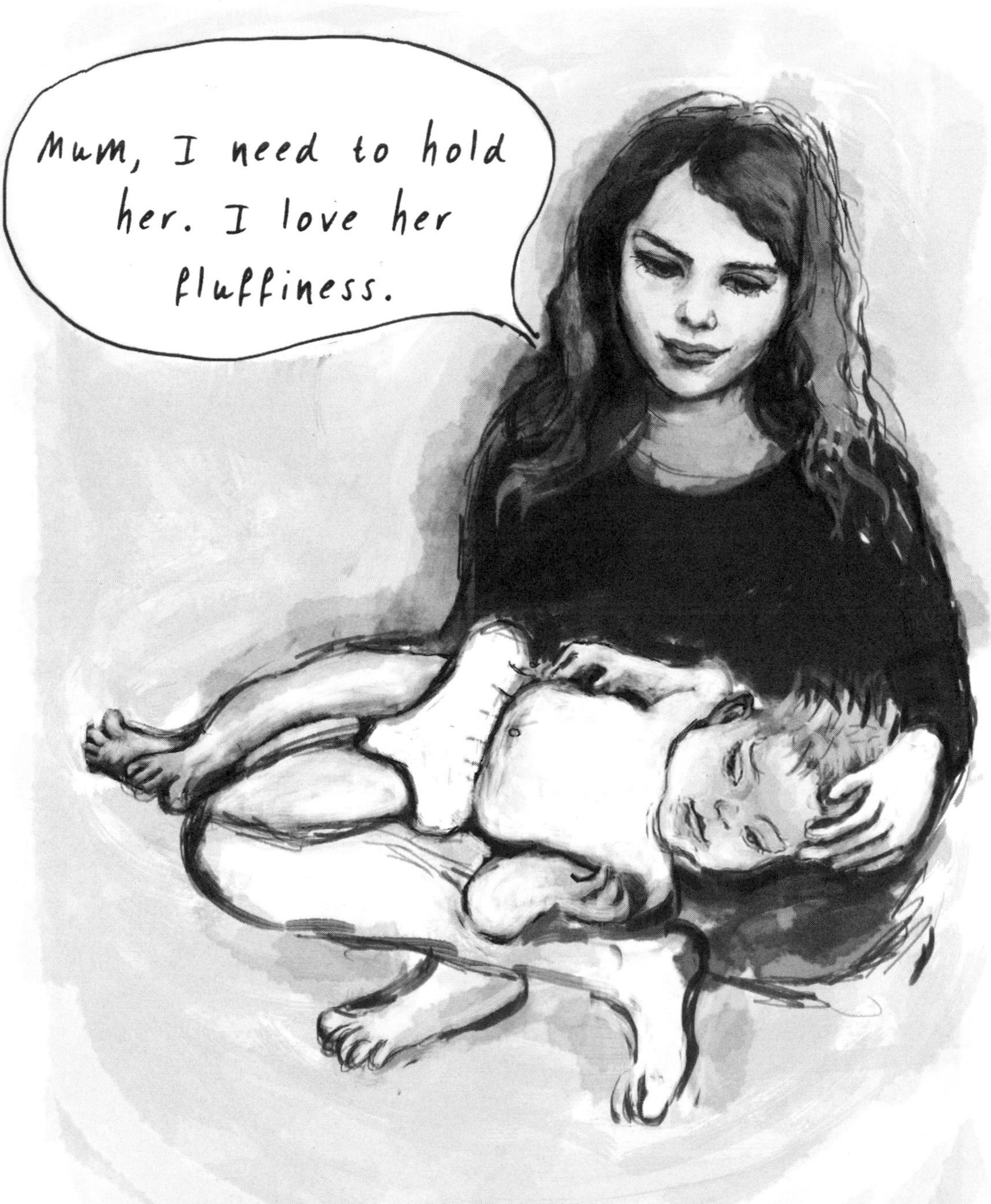
Mum, I need to hold her. I love her fluffiness.

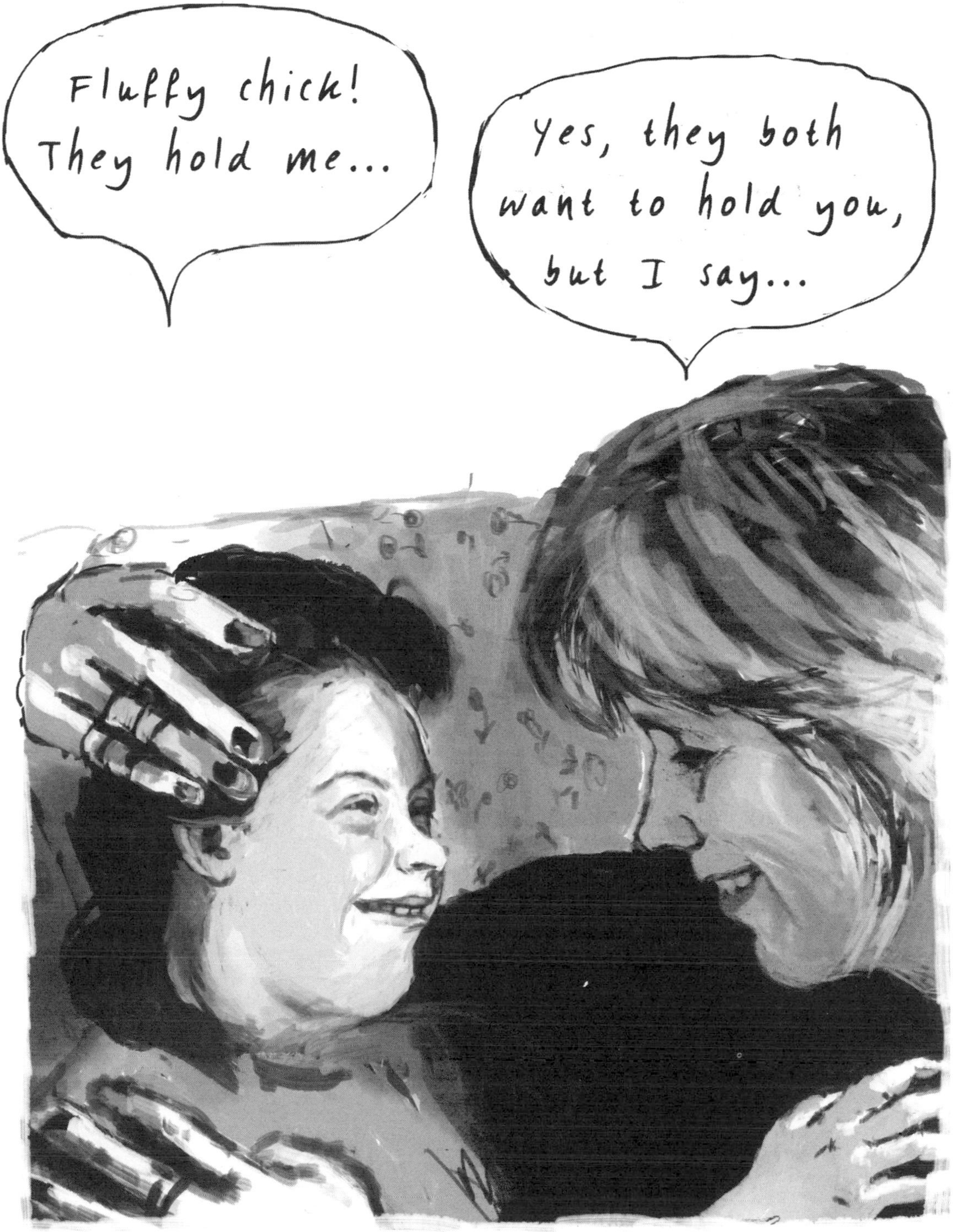
Fluffy chick! They hold me...
Yes, they both want to hold you, but I say...

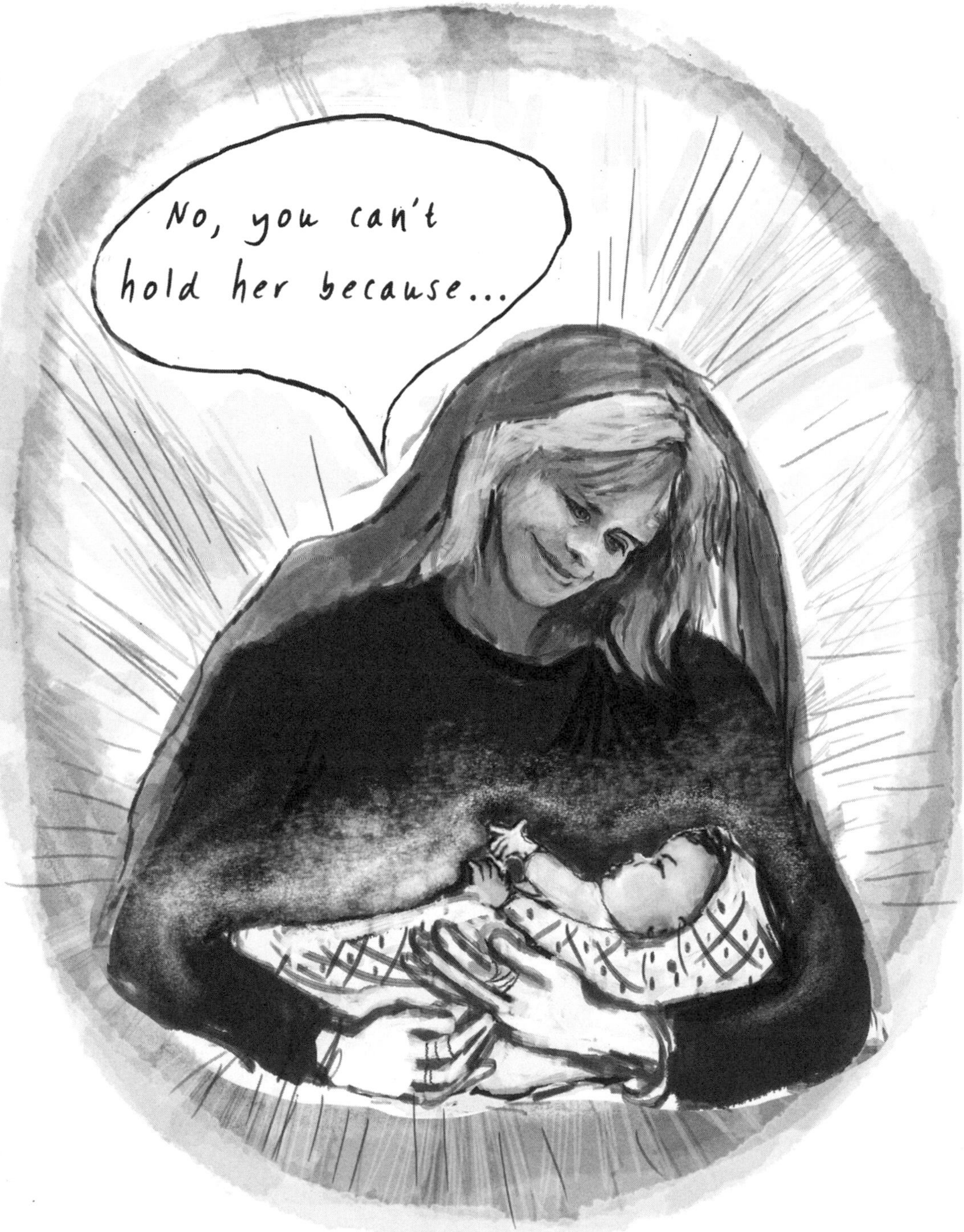
No, you can't hold her because...

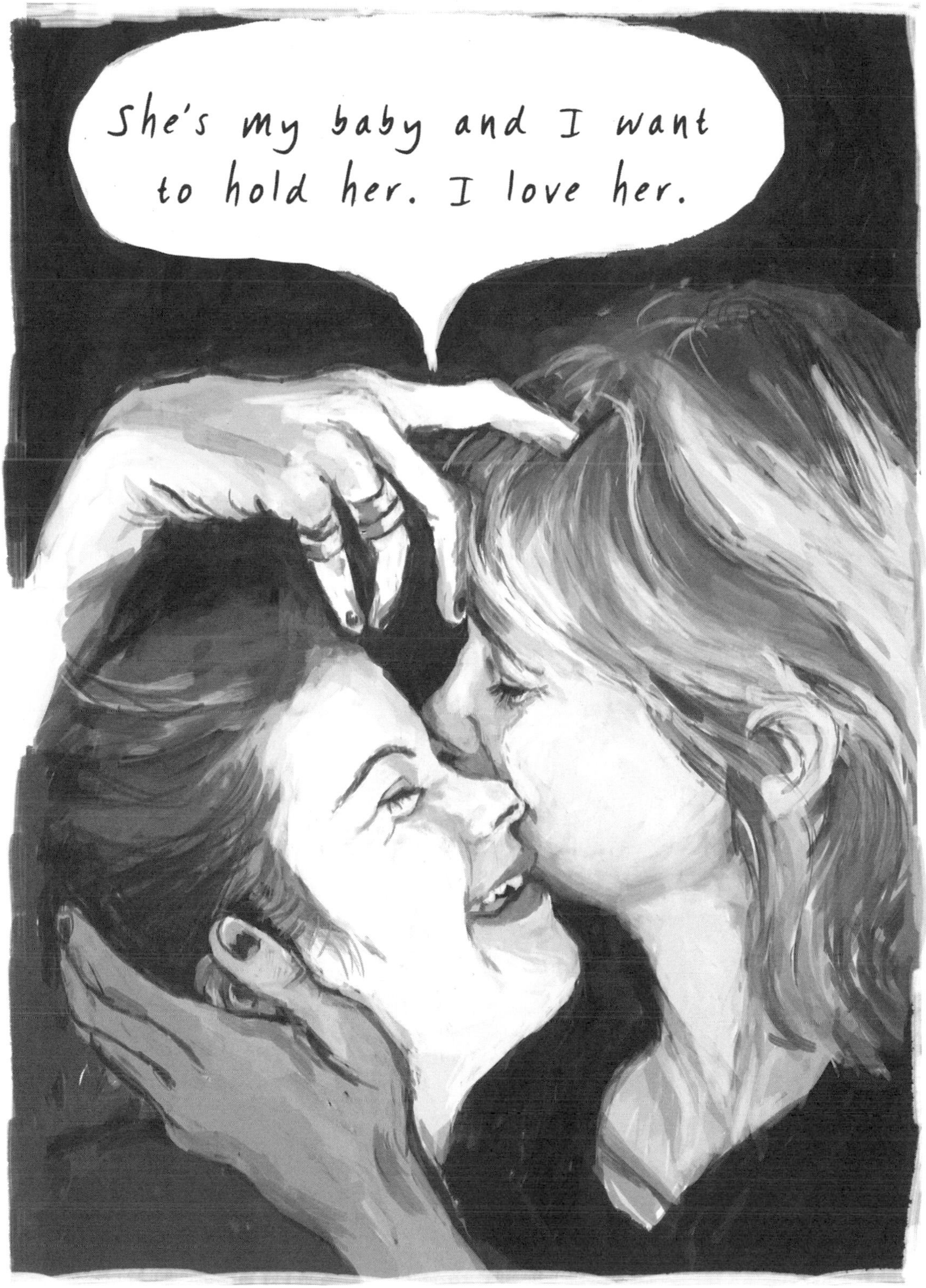
She's my baby and I want to hold her. I love her.

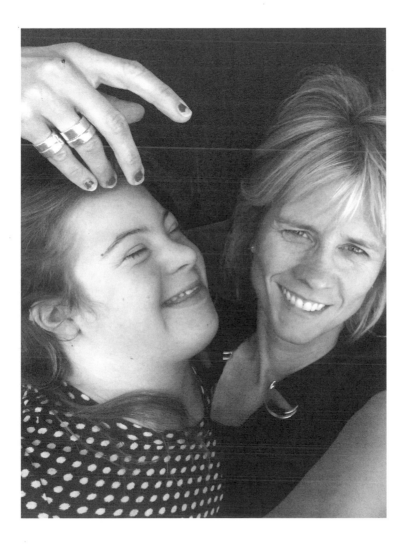

Acknowledgements

When I first started this book, I had no idea what a team effort it would become, and without the following people there would be no book.

Thank you to Myriad: Candida Lacey, Vicky Blunden, Emma Dowson, Dawn Sackett, Emma Grundy Haigh for all your invaluable help and advice. And thank you to Kendra Boileau at Penn State University Press for this North American edition.

My fantastic editor, Corinne Pearlman, for your unwavering patience, kindness and expertise.

Meg Rosoff for believing in and championing my work from the very beginning.

My agent, Rebecca Carter from Janklow and Nesbit, for being able to imagine that twenty drawings could become a book, and for your never-ending supply of support and wisdom, through every stage of the process.

To all my friends: Leslie Bookless for your unconditional love and humour, Brigit and Karen for the running and chats. Thank you: Philly Beaumont, Nick Coleman, Anna Hsiung, Juju Vail for looking at early drafts.

To Sophie Thomas and David Pearson for help with the cover.

Thank you to Lesley Caldwell.

To the Down's Syndrome Association and Great Ormond Street Hospital.

To Nicola Streeten and Laydeez Do Comics, Ian Williams and Graphic Medicine, for showing me the potential of graphic novels.

Thank you to my mum and dad.

To my siblings, Philly, Charlie and Chris, and my extended family for your love and support.

To my other editors, Matty and Bridie, for helping me decide what to include and leave out, and for always coming up with the best lines. Thank you both for your honesty, humour and wisdom.

To Karl, for religiously keeping a count of how many drawings I did each week and dividing it by the amount of days I had left to make my deadline.

To Steve, the biggest thank you for all your support, understanding and love over the last thirty years and for posing for drawings when you really didn't want to.

And Bethy, last but not least, I couldn't have done it without you: thank you for being yourself.

GRAPHIC MEDICINE

Aliceheimer's

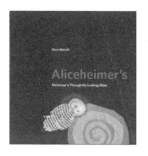

"A deeply moving, informative, and funny memoir by a woman watching her mother's descent into Alzheimer's disease."
—Roz Chast, author of *Can't We Talk About Something More Pleasant?*

My Degeneration
A Journey Through Parkinson's
Peter Dunlap-Shohl

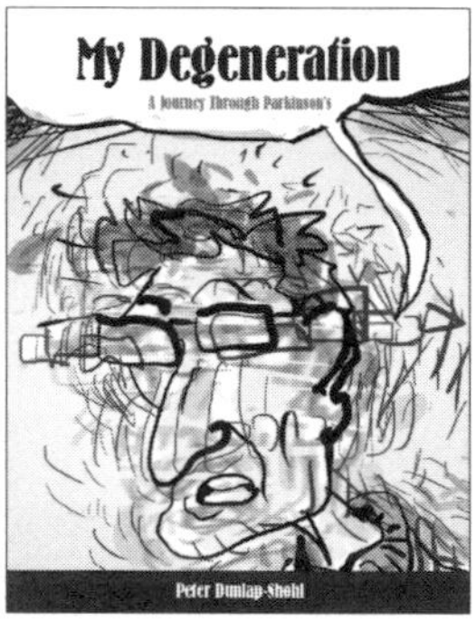

"*My Degeneration* opens up a powerful new purpose for comics—as an effective tool to educate doctors, patients, and others about both the clinical and the personal sides of living with a disease."
—*Foreword Reviews*

"A powerful debut with a deeply resonant story about living with the seemingly impossible."
—*Publishers Weekly*

THINGS
RETIREMENT
HOME
TRAILER
PARK
ANEURIN
WRIGHT
...When You're 29 and Unemployed

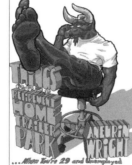

"The manifesto puts to the test its authors' belief in the ability of comics to forge connections—between medicine and humanities, between doctors and patients—that prose alone often makes impossible."
—Jared Gardner, *Public Culture/Public Books*

GRAPHIC
MEDICINE
MANIFESTO

The BAD DOCTOR
THE TROUBLED LIFE AND TIMES OF DR. IWAN JAMES
IAN WILLIAMS

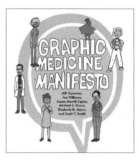

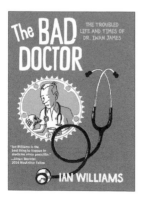

"Ian Williams is the best thing to happen to medicine since penicillin."
—Alison Bechdel, 2014 MacArthur Fellow

THE
WALKING
MED
ZOMBIES AND
THE MEDICAL IMAGE

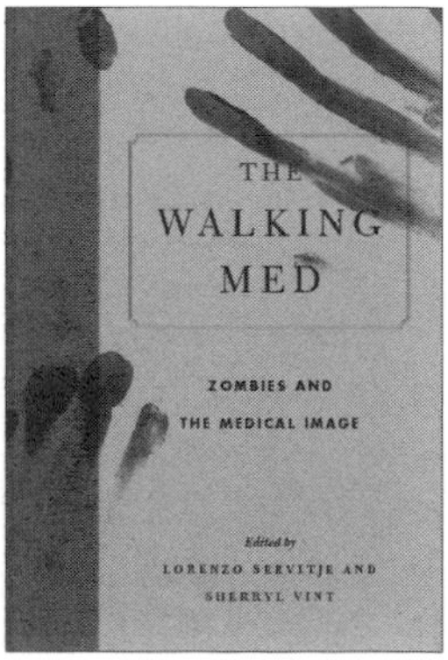

"*The Walking Med* convincingly argues that zombies are powerful and necessary symbols of medicine and its politics."
—Marina Levina, University of Memphis